Head and Neck Cancer

Cancer Treatment and Research

Lippman M.E., Dickson R. (eds): Breast Cancer: Cellular and Molecular Biology. 1988. ISBN 0-89838-368-4.

Kamps W.A., Humphrey G.B., Poppema S. (eds): Hodgkin's Disease in Children: Controversies and Current Practice. 1988. ISBN 0-89838-372-2.

Muggia F.M. (ed): Cancer Chemotherapy: Concepts, Clinical Investigations and Therapeutic Advances. 1988. ISBN 0-89838-381-1.

Nathanson L. (ed): Malignant Melanoma: Biology, Diagnosis, and Therapy. 1988. ISBN 0-89838-384-6.

Pinedo H.M., Verweij J. (eds): Treatment of Soft Tissue Sarcomas. 1989. ISBN 0-89838-391-9.

Hansen H.H. (ed): Basic and Clinical Concepts of Lung Cancer. 1989. ISBN 0-7923-0153-6.

Lepor H., Ratliff T.L. (eds): Urologic Oncology. 1989. ISBN 0-7923-0161-7.

Benz C., Liu E. (eds): Oncogenes. 1989. ISBN 0-7923-0237-0.

Ozols R.F. (ed): Drug Resistance in Cancer Therapy. 1989. ISBN 0-7923-0244-3.

Surwit E.A., Alberts D.S. (eds): Endometrial Cancer. 1989. ISBN 0-7923-0286-9.

Champlin R. (ed): Bone Marrow Transplantation. 1990. ISBN 0-7923-0612-0.

Goldenberg D. (ed): Cancer Imaging with Radiolabeled Antibodies. 1990. ISBN 0-7923-0631-7.

Jacobs C. (ed): Carcinomas of the Head and Neck. 1990. ISBN 0-7923-0668-6.

Lippman M.E., Dickson R. (eds): Regulatory Mechanisms in Breast Cancer: Advances in Cellular and Molecular Biology of Breast Cancer. 1990. ISBN 0-7923-0868-9.

Nathanson L. (ed): Malignant Melanoma: Genetics, Growth Factors, Metastases, and Antigens. 1991. ISBN 0-7923-0895-6.

Sugarbaker P.H. (ed): Management of Gastric Cancer. 1991. ISBN 0-7923-1102-7.

Pinedo H.M., Verweij J., Suit H.D. (eds): Soft Tissue Sarcomas: New Developments in the Multidisciplinary Approach to Treatment. 1991. ISBN 0-7923-1139-6.

Ozols R.F. (ed): Molecular and Clinical Advances in Anticancer Drug Resistance. 1991. ISBN 0-7923-1212-0.

Muggia F.M. (ed): New Drugs, Concepts and Results in Cancer Chemotherapy. 1991. ISBN 0-7923-1253-8.

Dickson R.B., Lippman M.E. (eds): Genes, Oncogenes and Hormones: Advances in Cellular and Molecular Biology of Breast Cancer. 1992. ISBN 0-7923-1748-3.

Humphrey G. Bennett, Koops H. Schraffordt, Molenaar W.M., Postma A. (eds): Osteosarcoma in Adolescents and Young Adults: New Developments and Controversies. 1993. ISBN 0-7923-1905-2.

Benz C.C., Liu E.F. (eds): Oncogenes and Tumor Suppressor Genes in Human Malignancies. 1993. ISBN 0-7923-1960-5.

Freireich E.J., Kantarjian H. (eds): Leukemia: Advances in Research and Treatment. 1993. ISBN 0-7923-1967-2.

Dana B.W. (ed): Malignant Lymphomas, Including Hodgkin's Disease: Diagnosis, Management and Special Problems. 1993. ISBN 0-7923-2171-5.

Nathanson L. (ed): Current Research and Clinical Management of Melanoma. 1993. ISBN 0-7923-2152-9.

Verweij J., Pinedo H.M., Suit H.D. (eds): Multidisciplinary Treatment of Soft Tissue Sarcomas. 1993. ISBN 0-7923-2183-9.

Rosen S.T., Kuzel T.M. (eds): Immunoconjugate Therapy of Hematologic Malignancies. 1993. ISBN 0-7923-2270-3.

Sugarbaker P.H. (ed): Hepatobiliary Cancer. 1994. ISBN 0-7923-2501-X.

Rothenberg M.L. (ed): Gynecologic Oncology: Controversies and New Developments. 1994. ISBN 0-7923-2634-2.

Dickson R.B., Lippman M.E. (eds): Mammary Tumorigenesis and Malignant Progression. 1994. ISBN 0-7923-2647-4.

Hansen H.H. (ed): Lung Cancer. Advances in Basic and Clinical Research. 1994. ISBN 0-7923-2835-3.

Goldstein L.J., Ozols R.F. (eds): Anticancer Drug Resistance. Advances in Molecular and Clinical Research. 1994. ISBN 0-7923-2836-1.

Head and Neck Cancer

Basic and Clinical Aspects

edited by

Waun Ki Hong, M.D.
The University of Texas
M. D. Anderson Cancer Center
Houston, Texas

Randal S. Weber, M.D.
The University of Texas
M. D. Anderson Cancer Center
Houston, Texas

RC280
H4
H3848
1995

1995 **KLUWER ACADEMIC PUBLISHERS**
BOSTON / DORDRECHT / LONDON

Distributors for North America:
Kluwer Academic Publishers
101 Philip Drive
Assinippi Park
Norwell, Massachusetts 02061, USA

Distributors for all other countries:
Kluwer Academic Publishers Group
Distribution Centre
Post Office Box 322
3300 AH Dordrecht, THE NETHERLANDS

Library of Congress Cataloging-in-Publication Data
Head and neck cancer: basic and clinical aspects/edited by Waun Ki Hong,
    Randal S. Weber.
        p.   cm. — (Cancer treatment and research; CTAR 74)
    Includes bibliographical references and index.
    ISBN 0-7923-3015-3 (alk. paper)
    1. Head — Cancer.   2. Neck — Cancer.   I. Hong, Waun
Ki.   II. Weber, Randal S.   III. Series: Cancer treatment and research;
v. 74.
    [DNLM: 1. Head and Neck Neoplasms.   W1 CA693 v. 74 1994/
WE 707 H43173 1994]
RC280.H4H3848   1994
616.99′491 — dc20
DNLM/DLC
for Library of Congress   94-27497
                                                                   CIP

Printed on acid-free paper.

Printed in the United States of America

Contents

Preface

Throughout the world, head and neck cancer is a major threat to public health and a significant challenge to both clinicians and basic scientists. Despite extensive efforts in primary prevention, screening, early detection, and therapy, long-term survival rates have not improved substantially in the last three decades. This book covers a wide range of exciting new findings in both clinical and basic sciences as they are relevant to head and neck cancer. These findings have recently enhanced our understanding of head and neck carcinogenesis at the genetic and molecular levels, offering the promise of improved preventive and therapeutic strategies. This book will also present information on the important clinical advances that have been made in chemoprevention, organ preservation, and the simultaneous use of chemotherapy and radiotherapy.

The first part provides an overview of the etiology and biology of head and neck cancer, including an examination of human papillomaviruses in both benign and malignant lesions. This section also discusses the carcinogenic process at the genetic and molecular levels, as well as aberrant squamous differentiation; increased understanding of these areas has great potential to translate into new strategies for cancer prevention. The second part describes recent advances in developing a risk model for head and neck cancer, as well as the application of genetic susceptibility data in chemoprevention. This section also includes overviews of the status of chemoprevention trials and of the process of invasion and metastasis in head and neck cancer.

The third part covers molecular studies of radioresistance, early detection of head and neck cancer, and the implications of photodynamic therapy, while the fourth section includes studies of the timing and sequencing of chemoradiotherapy. New strategies in this area have significantly increased the feasibility of laryngeal preservation in the treatment of advanced laryngeal cancer. The fifth and last part discusses the management of clinically negative neck disease, the role of adjuvant therapy in preventing distant metastasis, and new strategies for the treatment of recurrent tumors. Finally, we close with some intriguing predictions for the future of head and neck cancer therapy.

Our goal is to provide a summary of the state of the art in head and neck cancer, so that practicing physicians can determine how these findings will influence the management of their patients. The participation of the many specialties represented by the authors emphasizes the importance of multidisciplinary care for the head and neck cancer patient.

WAUN KI HONG
RANDAL S. WEBER

Acknowledgments

The editors would like to express their deep appreciation to the authors for submitting their manuscripts in a timely manner. We would also like to thank Arianne O'Loughlin for her efforts in editing the manuscripts and making this project a success.

Contributing Authors

BECKETT, MICHAEL A., Laboratory Manager, Department of Radiation and Cellular Oncology, University of Chicago Medical Center, 5841 South Maryland Avenue, MC0085, Chicago, IL 60637

BENNER, STEVEN E., M.D., Associate Professor of Medicine, Division of Medical Oncology, University of North Carolina, Chapel Hill, CB 7305, Chapel Hill, NC 27599

BOYD, DOUGLAS D., Ph.D., Assistant Professor of Tumor Biology, Department of Tumor Biology, The University of Texas M. D. Anderson Cancer Center, 1515 Holcombe Boulevard, Box 108, Houston, TX 77030

CALLENDER, DAVID L., M.D., Assistant Professor of Surgery, Department of Head and Neck Surgery, The University of Texas M. D. Anderson Cancer Center, 1515 Holcombe Boulevard, Box 69, Houston, TX 77030

CLAYMAN, GARY L., D.D.S., M.D., Assistant Professor of Surgery, Department of Head and Neck Surgery, The University of Texas M. D. Anderson Cancer Center, 1515 Holcombe Boulevard, Box 69, Houston, TX 77030

DIBB, CHARLES R., M.D., Medford Clinic, 555 Black Oak Drive, Medford, OR 97504

FORASTIERE, ARLENE A., M.D., Associate Professor of Medicine, The Johns Hopkins Oncology Center, Johns Hopkins University School of Medicine, 600 North Wolfe Street, Baltimore, MD 21287-8936

GLUCKMAN, JACK L., M.D., Professor and Chairman, Department of Otolaryngology — Head and Neck Surgery, University of Cincinnati Medical Center, Mail Location 0528, 231 Bethesda Avenue, Cincinnati, OH 45267-0528

GOEPFERT, HELMUT, M.D., Professor and Chairman, Department of Head and Neck Surgery; M.G. and Lillie A. Johnson Chair for Cancer Treatment and Research, Department of Head and Neck Surgery, The University of Texas M. D. Anderson Cancer Center, 1515 Holcombe Boulevard, Box 69, Houston, TX 77030

HALLAHAN, DENNIS, M.D., Assistant Professor, Department of Radiation and Cellular Oncology, University of Chicago Medical Center,

5841 South Maryland Avenue, MC0085, Chicago, IL 60637

HARAF, DANIEL., M.D. Assistant Professor, Department of Radiation and Cellular Oncology, University of Chicago Medical Center, 5841 South Maryland Avenue, MC0085, Chicago, IL 60637

HONG, WAUN K., M.D., Professor and Chairman, Department of Thoracic/Head, and Neck Medical Oncology, Charles A. LeMaistre Chair in Thoracic Oncology, The University of Texas M. D. Anderson Cancer Center, 1515 Holcombe Boulevard, Box 80, Houston, TX 77030

HUBER, MARTIN H., M.D., Assistant Internist and Assistant Professor of Medicine, Department of Thoracic/Head and Neck Medical Oncology, The University of Texas M. D. Anderson Cancer Center, 1515 Holcombe Boulevard, Box 80, Houston, TX 77030

JACOBS, CHARLOTTE, M.D., Senior Associate Dean for Education and Student Affairs, Vice President and Dean's Office, M121 School of Medicine, Stanford University, Stanford, CA 94505

KUFE, DONALD, M.D., Chief, Division of Cancer Pharmacology, Dana-Farber Cancer Institute, Division of Cancer Pharmacology, 44 Binney Street, Room D1730, Boston, MA 02115

LIPPMAN, SCOTT M., M.D., Associate Professor of Medicine, Chief of Section of Head and Neck Medical Oncology, Department of Thoracic/Head and Neck Medical Oncology, The University of Texas M. D. Anderson Cancer Center, 1515 Holcombe Boulevard, Box 80, Houston, TX 77030

LOTAN, REUBEN M., Ph.D., Professor of Tumor Biology, Deputy Chairman, Department of Tumor Biology, Abell-Hanger Foundation Professor, The University of Texas M. D. Anderson Cancer Center, 1515 Holcombe Boulevard, Box 108, Houston, TX 77030

NICOLSON, GARTH L., Ph.D., Professor of Tumor Biology, Chairman, Department of Tumor Biology, David Bruton, Jr. Chair in Cancer Research, The University of Texas M. D. Anderson Cancer Center, 1515 Holcombe Boulevard, Box 108, Houston, TX 77030

PINTO, HARLAN A., M.D., Assistant Professor of Medicine, Division of Medical Oncology, Room M211, Stanford University Medical Center, Stanford, CA 94505

PORTUGAL, LOUIS G., M.D., Assistant Professor of Medicine, University of Illinois Eye and Ear Infirmary, Department of Otolaryngology — Head and Neck Surgery, 1855 West Taylor Street, Chicago, IL 60612

SHIN, DONG M., M.D., Assistant Internist and Assistant Professor of Medicine, Department of Thoracic/Head and Neck Medical Oncology, The University of Texas M. D. Anderson Cancer Center, 1515 Holcombe Boulevard, Box 80, Houston, TX 77030

SPITZ, MARGARET R., M.D., M.P.H., Acting Chair, Department of Epidemiology, The University of Texas M. D. Anderson Cancer Center, 1515 Holcombe Boulevard, Box 189, Houston, TX 77030

STEINBERG, BETTIE M., Ph.D., Chief, Division of Otolaryngologic

Research, LIJMC, Associate Professor, Otolaryngology, Albert Einstein College of Medicine, Long Island Jewish Medical Center, Department of Otolaryngology and Communicative Disorders, New Hyde Park, NY 11042

TAINSKY, MICHAEL A., Ph.D., Associate Biologist, Associate Professor of Tumor Biology, Department of Tumor Biology, The University of Texas M. D. Anderson Cancer Center, 1515 Holcombe Boulevard, Box 79, Houston, TX 77030

URBA, SUSAN G., M.D., Assistant Professor of Medicine, Division of Hematology/Oncology, Department of Internal Medicine, University of Michigan Medical School, 3119 Taubman Center, Ann Arbor, MI 48109-0374

VOKES, EVERETT E., M.D., Associate Professor of Medicine, Department of Medicine, Section of Hematology/Oncology, University of Chicago Medical Center, 5841 South Maryland Avenue, MC2115, Chicago, IL 60637-1470

WEBER, RANDAL S., M.D., Associate Professor and Deputy Chairman, Department of Head and Neck Surgery, The University of Texas M. D. Anderson Cancer Center, 1515 Holcombe Boulevard, Box 69, Houston, TX 77030

WEICHSELBAUM, RALPH R., M.D., Harold H. Hines Jr. Professor and Chairman, Department of Radiation and Cellular Oncology, Director, Chicago Tumor Institue, Department of Radiation and Cellular Oncology, University of Chicago Medical Center, 5841 South Maryland Avenue, MC0085, Chicago, IL 60637

WOLF, GREGORY T., M.D., Professor and Chairman, Department of Otolaryngology, University of Michigan Medical School, 1500 East Medical Center Drive, Ann Arbor, MI 48109-0312

ZITSCH, ROBERT P., M.D., Assistant Professor of Surgery, University of Missouri Medical Center, Division of Otolaryngology, One Hospital Drive, Columbia, MO 65201

1. Role of human papillomaviruses in benign and malignant lesions

Bettie M. Steinberg

The human papillomaviruses (HPVs) are a large family of related DNA viruses. They are the etiologic agents of benign lesions (warts or papillomas) of the skin, genitalia, and respiratory tract, as well as some malignancies [for reviews see 1,2]. These viruses are very similar to the papillomaviruses that cause warts in other vertebrates, ranging from birds to cattle. All of the papillomaviruses have a similar genetic structure. The double-stranded circular DNA is approximately 8000 base pairs long. In benign lesions it exists as multiple copies of separate episomes or *mini-chromosomes*, not integrated into the cellular chromosomes. In malignant lesions, the viral DNA is frequently, but not always, integrated into the host DNA. In infectious viral particles, the DNA is packaged inside two viral coat proteins. The virus does not contain a lipid envelope. Lack of an envelope means that these viruses are resistant to drying and cannot be inactivated with alcohol or other solvents.

More than 60 HPV types are currently known. Typing is based on DNA homology, rather than on serotype. This is because virus particles for most HPV types are not available to develop serologic assays. The only types in which virus is readily available in abundance are HPV 1, extracted from plantar warts, and one isolate of HPV 11 which has been propagated in human foreskin tissue implanted into nude mice. Most mucosal lesions contain only small amounts of virus. Investigators have not been able to grow papillomaviruses in tissue cluture, and only cloned DNA is available for most types.

Biology of HPV infection

Human papillomaviruses are absolutely specific for squamous epithelium for their replication, although they are able to infect respiratory epithelium and the columnar cells of the endocervix. They also show specificity for parti-

Hong, Waun Ki and Weber, Randal S., (eds.), Head and Neck Cancer. © 1995 Kluwer Academic Publishers. ISBN 0-7923-3015-3. All rights reserved.

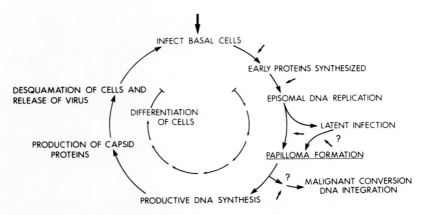

Figure 1. Life cycle of human papillomaviruses. This figure illustrates the overall life cycle of the HPVs, showing the alternate outcomes of infections. The inner broken circle represents the progressive differentiation of the stratified squamous epithelium. Thin arrows mark steps where interventions might be developed to prevent disease. Question marks indicate events that are only poorly defined to date. (Reprinted with permission from Auborn and Steinberg [38], Copyright CRC Press, Inc. Boca Raton, FL.)

cular types of epithelium. If the HPVs are grouped by their DNA sequences, the groupings show clear tissue specificity, with a major subdivision between mucosal and epidermal viruses [3,4]. The basis of the tissue specificity is only partly understood, but appears to involve regulatory sequences within the viral DNA that interact with proteins found in preferred epithelial tissues [5]. The mucosal virus can then be subgrouped into three groups: those with relatively rare association with malignancy in the genital tract (HPV 6 and 11, for example), those with intermediate malignant association (i.e., HPVs 30, 31, and 33), and those with high malignant association (HPVs 16 and 18).

Figure 1 shows the life cycle of the HPVs. Much of this information is based on analysis of clinical tissues and analogy with the bovine papillomavirus. There has been one system available for the propagation of HPV 11, using human epithelial tissues infected with the virus and implanted under the renal capsule of nude mice [6]. In this system, after a lag phase of weeks or months, the tissue will proliferate to form a benign papillomatous cyst expressing all the viral RNAs and proteins, and producing new virus. In situ hybridization of these cysts, as well as many different studies of pathology specimens of both papillomas and carcinomas, has helped us begin to understand the viral life cycle [7,8].

There are carefully controlled steps in the life cycle, coordinately regulated by the degree of differentiation of the epithelium. Synthesis of low levels of RNA coding for early proteins and low level episomal DNA replication occur in the parabasal and lower spinous layers. Only in the upper layers of the papillomatous tissues is there abundant expression of viral RNA and viral proteins and production of new viral particles.

There are three possible outcomes of HPV infection. First, and probably most common, is latent infection. In this state viral DNA is present, but there is no clinical or histological evidence of disease [9]. Latency can exist for years without any pathology. In Figure 1 latency is not shown as part of the main cycle, because there is no evidence for virus production during latency.

Our laboratory is currently studying the molecular biology of latency. We know that HPV RNA is in very low supply in latently infected tissues, much lower than in papillomas. While still preliminary, we have data that suggest that the RNAs made during latency are smaller than those made in active infection, and that at least some genes for early viral proteins are not expressed. We speculate that the absence of one or more critical viral gene products results in the lack of any phenotypic changes in the tissue. We know there is a lag period of several weeks to months between initial HPV infection and the appearance of HPV RNA and then a papilloma [8]. We also know that latent viral DNA can persist in tissues for years [9]. We do not know whether these two 'latent' states are biochemically the same. Are the same RNAs made in both cases? Are there any differences at the cellular level that are not detected histologically? We have long postulated that latent infection can be activated, leading to the formation of papillomas, and that latent infection is the source of recurrent disease, but this has not been proven. We are actively engaged in these studies, asking what cellular or environmental factor(s) might be important in activation.

The second possible outcome of infection is the formation of a benign papilloma or wart, which can be either markedly exophytic or rather flat. These benign lesions are the classical clinical manifestations of HPV infection. The tissue is hyperplastic, with a relatively normal basal layer and marked thickening of the spinous layer surrounding cores of connective tissue (Figure 2). New virus particles are produced in a subset of the uppermost papilloma cells. These particles are released as the surface cells shed. Comparatively little virus is produced in respiratory papillomas, and some papillomas produce no new virus.

One common characteristic of papillomas is increased capillary proliferation, with capillary loops in each connective core of the papillary fronds. To date, nothing is known about the mechanism of induction of capillary proliferation in these tissues. Intriguingly, recent studies have shown that interferon blocks capillary proliferation [10]. Interferon has also been shown to reduce or prevent papilloma recurrences [11,12]. The relationship between these two facts needs to be studied. Perhaps it is the inhibition of angiogenesis, rather than antiviral effects, that functions in interferon therapy.

Finally, conversion of a benign papilloma to a malignant carcinoma can occur. There are three lines of evidence linking HPVs to human cancer.

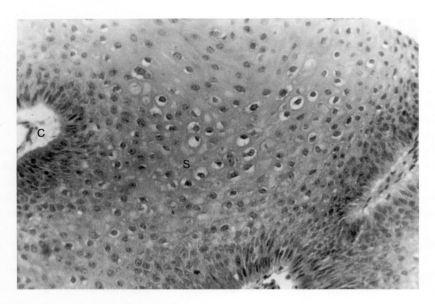

Figure 2. Histology of a papilloma. The hyperplasia of the spinous layer (S) and the connective tissue cores containing capillaries (C) are clearly seen in this cross section of a benign laryngeal papilloma. Hematoxylin-eosin stain.

First, over 90% of genital cancers contain HPVs [for extensive review see 2]. Second, laryngeal papillomas can convert to carcinomas after X-irradiation [13]. Third, cultured human keratinocytes can be immortalized with either intact HPV 16 or 18 DNA, or with subgenomic fragments [for review see 2]. The immortalized cells can gain the ability to form malignant tumors after prolonged passage in culture. Moreover, the fact that papillomas on domestic rabbits induced with the cottontail rabbit papillomavirus can convert to malignancy also supports the relationship between papillomaviruses and cancers.

Malignant conversion is a rare event, even with those HPV types such as HPVs 16 and 18 that are 'high risk.' It has been estimated that in the genital tract 10–15% of benign lesions progress to dysplastic premalignant lesions, and approximately 10% of these will develop into fully invasive carcinomas if not treated [for review see 2]. The risk of spontaneous progression of laryngeal papillomas is not known but is much lower. Such conversions are presented in the literature as scattered case reports.

New HPV particles are not produced in the malignant tumors. This outcome of infection is a dead end for the virus. The viral DNA is usually integrated in cancers, interrupting expression of the sequences for capsid proteins. In addition, there is absence of the epithelial differentiation required for the complete life cycle. Even those tumors classified as 'well differentiated' do not complete the full differentiation process.

4

Environmental factors play a significant role in the malignant conversion of an HPV infection. X-ray therapy, used in the 1930s to treat laryngeal papillomas, caused approximately one third of the patients to develop carcinoma of the larynx [13]. Tobacco smoking is postulated to be a risk factor for development of cervical cancer in patients with HPV 16 and HPV 18 infections [14]. Ultraviolet light is a cofactor for malignant conversion of flat skin warts caused by HPV 5 and HPV 8 in patients with the rare disease epidermodysplasia verruciformis [15]. In each case, a combination of HPV plus a carcinogen increases the probability of malignant conversion of the pre-existing benign lesion.

Functions of HPV proteins

HPV DNA can be divided into three functional areas. Figure 3 shows the HPV DNA drawn in linear form, to facilitate seeing the relative positions of the regions coding for viral proteins. Actually, the two ends are joined and the DNA exists as a circle. The upstream regulatory region contains the origin of replication and sequences that control expression in both positive and negative ways. It does not code for any known protein. The early region (E) contains the sequences that code for the early proteins: those involved in establishment of the virus within a host cell, viral replication, and transformation of the normal host cell to a papilloma or carcinoma. The late region (L) contains the coding sequences for the two capsid proteins.

Three of the early proteins are of particular interest because they are important in tumor formation. E5 is a small protein localized in the cell membranes [16]. It interacts with receptors for growth factors and in this way may alter the response of the cell to signals for growth and differentiation [17]. The E5 protein is not able to immortalize cells but can cause changes in growth characteristics. It may be the major protein inducing benign, hyperproliferative papillomas.

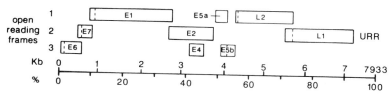

Figure 3. Organization of the HPV 11 molecule. The relative positions of upstream regulatory region (URR) and the open reading frames coding for the early (E) and late (L) proteins are shown. The DNA molecule is depicted as linear, opened at the beginning of the early region. In actuality, the molecule is circular, and the URR is positioned directly before the E6 open reading frame. Numbers above the line show the actual nucleotide sequence in kilobases (Kb), while numbers below the line indicate the percentage of the total viral DNA molecule.

5

E6 and E7 proteins are found in the nucleus, where they appear to have several functions. There is some evidence that E7 can alter gene expression [18]. In papillomas it has been postulated that the main function of these two proteins is to help maintain the cellular DNA replication machinery in the more superficial cells where the virus replicates (Dr. T. Broker, personal communication). In normal epithelium, the upper spinous cells are terminally differentiated. They have lost the complex set of enzymes and factors required to replicate cell DNA. The virus is dependent on these celluar proteins to replicate its DNA and therefore must have some mechanism to maintain that function.

E6 and E7 proteins from either HPV 16 or HPV 18 work together to cause complete transformation of human cells [19]. Epithelial cells infected in the laboratory with these two HPV proteins can become immortal, and a subset develop the ability to form carcinomas in animals. The HPV proteins form complexes with two very important cellular tumor suppressor proteins. E7 complexes with the retinoblastoma protein (Rb), while E6 binds to and facilitates degradation of p53 [20,21]. E6 and E7 proteins from the HPV types that normally do not cause cancers show reduced or absent binding to the p53 and Rb proteins. The current belief is that complexing with and inactivating these two proteins is at least part of the mechanism by which HPVs cause cancers. Integration of HPV DNA into the host cell in malignant tumors usually results in loss of regulation of E6 and E7 RNA synthesis, increasing the levels of these two proteins. Perhaps low levels are required and sufficient to induce benign papillomas, while overexpression of the oncogenic types leads to carcinomas.

The E1 protein is involved in replication of HPV DNA, interacting with cellular proteins in ways that are currently under study [22]. The E2 protein plays multiple regulatory roles. It interacts with the E1 protein in replication [23]. It also acts as both a positive and negative regulator of E6 and E7 expression, with its primary function to suppress expression [24]. Most carcinomas do not express E2, because integration of the viral DNA into the host chromosomes usually occurs at the end of E1 or the beginning of E2. This is probably the reason carcinomas overexpress the E6 and E7 genes. The function of E4 is still not clear.

Model systems to study HPV

Standard tissue culture systems are not well suited to study many aspects of HPV–host cell interactions. In order to understand why, we must understand the effect HPV infection has on host cell functions. Laryngeal papillomas are characterized by an abnormal type of differentiation [25]. Involucrin, a marker for squamous differentiation, is present in both normal and papilloma tissues (Figure 4a,b). In contrast, papillomas show marked reduction in the presence of differentiation-specific keratins and filaggrin

Normal **Papilloma**

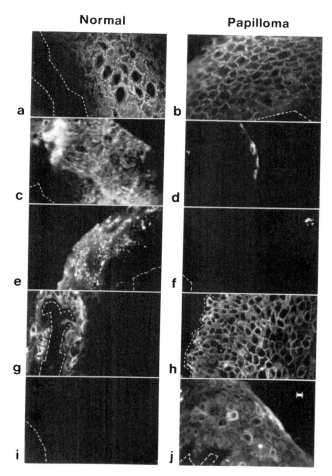

Figure 4. Differentiation of laryngeal papilloma compared to normal larynx. Frozen sections of both normal and papilloma tissues were stained by immunohistochemical techniques, using a panel of antibodies for differentiation markers, followed by a fluorescein-labeled second antibody. Peanut agglutinin (PNA) staining of the cell-surface glycoprotein was determined by binding frozen sections directly to fluorescein-labeled PNA. a, b: involucrin; c, d: keratin 13; e, f: filaggrin; g, h: PNA; i, j: psoriatic antigen psi-3, found in suprabasal hyperproliferative epidermis. (Reprinted with permission from Steinberg et al. [25].)

(Figure 4d,f) and the new appearance of markers of hyperproliferative epithelium (Figure 4j). The differentiation abnormality is the primary phenotypic marker for papillomas. Unfortunately, standard culture systems for epithelial cells do not permit normal differentiation. In these cultures, the normal cells display a hyperproliferative phenotype very similar to papilloma cells.

Papilloma cells do not divide more rapidly than normal cells. They do not have an expanded life span in culture and do not show any difference in cell size or shape. The fraction of basal and parabasal cells in papillomas that replicate their DNA is slightly lower than the normal cells [25]. Therefore, growth rates and proliferative capability, markers of basal cells, cannot be used to distinguish between normal and papilloma cells in culture.

Recently, a different method for the culture of epidermal cells has been developed [26]. This method cultures the epithelial cells on a collagen gel containing fibroblasts, which simulates the dermis. The entire culture is lifted to the air-liquid interface, so that the culture medium is only in contact with the bottom of the gel. In this way, the epithelial cells receive nutrients via their basal surface, in a manner much more analogous to the in vivo tissue. These 'raft' cultures permit much more faithful differentiation.

We have modified the raft culture system and optimized it for the growth of human laryngeal epithelial cells using a completely defined serum-free culture medium [27]. The histology of raft cultures of normal cells, grown in the presence of 10 nmol/l retinoic acid, is shown in Figure 5a. For comparison, the histology of normal vocal cord epithelium is shown in Figure 5b. The raft cultures showed very good histologic differentiation of the cells, with a well-defined basal layer, several layers of spinous cells, and some granular cells at the surface. All suprabasal cells synthesized the differentiation-specific keratin 13, and the upper half of the 'epithelium' was positive for involucrin, a marker of squamous differentiation. When the retinoic acid was increased to 100 nmol/l, the morphology of the cells changed to that of pseudostratified squamous respiratory epithelium with cilia on their surface (Figure 6). We were able to confirm the presence of cilia with electron microscopy [27]. We have thus shown that not only can human laryngeal cells differentiate normally in culture, but that the choice between the two normal differentiation pathways for this tissue can be modulated by retinoids in vitro.

This system also allowed us to begin to determine the effects of various hormones and biological modifiers on the papilloma cells. Treatment of cultured papilloma cells with retinoic acid altered both differentiation and persistence of the viral DNA [28]. These results are summarized in Table 1. At high concentrations of retinoic acid the papilloma cells did not show extensive cilia formation, but there was a clear shift away from squamous differentiation. This shift was accompanied by a reduction in the amount of episomal viral DNA persisting in the cells. At 1 nmol/l retinoic acid, when squamous differentiation was maximal, nearly all of the papilloma cells were still negative for keratin 13. Therefore, this raft culture reproduces the papilloma differentiation abnormality seen in vivo.

Most recently, we have evaluated the presence of the epidermal growth factor (EGF) receptor on normal and papilloma cells, and the effects of EGF on the raft cultures (manuscript in preparation). When cultured continuously in medium containing 1 ng/ml EGF, the normal cells showed faint

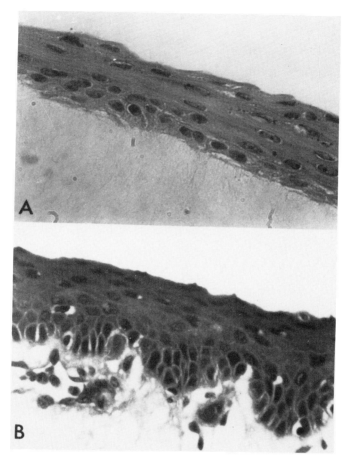

Figure 5. Histology of normal larynx cells cultured on collagen rafts. A: Cells were cultured at the air-liquid interface for 2 weeks in serum-free medium containing 10 nmol/l retinoic acid, then fixed with 0.37 mol/l formaldehyde and embedded in paraffin; 5-μm sections were cut and stained with hematoxylin-eosin. B. Histology of normal vocal cord tissue, for comparison to raft cultures. Hematoxylin-eosin stain. (Reprinted with permission from Mendelsohn et al. [27].)

immunohistochemical staining of the basal layer with an antibody to the EGF receptor. Staining increased when EGF was removed from the medium and diminished to undetectable levels if EGF was added at 50 ng/ml. This was expected, since binding of EGF to the receptor induces internalization and degradation of the complex [29]. In contrast, the papilloma cells stained intensely with the anti-EGF receptor antibody. The staining was only slightly diminished when 50 ng/ml EGF was present. These data, coupled with the report that the E5 gene product from the bovine papillomavirus can complex with the EGF receptor in fibroblasts [17], suggest that similar complexes might exist in the laryngeal papilloma cells.

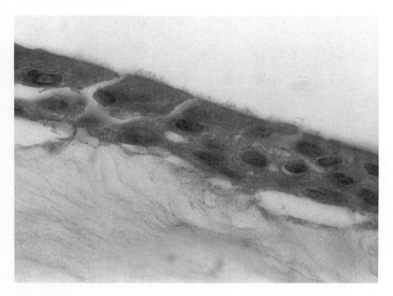

Figure 6. Effects of increased retinoic acid in morphology of normal larynx cells on collagen rafts. The same primary cell preparation used in Figure 5 was cultured in medium containing 100 nmol/l retinoic acid. Note the change in morphology to pseudostratified columnar epithelium and the appearance of cilia on the surface of many of the cells. (Reprinted with permission from Mendelsohn et al. [27].)

Table 1. Effects of retinoic acid on papilloma cells

Retinoic acid concentration	Squamous differentiation[a]	Relative HPV DNA content[b]
0	ND	1.0
1 nmol/l	++++	0.9
10 nmol/l	+++	0.4
100 nmol/l	+	0.2
1 µmol/l	—	0.1

Cells were cultured on collagen rafts at the air-liquid interface in serum-free medium supplemented with the specified concentration of retinoic acid.
[a] Determined by immunohistochemical staining for involucrin staining.
[b] Mean values of three experiments. Normalized to values obtained when cells were cultured in the absence of retinoic acid.
ND = not determined. The histology in the absence of retinoic acid was so poor that the antibody staining was not done.
Adapted from Reppucci et al. [28], with permission.

Changing the concentrations of EGF in the culture medium had marked effects on the papilloma cells (Table 2). Removal of EGF from the culture medium for 5 days induced normal differentiation of these cells, as measured by presence of keratin 13 in all suprabasal cells, but had no measurable

Table 2. Effects of epidermal growth factor on papilloma cells

EGF concentration[a]	Keratin 13 staining	Relative HPV RNA content[b]
1 ng/ml[c]	+/−	1.0
0 ng/ml	+ + + + +	14.0
1 ng/ml	+ + +	8.4
50 ng/ml	+ +	2.7

[a] Cells were grown on collagen rafts at the air-liquid interface. EGF was either maintained continuously in the medium or removed for 48 hours, then replaced at the indicated concentration for 72 hours. Cells were then prepared for frozen sections, or RNA was extracted and analyzed by dot blot hybridization with full-length ^{32}P-labeled HPV probe, followed by rehybridization with an actin probe.
[b] Autoradiographic signals were quantified by densitometry, corrected for actin signal to adjust for the amount of total RNA in each sample, and normalized to the value obtained for cells cultured continuously in 1 ng/ml EGF.
[c] Culture maintained continuously in the presence of EGF.

effect on differentiation of normal cells. Removal of EGF also induced a 14-fold increase in the amount of HPV-specific RNA in the cells, consistent with the fact that squamous differentiation is required for high-level expression of viral proteins and viral replication. Meyers et al. [30] and Dollard et al. [31] recently reported that raft cultures can be used to induce HPV replication and virion production in infected genital cells, permitting HPV production in cultured cells for the first time. We are currently investigating the possibility that removal of EGF induces HPV production in laryngeal papilloma cells.

Role of HPV in benign tumors

The most clearly defined role of HPVs in head and neck tumors is in laryngeal papillomas. These lesions are characterized by large recurrent exophytic masses (see Figure 2) located primarily on the vocal folds. They frequently involve the epiglottis and false vocal folds, and occasionally involve the subglottis, trachea, bronchi, and lung parenchyma. Involvement of the lower respiratory tract is usually fatal, due to airway obstruction and destruction of lung function.

All laryngeal papillomas analyzed to date contain HPV DNA. The HPV types usually found, types 6 and 11, are the same as those found in exophytic genital papillomas [32]. These two closely related HPV types show a marked tissue preference for mucosal epithelium, also causing papillomas of the oropharynx and nasopharynx and conjunctiva of the eye. The relationship between HPV 11 and laryngeal papillomas is more than circumstantial. Kreider et al. [6] have satisfied Koch's postulates by infecting fragments of laryngeal tissue with purified HPV 11, implanting the tissue under the

11

renal capsule of immunodeficient mice, and observing the formation of papillomatous cysts that have all the histological features of laryngeal papillomas.

HPVs have also been found in other benign and premalignant lesions of the head and neck. Many oral lesions, including papillomas, focal epithelial hyperplasia, and leukoplakia, have been positive for HPV 2, 6, 11, 13, 32, or 16 [32]. Fungiform papillomas of the nose frequently contain HPV 6 or 11, and several reports describe HPVs 11 and/or 16 in some inverting papillomas [34–36]. Papillomaviruses probably play a role in the etiology of many of these lesions. However, it is difficult to determine what that role is. Not all lesions contained detectable HPV DNA, and a substantial fraction of normal biopsies from the nasopharynx also contained viral DNA [37].

Standard treatment for laryngeal papillomas is surgical excision with the carbon dioxide laser. Many other therapies have been tried, most with minimal success [for review see 38]. Removal of papillomas during surgery does not result in cure. Some patients require surgery as frequently as every 2 weeks to maintain the airway, while others will have one or two widely separated recurrences, and then go into a remission that can last for months, years, or the life of the patient. Latent HPV can be detected in clinically and histologically normal respiratory tissues in papilloma patients [9]. Activation of latent HPV, rather than spread of infection during surgery, is postulated to be the source of recurrent disease. Our institution is currently conducting a clinical trial of photodynamic therapy for laryngeal papillomas to determine whether this treatment will reduce the frequency of recurrence. Results from the first part of the study, using a relatively low dose of activating drug, are encouraging [39].

HPV and malignant tumors

There are a few cases of head and neck carcinomas that are clearly HPV related. These are in patients with long-standing recurrent respiratory papillomatosis in which one of the papillomas has undergone malignant conversion. Radiation exposure induced malignant conversion in approximately one third of the patients after a period of 10–20 years [13]. Spontaneous malignant conversion of papillomas also can occur, although with a much lower frequency. The cofactors in these cases are less clearly defined. Smoking is strongly implicated in several instances, while other patients have been nonsmokers. The carcinomas from papilloma patients contain the same HPV 6 or 11 found in the papillomas [40–42], but the molecules have frequently undergone rearrangements that might contribute to their increased malignant potential [41,42].

One other type of head and neck tumor with a strong association with HPV is verrucous carcinoma of the larynx. These extremely well-differentiated tumors share many histologic features with papillomas, and

Table 3. Prevalence of HPV in head and neck carcinomas

Location of tumor	Number pos./total number	HPV type	Method used	Ref.
Oral cavity, oropharynx	3/7	2,16	Southern	46
	3/9	2	In situ	47
	3/4	11	In situ	48
	8/24	16,18	PCR	49
	5/36	16	Southern	50
Nose and nasopharynx	7/60	16,18	PCR	51
	0/16	NA	PCR	52
	3/3	16	In situ	53
Larynx	7/34	6,16	PCR	54
	3/60	11,16	Southern	50
	26/48	16	PCR	44

thus it might not be too surprising to find them HPV positive. Brandsma et al. [43] found six out of six tumors, and Perez-Ayala [44] found three out of three tumors positive for sequences related to HPV 16. McLachlin et al. [45] found 10 of 21 lesions positive for either HPV 16 or 18.

The role of HPV in other malignant tumors of the head and neck is more difficult to determine. HPV DNA is found in a subset of squamous carcinomas. A number of case reports describe an individual positive tumor, but no prevalence information can be derived from such reports. However, larger series have also been conducted. Table 3 summarizes some of those findings and illustrates the extent of variability from one study to the next.

Although some carcinomas did contain HPV DNA, there is no consensus about the fraction that are positive. If data from all of the studies are pooled, 23% of the tumors analyzed were positive. However, from these data we do not know with certainty whether HPV plays any role in the etiology of the carcinomas. Since HPVs can form latent infection, it is very possible that at least some of these infections simply reflect latent virus that happened to be in the tumor. Brandsma et al. [50] detected 4% latency by Southern blot of laryngeal tissues, and Bryan et al. [37] found 64% latent infection in nasopharyngeal tissues using PCR detection.

Detection of HPV

The presence of HPV in benign or malignant tumors can be determined in several different ways. Each has advantages and disadvantages, and different sensitivities and specificities. The various methods that have been used have contributed to the confusion surrounding the role of HPVs in head and neck tumors.

Early studies to detect HPVs used an antibody that crossreacts with a

13

viral protein present on most animal and human papillomavirus particles. Use of this antibody has the advantage that the HPV type does not have to be known. Moreover, it can readily be used on tissue sections from archival specimens. Unfortunately, not all HPV-induced papillomas make virus particles. This limitation is even more true for carcinomas, which rarely if ever make virus particles.

Detection of viral DNA by one of several methods is more sensitive and is able to distinguish specific HPV types but is associated with other problems. All of these methods require the use of probes that are generally specific for just one type of HPV. Mixed probes can detect several types, but only those types represented in the mixture. If the HPV in the tissue being studied is of a different and perhaps undiscovered type, the assay will be negative. Use of less stringent conditions permits detection of related but not identical types, but use of these conditions results in loss of sensitivity and increased background. Therefore, there might well be unique HPVs associated with head and neck tumors that have not yet been identified.

Dot blot assays, used because they are simple to perform, are relatively insensitive and somewhat prone to false-positive results. They have a minimum detection level of approximately 1 million copies of HPV DNA, and thus require many copies of viral DNA per cell or large numbers of infected cells. Southern blots are slightly more sensitive (100,000–500,000 copies). This procedure is the current gold standard, but it is technically demanding. Southern blots cannot be done on paraffin-embedded material, necessitating the use of fresh tissue. In situ hybridization can be done on archival tissues. It also has the advantage that it permits correlation between positive signal and histology. Even a few positive cells can be detected if they have 50–100 copies of HPV per cell. However, many cancer cells and some papillomas do not contain such high copy numbers of virus. The newest method, polymerase chain reaction (PCR), can be done on archival tissue and is exquisitely sensitive, able to detect as few as 10 molecules of viral DNA! Unfortunately, its very sensitivity can be a problem. Trace contamination of samples in the laboratory is difficult to prevent, especially in laboratories that frequently process tissues known to contain HPVs. Even if the detected virus is not a contaminant, it may be unrelated to the disease process. We live in a sea of viruses, most of which do not cause disease. The simple presence of a few molecules of virus in one or a few cells does not mean that it is the etiologic agent of the tumor.

Conclusions

We have presented a review of the evidence linking HPVs to head and neck lesions. Clearly, they are the etiologic agents of papillomas, and this is not debated. With papillomas, the questions to be addressed involve regulation of viral expression and the interactions between the virus and the host cell.

14

Four types of studies are needed to better determine whether HPVs have an active role in head and neck carcinomas. First, studies must be done to determine whether the HPV-positive tumors contain HPV RNA and protein. Neither is readily detectable in latent infection, but they can be detected in genital carcinomas. Second, more studies analyzing normal tissues are needed to provide a true prevalence rate for latency. Third, additional studies should continue to look for the presence of novel HPV types that might be associated with a large fraction of head and neck tumors. These types of studies are currently in progress in several laboratories. Finally, we need to understand the relationship between HPV presence and environmental factors that could activate latent infection and contribute to malignant progression. With this information, perhaps the role of HPV in head and neck malignancies will no longer be in question.

Acknowledgment

This work was supported in part by grant DC00203 from the National Institute on Deafness and Other Communication Disorders, and a grant from the Irving and Helen Schneider family.

References

1. Salzman NP, Howley PM, ed. The Papovaviridae, The Papillomaviruses. New York: Plenum Press, 1987.
2. Pfister H, ed. Papillomaviruses and Human Cancer. Boca Raton, FL: CRC Press, 1990.
3. Pfister H. In: G Gross, S Jablonska, H Pfister, H Stegner, eds. Genital Papillomavirus Infections. Berlin: Springer-Verlag, 1990, pp 38–49.
4. Chan SY, Bernard HU, Ong CK, et al. J Virol 66:5714–5725, 1992.
5. Steinberg BM, Auborn K, Brandsma J, Taichman L. J Virol 63:957–960, 1989.
6. Kreider JW, Howett MK, Stoler M, Zaino R, et al. Int J Cancer 39:459–465, 1987.
7. Stoler MH, Wolinsky SM, Whitbeck A, et al. Virology 172:331–340, 1989.
8. Stoler MH, Whitbeck A, Wolinsky SM, et al. J Virol 64:3310–3318, 1990.
9. Steinberg BM, Topp WC, Schneider P, Abramson AL. N Engl J Med 308:1262–1264, 1983.
10. Sidkey YA, Borde EC. Cancer Res 47:5155–5161, 1987.
11. Weck PK, Whisnant JK. In: BM Steinberg, JL Brandsma, LB Taichman, eds. Cancer Cells V, Papillomaviruses. Cold Spring Harbor, NY: Cold Spring Harbor Laboratory Press, 1987, pp 393–402.
12. Kashima H, Leventhal B, Clark K, et al. Laryngoscope 98:334–340, 1988.
13. Galloway TC, Soper GR, Elsen G. Arch Otolaryngol 72:289–293, 1960.
14. Brinton LA. In: N Munoz, FX Bosch, KV Shah, A Meheus, eds. The Epidemiology of Human Papillomavirus and Cervical Cancer. Lyon, France: International Agency for Research on Cancer, 1992, pp 3–22.
15. Jablonska S. In: H Pfister, ed. Papillomaviruses and Human Cancer. Boca Raton, FL: CRC Press, 1990, pp 45–71.
16. Schlegel R, Wade-Glass M, Rabson MS, Yang Y-C. Science 233:262–267, 1986.
17. Martin M, Vass WC, Schiller JT, Lowy DR, Velu TJ. Cell 59:21–32, 1989.

18. Munger K, Phelps WC, Bubb V, et al. Cell 53:539–547, 1988.
19. Munger K, Phelps WC, Bubb V, Howley PM, et al. J Virol 63:4417–4421, 1989.
20. Munger K, Werness BA, Dyson N, Howley PM, et al. EMBO J 8:4099–4105, 1989.
21. Werness BA, Levine AJ, Howley PM. Science 248:76–79, 1990.
22. Ustav M, Stenlund A. EMBO J 10:4321–4329, 1991.
23. Mohr IJ, Clark R, Sun S, et al. Science 250:1694–1699, 1990.
24. Chin MT, Hirochika R, Hirochika H, et al. J Virol 62:2944–3002, 1988.
25. Steinberg BM, Meade R, Kalinowski S, Abramson AL. Arch Otolaryngol Head Neck Surg 116:1167–1171, 1990.
26. Asselineau D, Bernhard B, Bailly C, et al. Exp Cell Res 159:536–539, 1985.
27. Mendelsohn MG, DiLorenzo TP, Abramson AL, Steinberg BM. In Vitro Cell Devel Biol 27A:137–141, 1991.
28. Reppucci AD, DiLorenzo TP, Steinberg BM. Otolaryngol Head Neck Surg 105:528–532, 1991.
29. Carpenter G. Annu Rev Biochem 56:881–914, 1987.
30. Meyers C. Frattini MG, Hudson JB, Laimins LA. Science 257:921–972, 1992.
31. Dollard SC, Wilson JL, Demeter LM, et al. Genes Dev 6:1131–1142.
32. Gissmann L, Diehl V, Schultz-Coulon H, zur Hausen H. J Virol 44:393–400, 1982.
33. Chang F, Syrjanen S, Kellokoski J, Syrjanen K. J Oral Pathol 20:305–317, 1991.
34. Respler D, Jahn A, Pater A, Pater, M. Ann Otol Rhinol Laryngol 96:170–172, 1987.
35. Brandsma J, Abramson A, Sciubba, Shah K, et al. In: BM Steinberg, JL Brandsma, LLB Taichman, eds. Cancer Cells 5/Papillomaviruses. Cold Spring Harbor, NY: Cold Spring Harbor Laboratory Press, 1987, pp 301–308.
36. Judd R, Zaki SR, Coffield LM, Evatt, BL. Hum Pathol 22:550–556, 1991.
37. Bryan RL, Bevan IS, Croker J, Young LS. Clin Otolaryngol 15:177–180, 1990.
38. Auborn KJ, Steinberg BM. In: H Pfister, ed. Papillomaviruses and Human Cancer. Boca Raton, FL: CRC Press, 1990, pp 203–223.
39. Abramson AL, Shikowitz MJ, Mullooly VM, Steinberg BM, et al. Arch Otolaryngol Head Neck Surg 118:25–29, 1992.
40. Byrne JC, Tsao M-S, Fraser R, Howley PM. N Engl J Med 317:873–878, 1987.
41. DiLorenzo T, Tamsen A, Abramson A, Steinberg B. J Gen Virol 73:423–428, 1992.
42. Lindeberg H, Surjanen S, Karja J, Syrjanen K. Acta Otolaryngol 107:141–149, 1989.
43. Brandsma J, Steinberg B, Abramson A, Winkler B. Cancer Res 46:2185–2188, 1986.
44. Perez-Ayala M, Ruiz-Cabello F, Esteban F, et al. Int J Cancer 46:8–11, 1990.
45. McLachlin CM, Noble-Topham S, Fliss D, Andrulis I, et al. Lab Invest 66:A72, 1992.
46. DeVilliers EM, Weidauer H, Otto H, zur Hausen H. Int J Cancer 36:575–578, 1985.
47. Adler-Storthz K, Newland JR, Tessin BA, Yeudall WA, et al. J Oral Pathol 15:472–475, 1986.
48. Dekmezian RH, Batsakis JG, Goepfert H. Arch Otolaryngol Head Neck Surg 113:819–821, 1987.
49. Shindoh M, Sawada Y, Kohgo T, Amemiya A, et al. Int J Cancer 50:167–171, 1992.
50. Brandsma J, Abramson A. Arch Otolaryngol Head Neck Surg 115:621–625, 1989.
51. Furuta Y, Takasu T, Asai T, Shinohara T, et al. Cancer 69:353–357, 1992.
52. Dickens P, Srivastava G, Liu YT. J Clin Pathol 45:81–82, 1992.
53. Syrjanen S, Happonen R-P, Virolainen E, Siivonen L, et al. Acta Otolaryngol 104:334–341, 1987.
54. Hoshikawa T, Nakajima T, Uhara H, Gotoh M, et al. Laryngoscope 100:647–650, 1990.

2. Molecular phenotyping of head and neck cancer

Dong M. Shin and Michael A. Tainsky

Squamous cell carcinoma of the head and neck accounts for 5% of all cancers in the United States, where approximately 45,000 new cases of head and neck cancer were expected in 1992 [1]. However, the estimated international incidence of cancers of this region is significantly higher than in the United States. For example, nasopharyngeal carcinomas occur 25 times more frequently in Southern China than in the Caucasian population [2], and India records 30% of all its cancers to be in the oropharyngeal region [3].

The leading known etiologic factors in head and neck cancer are tobacco and alcohol consumption [4–7]. It has also been suggested that vitamin A deficiency and the resulting squamous metaplasia might be a promoting factor [8,9]. However, the mechanisms by which these agents change normal cells into malignant cells really are the crux of the problem. A better understanding of the molecular basis of malignant transformation is essential if there is to be hope of early detection or better treatment, prognostication, or preventive measures.

The techniques of molecular biology are beginning to shed new light on the subcellular pathobiology of malignancy. The crucial events of carcinogenesis, tumor progression, and metastatic spread are coming into focus at a molecular level. However, despite the fact that the flow of important observations from many investigators is accelerating, understanding of their complexity is far from complete. These advances in laboratory research, therefore, have not yet been applied at the bedside. Profound and fundamental insights into the molecular biology of cancer are, in large part, an unfulfilled promise to clinical oncologists and their patients. In the near future, however, molecular biology will provide useful predictive information and may guide therapeutic strategy in a variety of malignancies.

The concept of a genetic basis for cancer dates back to the turn of the century, when it was contended that chromosomal changes play a major role in cancer development. Support for this contention was enhanced by the discovery of cellular oncogenes, and these genes have formed the basis for

Hong, Waun Ki and Weber, Randal S., (eds.), Head and Neck Cancer. © 1995 Kluwer Academic Publishers.
ISBN 0-7923-3015-3. All rights reserved.

our understanding of the genetic events in cancer [10–13]. When normal cellular proto-oncogenes become activated to potential tumorigenic oncogenes, they can play a direct role in tumorigenesis. It is obvious that cells of all vertebrates and invertebrates as diverse as humans, fish, frog, and *Drosophila*, as well as lower single-cell eukaryotes such as yeast, contain proto-oncogenes. These genes possess a high degree of interspecies homology, even in totally unrelated species [14]. Certain proto-oncogenes are transcribed in particular cell types at specific times during normal embryogenesis and transiently when cells are stimulated by mitogens to proliferate [15,16]. Alterations in the expression or function of proto-oncogenes are widely considered to be contributing causes of cancer development [17]. It is thought that groups of functionally diverse proto-oncogenes play a critical role, perhaps cooperatively, in governing normal cellular proliferation and/or differentiation by functioning at distinct steps in intracellular signal transduction of growth factor cascades.

Proto-oncogenes can be classified into groups by the location and biological activity of their products: These include secreted growth factors, cell surface receptors with the associated kinase activity, cytoplasmic kinase activity, and nuclear proteins with transcription factor activity. The groups are shown in Table 1. For example, the c-*sis* gene product has been identified as the beta-subunit of platelet-derived growth factor (PDGF) [18]; the products of the c-*erb*B and c-*fms* genes have been identified as the cell surface receptors of epidermal growth factor (EGF) and monocyte colony stimulating factor 1, respectively [19,20]; and the erbA protein has been identified as thyroid hormone nuclear receptor [21]. It has been demonstrated that growth factors such as PDGF are able to induce expression of nuclear proto-oncogenes *myc*, *fos*, and *jun* [22–24] and that c-*mos* is able to induce mitotic maturation [25]. Therefore, proto-oncogene protein products seem to be involved in many steps of the growth factor receptor–mediated intracellular signalling pathway.

In view of these complexities, this chapter describes the concept of oncogenes and their possible role in the development of neoplasia, specifically head and neck squamous cell carcinomas.

Animal models

The cheek pouch of the Syrian hamster is an excellent target tissue for the chemical induction of squamous cell carcinoma [28]. The gross appearance, histopathologic characteristics, and, presumably, pathogenesis of these squamous cell carcinomas closely resembles those of human oral cancer. One of the advantageous features of this animal carcinogenesis model is that consistent and reproducible histopathologic changes in the chemically transformed oral epithelium can be easily monitored. Polycyclic aromatic hydrocarbons, such as dimethyl-benz(*a*)anthracene (DMBA), are widespread

Table 1. Types of proto-oncogenes

Gene	Origin	Function	Location on human chromosome
Growth factor related			
c-sis/PDGF	Simian sarcoma virus	Platelet-derived growth factor	22q
TGF-α	Not known	Tumor enhancing growth factors	2p
TGF-β	Not known	Epidermal growth factor	19q
EGF		Fibroblast growth factor	4q25
FGF			
Growth factor receptor related			
erbB-1	Avian erythroblastosis virus	Receptor for EGF and TGF-α	7p11.2
erbB-2	Rat neuroglioblastoma	Receptor for?	17q11.2
fms	McDonough sarcoma virus	Receptor for CSF-1	5q33
Tyrosine kinase related			
src	Rous sarcoma virus	Protein tyrosine kinase activity/	20q13.3
abl	Abelson mouse leukemia virus	certain types of growth factors	9q34.1
fes/fps	Feline sarcoma virus		15p26.1
fgr	Gardner feline virus		1p36.1
mos	Moloney sarcoma virus		8q
yes	Yamaguchi sarcoma virus		18q
Serine threonine kinase related			
ros	Chicken simian virus	Protein serine + threonine activity	6q
raf	Mouse sarcoma virus		3p25.4
rel	Reticuloendotheliosis virus		3
G-protein related			
Ha-ras	Harvey sarcoma virus	p21 protein/GTP binding protein	11p15
K-ras	Kirstein sarcoma virus		12p12ter
N-ras	Human colonic DNA		1p13.1
Nuclear protein related			
myc	Avian myelocytoma virus	DNA binding	8q24
N-myc	Human neuroblastoma	DNA binding	2p24.2
fos	Osteosarcoma virus	Transcription factor	14q
jun	Avian myeloblastosis virus	Transcription factor	1p
myb		Transcription factor	6q
ski		Transcription factor	1q
sno		Related to ski	?

EGF = epidermal growth factor; TGF = transforming growth factor; GTP = guanosine triphosphate; CSF = colony stimulating factor.

environmental pollutants and are powerful carcinogens in this experimental animal system [29]. In the last 25 years, Shklar and others have extensively studied the model demonstrating the experimental efficacy of a variety of chemopreventive and therapeutic agents [31–40].

Many investigators have begun using this animal model system to search for altered molecular events during tumor development. Epidermal growth factor receptor (EGFR) is an M_r 170,000 glycoprotein with an intrinsic tyrosine-specific protein kinase activity stimulating EGF binding [41]. The sequence homology between the v-erbB oncogene product and the cytoplasmic and membrane domains of the EGFR has been reported previously [41]. EGF itself has a potent mitogenic activity that stimulates proliferation of target cells in an autocrine fashion through its surface receptor [42]. Amplification or overexpression of the EGFR gene has been observed in A431 human vulva squamous cell carcinoma cells, human glial tumors, human squamous cell carcinoma cell lines [43–47], DMBA-induced tumor tissues, and a hamster cheek pouch carcinoma cell line (HCPC-1) established from one of these tumors [48–50]. Specifically, the expression of the c-erbB gene can be detected in cheek pouch tissue at an early stage (8 weeks) of tumor development and in all tumor-bearing tissues of subsequent stages [50]. Transforming growth factor-α (TGF-α) was not detected in normal hamster tissue, although its expression had been induced in tumor tissues [51]. The expression of both TGF-α and EGFR by the same tumor type supports the hypothesis that the autocrine growth mechanism may be operative in this chemically induced hamster tumor model.

To elucidate the role and timing of changes in different growth and differentiation markers during DMBA-induced carcinogenesis, we assessed the expression of EGFR, transglutaminase type 1, and polyamines (putrescine, spermidine, and spermine), ornithine decarboxylase activity, and the frequency of micronuclei in this animal model [52]. DMBA (0.5%) in heavy mineral oil was applied to the right buccal pouch three times per week for up to 16 weeks; control animals received mineral oil alone. Hamsters were killed at 0, 4, 8, and 16 weeks. Histologic assessment showed that hyperplasia was detected at 4 weeks, dysplasia with or without papillomatous changes at 8 weeks, and squamous cell carcinoma at 16 weeks. EGFR was expressed not at all in the normal epithelial layer, at a moderate level in hyperplastic epithelium, and at very high levels in both dysplasia and squamous cell carcinoma. Transglutaminase type 1 levels also increased sequentially in a similar fashion. Putrescine and spermidine levels, and ornithine decarboxylase activity, increased dramatically after 8 and 16 weeks of exposure to DMBA. Micronucleated cell frequency increased after 4 weeks of DMBA treatment, and that high frequency was sustained during all stages of carcinogenesis. We conclude that these biological markers could be excellent intermediate end points in assessing the effects of various chemopreventive agents to be tested in the hamster buccal pouch model [52].

In vivo DNA-mediated transformation studies have led several investigators to propose that cooperative interaction of more than one cellular proto-oncogene, such as *ras* and *myc*, is involved in the carcinogenesis process [53–60]. The activation and overexpression of the rat sarcoma virus (*ras*) family of genes in chemically induced benign growths or growths that ultimately self-regress [61,62] suggest a possible role for these genes in the chemical carcinogenesis process. It has been proposed that activation of the *ras* gene may generate the signal necessary for the subsequent activation of cell proliferation-associated proto-oncogenes and that the latter genes are involved in the progression of the *ras*-initiated cells to malignancy [63]. Besides the systems such as DMBA-induced skin carcinoma [64] and rabbit keratoacanthomas [63], in which aberrant expression of cellular proto-oncogenes are studied, there are very few in vivo carcinogenesis systems in which stepwise molecular analysis of the transformation process is conducted from the very early stage to the last stages of tumor development. In the DMBA-induced hamster cheek pouch tumor model, overexpression of the Harvey-*ras*, or Ha-*ras*, gene occurred at a very early stage of tumor development and persisted throughout the tumorigenesis process [65]. The expression of c-*erb*B, on the other hand, was detected only after 8–10 weeks of DMBA exposure and increased with the progression of the disease. Hussain et al. concluded that the overexpression of Ha-*ras* alone was not sufficient to induce tumors, whereas expression of the Ha-*ras* and *erb*B genes at later stages of tumor development induced histopathologically defined epithelial cell carcinoma. This study demonstrated the sequential overexpression of Ha-*ras* and *erb*B in a stage-specific manner and their cooperative interaction in DMBA-induced in vivo oral carcinogenesis [65].

Kirsten-*ras* (K-*ras*) mRNA was also studied in the experimental oral model. No K-*ras* mRNA was found in normal hamster cheek pouch epithelium, whereas all DMBA-induced tumors expressed detectable levels of K-*ras* mRNA [66]. Cellular synchronization experiments using a cell line derived from hamster cheek pouch carcinoma revealed that the K-*ras* proto-oncogene was expressed during the G_1 phase of the cell cycle. Serum starvation and RNA synthesis inhibition experiments using hamster cheek pouch carcinoma cells suggested that whereas the K-*ras* proto-oncogene is indeed quiescent in the normal hamster cheek pouch epithelium [66], it is expressed at a high level in a cycle-dependent manner in the chemically transformed counterpart.

It is interesting to note that EGF may control expression of the K-*ras* gene [67]. A closely associated mitogenic peptide, TGF-α, is consistently expressed in these chemically transformed oral tumors [51]. Thus, the tumor-specific expression of the K-*ras* proto-oncogene in these hamster oral tumors might be a consequence of the aberrant expression of TGF-α. Whether the tumor-associated expression of K-*ras* is due to the direct action of DMBA, the tumor-associated expression of TGF-α or EGFR, or another mechanism is far from clear. Nevertheless, the hamster cheek pouch model of oral cancer represents an excellent model for the study of these possible molecular interactions.

There have also been some biochemical studies in this animal model. Probably the best study event has been the induction of gamma-glutamyl-transpeptidase (GGT), an enzyme that is not normally expressed in the hamster cheek pouch. Solt and Shklar showed that individual GGT-positive cells are detected histochemically as early as 3 days after the first DMBA treatment. After 3 weeks of treatment, they were able to detect GGT-positive intraepithelial cell clones (plaques), which appeared to be of clonal origin [68,69]. GGT activity has also been demonstrated histochemically in dysplasias, papillomas, and well-differentiated squamous cell carcinomas. These results led to speculation that the early GGT-expressed cell populations are preneoplastic in nature [70].

The expression of different keratins has also been explored in this model. An immunohistochemical technique was used to profile several keratins during experimentally induced carcinogenesis in hamster cheek pouch mucosa [71,72]. The antibodies used in the experiments were capable of identifying several groups of keratins, but they were unable to recognize individual keratins. We recently investigated the immunohistochemical and immunoblotting patterns of differentiation-associated keratins K1 (M_r 67,000), K13 (M_r 47,000), and K14 (M_r 55,000). The normal hamster cheek pouch epithelium expressed K14 in the basal layer and K13 in the suprabasal layer, whereas K1 was not detected [73]. In contrast, after 2 weeks of DMBA treatment, K1 expression started as a weak and patchy pattern in the suprabasal layer, becoming stronger and more homogeneous at 8 and 16 weeks of carcinogen exposure. However, K1 was almost absent in squamous cell carcinoma, where only small, very well-differentiated areas were preserved. Concomitant with DMBA-induced hyperplasia were some topographical alterations in the distribution of K14. K14 was no longer restricted to the basal layer but was expressed in differentiated areas. The same pattern was also observed in dysplastic lesions and in squamous cell carcinoma. Furthermore, expression of K13 was preserved in this hyperplastic epithelium during all stages of carcinogenesis. We concluded from this study that alterations in the pattern of keratin expression appear to be common during the different stages of development of squamous cell carcinoma and could be an excellent tool to study carcinogenesis in this system [73].

Gene alterations in human head and neck carcinoma

Alteration of ras gene family

A significant proportion of human tumors from various sites in the body have been shown to contain activated oncogenes from the *ras* family: Ha-*ras*, K-*ras*, and N-*ras* [74–76]. Oncogenes in the *ras* family are forms of the germline proto-oncogenes with specific point mutations that, when transfected into NIH/3T3 murine fibroblasts, induce foci of morphologically altered cells [12,13,77–80]. The normal *ras* genes code for proteins of molecular weight of approximately 21,000; they have guanine nucleotide binding activity and are able to hydrolyze guanosine 5'-triphosphate (GTP) [81]. Two different mechanisms of *ras* gene activation have been described: (1) point mutations, particularly at codons 12, 13, and 61, which result in mutated forms of p21*ras*; and (2) overexpression of normal cellular p21*ras* due to amplification or defective regulation [82–89]. Moreover, it has been suggested that the activation of *ras* genes in certain tumors, such as adenocarcinoma of the colon or bladder carcinoma, is related to the induction of invasiveness and metastatic potential [90–93].

A Ha-*ras* mutation at codon 12 was shown to be associated with cervical cancers of poor prognosis [94,95]. A Ha-*ras* restriction fragment length polymorphism has been linked to susceptibility of individuals to cancers [96], and the Ha-*ras* locus is known to be deleted in a variety of human cancers [97]. Studies on the expression of *ras* genes indicated that high levels of *ras*-specific mRNA and p21 *ras* protein were associated with tumor progression in human cancers of different origins [98].

Azuma et al. used immunohistochemical techniques to analyze p21 *ras* expression in paraffin-embedded squamous cell head and neck carcinoma tissues, and found that it was correlated with the degree of tumor differentiation, clinical staging, and clinical outcome [99]. In this study, 59 of 121 tumor samples reacted to the monoclonal antibody Y13-259 raised against the p21 encoded by the V-*ras* gene of the Harvey murine sarcoma virus [100], whereas oral leukoplakia and normal mucosa did not express p21*ras*. They also reported that the patients who expressed *ras* had a poor prognosis.

Two cell lines were established from untreated squamous cell carcinoma of the head and neck. Line 1483 is more aggressive in nude mice, has a high efficacy for anchorage-independent growth, expresses p21*ras* at a higher level, and is more aneuploid than the other line, 183 [101]. On the other hand, the Ha-*ras* gene was shown to have low incidence of *ras* activation in human squamous cell carcinomas. Of 37 squamous cell carcinomas of the head and neck, only two had mutations in codon 12 of the Ha-*ras* gene [102]. Total RNA was prepared from 79 of these tumor specimens and analyzed by northern and slot blot hybridization. Ha-*ras* transcript levels were found in 18% of lymph node metastases and in 21% of primary tumors, indicating that there are no significant differences between these cancers [103]. A study was also undertaken to determine whether the variation in the increased expression of three oncogenes (Ha-*ras*, K-*ras*, and *myc*) could be correlated with various clinicopathologic parameters of squamous cell carcinoma of the head and neck region. No correlation was found with sex, age, site of primary tumor, or level of differentiation of the tumor [104]. More sensitive techniques, such as polymerase chain reaction

(PCR), should be used, however, to explore the relationship between mutation or overexpression of *ras* family genes and clinical characteristics of head and neck carcinomas.

Int-*2*/Hst-*1 genes*

The *hst*-1 (*hst*F1) gene was the most frequently detected transforming gene in these cancers after the *ras* gene family [105,106]. Because this gene encodes a protein that is homologous to a fibroblast growth factor (FGF) and a protein encoded by the *int*-2 gene, it is assumed to be a new member of the gene family that is involved in cell growth [107,108]. Moreover, hst-1 transforming protein has been shown to be a novel heparin-binding growth factor [109]. Both the *hst*-1 and *int*-2 genes are mapped to chromosome 11q13 [110]. Coamplification of these genes has been reported in urinary bladder carcinoma [111], esophageal carcinoma [112], melanoma [113], and gastric carcinoma [106]. Coamplification of *hst*-1 and *int*-2 genes in a hepatocellular carcinoma was accompanied by amplification of integrated hepatitis B virus DNA [114]. Moreover, coamplification of the *hst*-1 and *int*-2 genes was reported in 17 of 110 (15%) breast tumors [115].

The biological significance of the coamplification of the *hst*-1 and *int*-2 genes is presently unclear. In head and neck carcinoma, the *int*-2 gene was amplified threefold to fivefold in 5 (50%) of 10 laryngeal carcinomas and twofold to threefold in 5 (45%) of 11 nonlaryngeal carcinomas of head and neck [116]. Adjacent histologically normal tissue from the same patients had only a single copy. In a survey of head and neck tumor–derived cell lines, *int*-2 was amplified ninefold in a hypopharyngeal tumor cell line (FaDu) but was not amplified in three laryngeal cell lines [116]. In another report, *int*-2 was found to be amplified in 2 of 8 head and neck carcinomas [117]. Although there was a suggestion that amplification of *int*-2 is correlated with tumor recurrence and clinical disease progression [116], a large patient population will be required to determine more precisely the significance of amplification of this gene or overexpression of any genes in head and neck carcinomas. We analyzed for the *int*-2 gene in head and neck squamous cell lines; 3 of 10 showed amplification, ranging from 5-fold to 50-fold (unpublished data). The significance of this gene amplification is currently being investigated.

myc *gene family*

The *myc* family of cellular oncogenes — c-*myc*, N-*myc*, and L-*myc* — encodes three highly related nuclear phosphoproteins. Although the exact function of *myc* family proteins has not been determined, they are thought to be important in the regulation of normal cellular growth and differentiation, and in dysregulation in many different types of malignancies [118].

The first member of this family to be discovered, c-*myc*, was identified as

24

the cellular homologue of the retroviral v-*myc* oncogene responsible for leukemia in chickens [119,102]. Additional *myc* family members were subsequently identified in human tumors as highly expressed and amplified genes with homology to c-*myc*. The N-*myc* and L-*myc* genes were isolated from human neuroblastomas [121,122] and small cell lung carcinomas [123], respectively, and were subsequently found to be capable of transforming primary cultured cells and producing tumors in transgenic mice. Thus, the aberrant structure and expression of *myc* family genes in a variety of neoplasia clearly indicate that *myc* gene activation can play a role in tumorigenesis. Reciprocal translocation between the c-*myc* gene and the immunoglobulin loci occurs in Burkitt's lymphomas [124,125] and human B-cell lymphomas [126]. Gene amplification is another mechanism by which *myc* expression is often activated in various tumors. Amplification of N-*myc* is a common feature of neuroblastomas, retinoblastomas, small-cell lung cancers, and other tumors of neuronal or neuroendocrine origin [121–123,127]. Of interest is the finding that *myc* gene amplification correlates well with clinical prognosis of a number of tumors [128]. For example, advanced stage III or IV neuroblastoma generally exhibits significant N-*myc* gene amplification, whereas amplification is limited in stage I and II tumors and absent in spontaneously regressing stage IV-S tumors [129]. Amplification of the N-*myc* gene correlates with progression-free survival rates as well, and thus provides a useful biomarker for determining neuroblastoma tumor stage and predicting clinical outcome. Levels of c-*myc* amplification often correspond with degree of tumorigenic potential [130]. The mixed-cell type of small-cell lung carcinoma also exhibits greater amplification of c-*myc* than the classic types and correlates with poor prognosis [130].

Field et al. quantitated c-*myc* oncoprotein in 44 squamous cell carcinomas of the head and neck using an enzyme-linked immunosorbent assay. The survival periods of patients with tumors with elevated levels of c-myc protein were found to be statistically shorter than those of patients whose tumors expressed lower levels of c-*myc* [131]. This indicates that c-myc expression may be an effective prognostic indicator in head and neck cancer. Amplification of the c-*myc*, N-*myc*, and K-*ras* genes was demonstrated in 20–40% of oral cancer tissues; almost 56% showed at least one of the oncogenes amplified [132]. The molecular mechanisms causing elevated levels of the c-myc protein in more aggressive squamous cell carcinoma of the head and neck are unknown. Nonetheless, the level of c-myc protein does appear to be a prognostic indicator, even within the somewhat limited follow-up for some of the patients studied [132]. This finding suggests that clinical trials incorporating measurements of c-myc protein expression may be valuable. Prospective studies should consider the measurement of c-myc protein to establish the significance of this gene in head and neck cancer.

Epidermal growth factor receptor

A role for elevated expression of the EGFR in tumorigenesis is suggested by consistent observations of augmented levels of the EGFR in several types of malignancies. For example, amplification of the glycosylated M_r 170,000 EGFR has been found in primary brain tumors of glial origin [44] as well as in the epidermoid cell line A431 [43]. High numbers of EGFR occur in several types of malignancies, including bladder tumors [133], breast carcinomas [134,135], and squamous cell carcinoma cells derived from human head and neck cancers [46,136]. Many studies have demonstrated that the receptors for EGF [137–140] have protein kinase activity specific for tyrosine residues. Upon binding their respective ligands, the tyrosine kinase activity becomes stimulated severalfold, as indicated by enhanced autophosphorylation of the receptor, increased phosphorylation of exogenous substrates in vitro, and elevated phosphorylation of the tyrosine residues of several proteins in vivo. Two cell lines established from tumors of the head and neck area at different clinical stages were found to differ in the expression and the tyrosine kinase activity of the EGFR [101]. The 1483 cells displayed a higher plating efficiency and clonogenicity in soft agar, suggesting that they have a more tumorigenic phenotype than the 183A cells. Analyses of EGFR levels using R1 anti-EGFR serum indicated that the 1483 cells expressed fivefold more receptor than the 183A cells. Autophosphorylation activity of both receptors was stimulated by the addition of EGFR to isolated membrane preparations and intact cells. The EGFR of the 1483 cells was much less responsive to EGF than the EGFR from 183A cells [141].

To examine whether EGFR expression could be of clinical value in head and neck squamous cell carcinoma, Santino et al. measured the EGFR levels of these tumors [142]. In 59 of 60 samples, EGFR levels were higher in the tumor than in the corresponding controls. They also found a significant correlation between EGFR levels and tumor size and stage. Using a cut-off EGFR value of 100 fmol/mg protein, which separated controls from tumors, EGFR-positive tumors had a greater probability of response to chemotherapy than EGFR-negative tumors [142]. Using immunohistochemical and cytometric techniques, expression of the Ki-67 antigen, EGFR, the transferrin receptor (TFR), and DNA ploidy were studied in 42 fresh samples of head and neck carcinomas. This study suggested that EGFR and TFR are widely distributed, especially on proliferating cells at the invading tumor margin. In addition, there is a close spatial relationship between cells expressing EGFR and TFR and those expressing Ki-67 antigen. Further follow-up will be necessary to determine whether these parameters will be important prognostic values [143].

EGFR gene amplification and expression were also studied in 11 early passage head and neck carcinoma cell lines. Three cell lines demonstrated *EGFR* gene amplification and 10 lines showed higher levels of *EGFR* mRNA than normal keratinocytes [144]. Therefore, increased expression and/or amplification of *EGFR* may be important in the development or progression of head and neck carcinoma, although the mechanisms and clinical significance need to be elucidated by further study.

p53 gene alteration

The p53 gene, which has been shown to act as a dominant oncogene in tumor cells [145–148], has been recently shown to also function as an anti-oncogene [149–151]. This paradox may be related to the fact that the wild-type p53 protein suppresses the outburst of the malignant phenotype. This complexity, however, makes it an attractive model for investigating the interrelationship between either oncogene or anti-oncogene activity and the neoplastic processes. In accord with the concept that malignant transformation is a multistage process, it is plausible to assume that the p53 protein, stimulated by various cellular signals, may in turn induce or suppress the expression of other cellular genes involved in this chain of events. The *p53* gene is highly conserved in diverse organisms such as *Xenopus laevis*, chickens, mice, and humans [152–155], suggesting that the encoded protein plays a central role in the cell and therefore is tightly conserved in evolution.

Mercer et al. [156] showed that microinjection of anti-p53 monoclonal antibodies into the cells inhibited DNA synthesis in quiescent nontransformed NIH/3T3 cells stimulated with serum, suggesting that p53 is synthesized as a late G_0 protein [156]. A similar observation was made by Reich and Levine [157] when they examined the steady-state levels of *p53* mRNA and p53 protein synthesis in a synchronous population of NIH/3T3 fibroblasts obtained by releasing a culture from density-dependent growth inhibition. Using the antisense methodology, shut-off of *p53* expression was shown by introduction of p53 synthesis, which ultimately caused cell death [158]. That wild-type *p53* functions as a growth-arrest gene was initially concluded from the observation that the p53 protein failed to enhance malignant transformation in an in vitro assay [159,160] and was further supported by the fact that the protein actively suppresses the transforming activity of other oncogenes [149]. Comparison of the transforming activity of the various *p53*-encoded proteins, as evaluated by their ability to transform primary embryonic cells in conjunction with the *ras* oncogene, have indicated that whereas the mutated p53 protein forms induce the appearance of foci, the wild-type cDNA codes for an inactive p53 protein [159,160].

Further support for the idea that *p53* may function as an anti-oncogene comes from previous cytogenetic and restriction fragment-length polymorphism studies that have shown that one allele of chromosome 17 is deleted in at least 60% of tumors of the colon, breast, lung, ovaries, cervix, adrenal cortex, and bone [161–166]. Thus, at the cellular level *p53* gene mutations may function as dominant negative [167] rather than recessive mutations. This dominant negative effect may in part be explained by oligomerization of the *p53* gene product [168,169]. A mutant *p53* gene product may inactivate the wild-type gene product by binding to it and preventing its normal association with other cellular constituents.

As the normal p53 protein has a very short half-life (6–20 minutes), it may be inferred that detection of the p53 protein is synonymous with mutation, because the mutant form has a half-life of up to 6 hours, probably due to stabilization of the protein [170]. In addition, Iggo et al. [171] found increased p53 oncoprotein staining in those lung cancers that are associated with smoking. They reported elevated p53 protein levels in 14 of 17 (82%) squamous cell carcinomas compared with 8 of 21 (38%) nonsquamous cell carcinomas. Similarly, Chiba et al. [172] reported that 65% of the lung squamous cell carcinomas had *p53* mutations, whereas only 36% of the nonsquamous tumors did. The association between smoking and squamous cell carcinomas of the lung provides further evidence for a link between *p53* mutations and smoking.

Using monoclonal antibodies (JG8, CM-1, and 1081) directed to the p53 protein, we found 34% (16/47) of squamous cell carcinomas of the head and neck and two squamous cell carcinoma lines to be strongly positive for the protein. The presence of the mutant *p53* was confirmed in the cell lines as substitutions in exon 7 (codon 238) and exon 5 (codon 152) [173]. Six of seven nonsmokers did not express p53, whereas 29 of 37 heavy smokers were found to have elevated p53 expression (p < 0.005). Also, of a group of 10 patients who had given up smoking more than 5 years ago, nine had elevated p53 expression [173]. Whether p53 has a significant impact on prognosis or survival of patients with head and neck carcinoma has not been well documented, however. This important issue should be addressed in future studies.

Phenotyping tumors with differentially expressed genes

Another experimental approach to developing a molecular phenotype of certain cancers is to directly clone genes that have a particular expression pattern during carcinogenesis. The technique of differential cDNA library screening can be used to isolate cDNA of genes that are expressed in one cell or tissue but not another or are induced by a particular oncogene. Clones are isolated that selectively hybridize to one cDNA probe prepared against total RNA from each cell. Most often this strategy generates cDNA clones of genes that are changed as a result of some oncogenic event other than those generated by the oncogenes themselves, though it is possible to isolate effector genes if their oncogenic activation is due to increased mRNA expression. Differential screening of a cDNA library was used to isolate

28

genes differentially expressed by a nontumorigenic clone and a N-*ras*-transformed variant of the human ovarian teratocarcinoma cell line PA-1. The RNA transcript for one of the cDNA clones that we identified was expressed at a 25-fold higher level in the *ras* oncogene-transformed PA-1 cells than in the nontumorigenic PA-1 cells. DNA sequence analysis of this clone showed that it codes for the human ribosomal S2 protein [174]. The S2

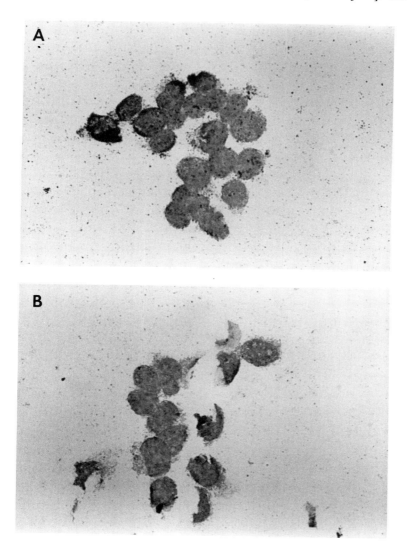

Figure 1. In situ hybridization of head and neck squamous cell carcinoma cell lines. (A) 1483 cells, (B) MDA 886 Ln Cells, (C) 183 cells, and (D) normal oral keratinocytes. The fixed sections were hybridized with clone 12 DNA labeled with digoxigenin-11-dUTP. (From Chiao et al. [174], with permission.)

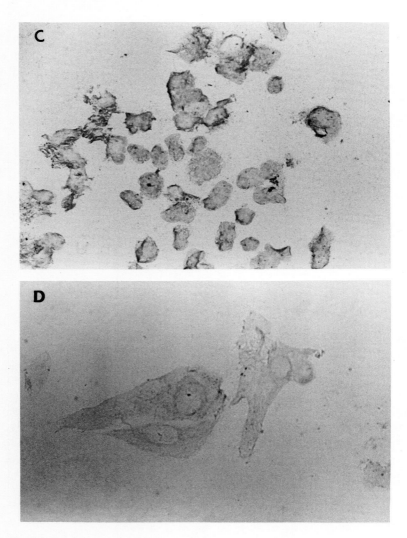

Figure 1. Continued

protein is part of the complex array of proteins that associate with the small ribosomal subunit and may play a role in the fidelity of protein synthesis.

Expression of the *S2* gene mRNA in head and neck tumors

The expression of *S2* in human tumor samples was analyzed by in situ hybridization using the *S2* clone cDNA labeled by the nonradioactive digoxigenin-112[-deoxyuridine-5''-triphosphate] (dUTP) method. We analyzed mRNA in three human squamous cell carcinoma cell lines (MDA 886 Ln, 1483, 183A) and normal oral keratinocytes [174]. The 1483 and 183A cell lines are derived from tumors whose histologic characteristics are identical to those of well-differentiated squamous cell carcinoma. However, 1483 cells are known to be more tumorigenic in nude mice and have a higher level of p21*ras* proteins than 183A cells [101]. *S2* mRNA was very highly expressed in 1483 (Figure 1A) and 886 cells (Figure 1B); 183A cells expressed considerably less of the *S2* gene (Figure 1C). The normal oral keratinocytes expressed the *S2* gene at a minimal level (Figure 1D). Therefore, expression of *S2* gene sequences may be related to malignancy.

We next analyzed histologic sections from 10 head and neck squamous cell carcinoma samples. Six expressed a significant level of *S2* mRNA in tumor cell nests (Table 2), whereas the collagen tissue adjacent to tumor cell nests and the adjacent normal mucosa did not express the *S2* gene (Figure 2A,B). The negative control of this experiment was a section from the same tumor sample that was hybridized to a digoxigenin-11-dUTP-labeled pBR328 DNA probe; this control showed only a minimal signal (Figure 2C). Interestingly, 1 of 3 premalignant dysplastic leukoplakias also expressed a detectable level of *S2* mRNA, although the level was lower than that expressed by the squamous cell carcinoma (Figure 2D). This probe may, therefore, identify dysplastic lesions that are more likely to undergo conversion to a carcinoma. From this result we can hypothesize that this marker may be useful to identify malignant cells within a premalignant lesion. It appears that *S2* gene expression is a good marker for oral epithelial tumors and may provide prognostic data by analysis of histologic sections. Because sections that appear histologically similar react differently to the *S2* probe,

Table 2. S2 mRNA expression by in situ hybridization in oral carcinomas

Case no.	mRNA Differentiation	S2	Site
1	Moderate	−	Base of tongue
2	Moderate	−	Hypopharynx
3	ND	+	Base of tongue
4	Moderate	+ +	Base of tongue
5	Moderate	+ +	Base of tongue
6	ND	+ + +	Pharynx
7	Moderate	+ +	Base of tongue
8	Moderate	−	Base of tongue
9	Moderate	−	Base of tongue
10	Moderate	+	Floor of mouth

ND = not determined.
From Chiao et al. [174], with permission.

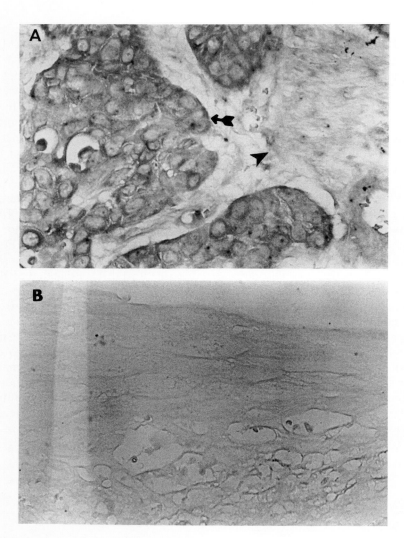

Figure 2. In situ hybridization to histologic sections of a human head and neck squamous cell carcinoma. (A) Human head and neck squamous cell carcinomas (the arrow indicates the tumor cells and arrow head indicates the adjacent collagen tissue); (B) normal mucosa; (C) the control, a section from the same tumor sample hybridized to pBR328 DNA labeled with digoxigenin-11-dUTP; (D) premalignant dysplastic leukoplakias. The sections in A, B, and D were hybridized with a digoxigenin-11-dUTP-labeled clone 12 cDNA probe. (From Chiao et al. [174], with permission.)

this analysis may reveal proliferative differences in tumors that appear otherwise identical.

In summary, using in situ hybridization experiments we have found that expression of the ribosomal protein S2 was higher in cultured human

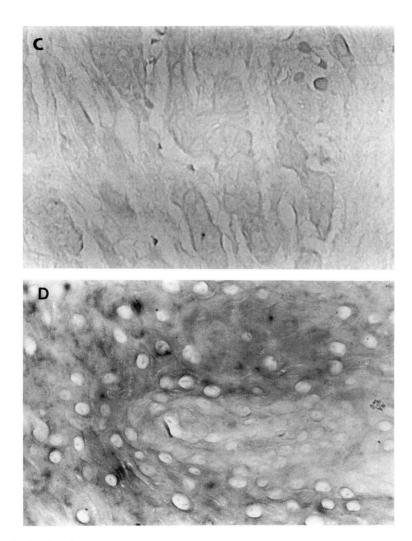

Figure 2. Continued

head and neck squamous cell carcinomas that in normal keratinocytes. In situ hybridization experiments also demonstrated that expression of this gene was selectively higher in histologic sections of human premalignant leukoplakia, head and neck squamous cell carcinomas, and colon and breast cancers than in the adjacent normal tissues [174]. Overexpression of another human ribosomal protein, L31, in 23 of 23 colorectal tumors has also been reported [175]. The levels of that human ribosomal protein increase co-ordinately fivefold to sixfold during estrogen-stimulated cell growth [176].

Pogue-Geile et al. have shown that additional ribosomal proteins S6, S8, S12, L5, and P0 are overexpressed in all colon cancers examined and in adenomatous polyps as compared to normal mucosa [177]. Our results indicate that elevation of levels of expression of the ribosomal protein *S2* gene may be more selective [174] than that of these other ribosomal protein genes, possibly reflecting differences associated with uncontrolled growth, suggesting a role for *S2* in proliferation and transformation. Ribosomal protein S2 may also be potentially useful as a marker for certain tumors in clinical diagnosis or as a prognostic indicator.

An important goal for cancer research is to recognize cancers at their earliest and most treatable stage. There are many tumor markers for both clinical and research use. The tumor markers presently in use generally meet only one or two of the criteria for the ideal marker, which are tumor specificity, correlation with tumor bulk and stage of the disease, and expression levels that decrease to normal after successful treatment and that rise prior to clinical manifestations of recurrence. Another use of a marker is to contrast benign lesions with those with malignant foci. We need to investigate the value of the *S2* gene probe for these analyses.

References

1. Boring CC, Squires TS, Tong T. Cancer statistics, 1992. CA Cancer J Clin 41:19–38, 1992.
2. Pillai R, Reddiar KS, Balaram P. Oncogene expression and oral cancer. J Surg Oncol 47:102–108, 1991.
3. Mehta FS, Gupta MB, Pindborg JJ, Bhonsle RB, Jalnawalla PN, Sinor PN. An intervention study of oral cancer and precancer in rural Indian population: A preliminary report. Bull World Health Org 60:441–468, 1982.
4. Fraumeni JF. Respiratory carcinogenesis: An epidemiologic appraisal. J Natl Cancer Inst 55:1039–1046, 1975.
5. Decker J, Goldstein JC. Risk factors in head and neck cancer. N Engl J Med 306:1151–1155, 1982.
6. Binnie WH, Rankin KV, Mackenzie IC. Etiology of squamous cell carcinoma. J Oral Pathol Med 12:11–29, 1983.
7. Miller AB. Trends in cancer mortality and epidemiology. Cancer 51:2413–2418, 1983.
8. Bollag W. Vitamin A and retinoids from nutrition to pharmacotherapy in dermatology and oncology. Lancet 1:860–863, 1983.
9. Goodman DS. Vitamin A and retinoids in health and disease. N Engl J Med 310:1023–1031, 1984.
10. Bishop JM. Retroviruses. Ann Rev Biochem 47:35–88, 1978.
11. Chang E, Furth M, Scolnick E, Lowy D. Tumorigenic transformation of mammalian cells by a normal human gene homologous to the oncogene of Harvey Murine Sarcoma Virus. Nature 297:479–483, 1982.
12. Parada LF, Tabin CJ, Shih C, Weinberg RA. Human EJ bladder carcinoma oncogene is a homologue of Harvey Sarcoma Virus *ras* gene. Nature 297:474–478, 1982.
13. Santos E, Tronick SR, Aaronson SA, Pulciani S, Barbacid M. T24 human bladder carcinoma oncogene is an activated form of the normal human homologue of *BALB*- and Harvey-MSV transforming gene. Nature 298:343–345, 1982.

14. Levine AS. Fruit flies, yeast, and oncogene: Developmental biology and cancer research come together. Med Pediatr Oncol 12:357–374, 1984.
15. Muller R, Slamon DJ, Tremblay JM, Cline MJ, Verma IM. Differential expression and postnatal development of the mouse. Nature 299:640–644, 1982.
16. Goyette M, Petropoulos CJ, Shank PR, Fanso N. Expression of a cellular oncogene during liver regeneration. Science 219:510–512, 1983.
17. Klein G, Klein E. Evolution of tumors and the impact of molecular oncology. Nature 315: 190–195, 1985.
18. Waterfield MD, Scare GT, Whittle N. Platelet derived growth factor is structurally related to the putative transforming protein p28 of Simian sarcoma virus. Nature 304:35–39, 1983.
19. Downward J, Yarden Y, Mayes E. Close similarity of epidermal growth factor receptor and v-erb B oncogene protein sequence. Nature 137:521–527, 1984.
20. Sherr CJ, Rettenmier CW, Sacca R, Roussel ME, Look AT, Stanley ER. The c-fms proto-oncogene product is related to the mononulcear phagocyte growth factor, CSF-1. Cell 41:665–676, 1985.
21. Donner P, Freiser-Wilke I, Moelling K. Nuclear localization and DNA binding of the transforming gene product of avian myelocytomatosis virus. Nature 296:262–264, 1982.
22. Kelly K, Cochran BH, Stiles CS, Leder P. Cell-specific regulation of the c-myc gene by lymphocyte mitogen and platelet derived growth factor. Cell 35:603–610, 1983.
23. Kruijer W, Cooper JA, Hunter T, Verma IM. Platelet derived growth factor induces rapid but transient expression of the c-fos gene and protein. Nature 312:711–720, 1984.
24. Quantin B, Breathnach R. Epidermal growth factor stimulates transcription of the c-jun proto-oncogene in rat fibroblasts. Nature 334:538–539, 1988.
25. Sagata N, Daar J, Oskarsson M, Shonulter SD, Vande Wood GF. The product of the mos proto-oncogene as a candidate "initiator" for oocyte maturation. Science 245:643–646, 1989.
26. Eagle H. Propagation in a fluid medium of human epidermoid carcinoma strain KB. Proc Soc Exp Biol Med 89:362–364, 1955.
27. Moore AE, Sabachewsky L, Toolan HW. Culture characteristics of four permanent lines of human cancer cells. Cancer Res 15:598–602, 1955.
28. Shklar G. Experimental pathology of oral cancer. In: G Shklar, ed. Oral Cancer. Philadelphia: WB Saunders, 1988, pp 41–54.
29. Harvey GR. Synthesis of the dihydrodiol and diol epoxide metabolites of carcinogenic polycyclic hydrocarbons. In: GR Harvey, ed. Polycyclic Hydrocarbon and Carcinogenesis. Washington, DC: American Chemical Society, 1985, pp 36–62.
30. Odukoya D, Schwartz J, Weichselbaum R, Shklar G. An epidermoid carcinoma cell line derived from hamster 7, 12-dimethylbenz(a)anthracene-induced oral buccal pouch tumors. J Natl Cancer Inst 71:1253–1264, 1983.
31. Silverman S, Shklar G. The effect of a carcinogen (DMBA) applied to the hamster cheek pouch in combination with croton oil. Oral Surg 16:1344–1355, 1963.
32. Rowe NH, Gorlin RJ. The effect of vitamin A deficiency upon experimental carcinogenesis. J Dent Res 38:72–83, 1959.
33. Santis H, Shklar G, Chauncey HH. Histochemistry of experimentally induced leukoplakia and carcinoma of the hamster buccal pouch. Oral Surg 17:307–318, 1964.
34. Shklar G. Metabolic characteristics of experimental hamster pouch carcinomas. Oral Surg 20:336–339, 1965.
35. Tsiklakis K, Papadakou A, Angelopoulos AP. The therapeutic effect of an aromatic retinoid (RO-109359) on hamster buccal pouch carcinomas. Oral Surg 64:327–332, 1987.
36. Suda D, Schwartz J, Shklar G. Inhibition of experimental oral carcinogenesis by topical beta-carotene. Carcinogenesis 7:711–715, 1986.
37. Shwartz J, Shklar G. Regression of experimental oral carcinogenesis by local injection of beta-carotene and canthaxanthine. Nutr Cancer 11:35–40, 1988.

38. Shklar G. Oral mucosal carcinogenesis in hamster: Inhibition by vitamin E. J Natl Cancer Inst 68:791–799, 1982.
39. Trickler D, Shklar G. Prevention by vitamin E of experimental oral carcinogenesis. J Natl Cancer Inst 78:165–169, 1989.
40. Schwartz J, Shklar G, Reid S, Trickler D. Prevention of oral cancer by extracts of Spirulina-Dunaliella algae. Nutr Cancer 11:127–134, 1988.
41. Downward J, Yarden Y, Mayes E, Scrace G, Toffy N, Stockwell P, et al. Close similarity of epidermal growth factor receptor and V-*erb*-B oncogene protein sequences. Nature 307:521–527, 1984.
42. Hunter T. The epidermal growth factor receptor gene and its products. Nature 311:414–416, 1984.
43. Ullrich A, Coussens L, Hayflick JS, Dull TJ, Gray A, Tam AW, et al. Human epidermal growth factor receptor cDNA sequence and aberrant expression of the amplified gene in A431 human carcinoma cells. Nature 309:418–425, 1984.
44. Libermann TA, Razon N, Bartal AD, Yarden Y, Schlessinger J, Soreq H. Expression of epidermal growth factor receptors in human brain tumors. Cancer Res 44:753–760, 1984.
45. Merlino GT, Xu Y-H, Ishii S, Clark AJL, Semba K, Toyoshima K, et al. Amplification and enhanced expression of the epidermal growth factor receptor gene in A431 human carcinoma cells. Science 224:417–419, 1984.
46. Cowley G, Smith JA, Gusterson B, Hendler F, Ozanne B. The amount of EGF receptor is elevated in squamous cell carcinomas. In: JL Arnold, GF van de Woode, WC Topp, JD Watson, eds. Cancer Cells I. Cold Spring Harbor, NY: Cold Spring Harbor Laboratory Press, 1984, pp 5–10.
47. Yamamoto T, Kamata N, Kawano H, Shimizu S, Kuroki T, Toyoshima K, et al. High incidence of amplification of the epidermal growth factor receptor gene in human squamous carcinoma cell lines. Cancer Res 46:414–416, 1986.
48. Wong DTW, Biswas DK. Activation of the C-*erb* B1 oncogene during DMBA-induced carcinogenesis in the hamster cheek pouch. J Dent Res 65:221, 1986.
49. Wong DTW. Amplification of the C-*erb* B1 oncogene in chemically-induced oral carcinomas. Carcinogenesis 8:1963–1965, 1987.
50. Wong DTW, Biswas DK. Expression of C-*erb* B proto-oncogene during dimethyl-benzanthracene-induced tumorigenesis in hamster cheek pouch. Oncogene 2:67–72, 1987.
51. Wong DTW, Gallagher GT, Gertz R, Chang ALC, Shklar G. Transforming growth factor-α in chemically transformed hamster oral keratinocytes. Cancer Res 48:3130–3134, 1988.
52. Shin DM, Gimenez IB, Lee JS, Nishioka K, Wargovich MJ, Thacher S, et al. Expression of epidermal growth factor receptor, polyamine levels, ornithine decarboxylase activity, micronuclei, and transglutaminase I in a 7,12-dimethylbenz(*a*)anthracene-induced hamster buccal pouch carcinogenesis model. Cancer Res 50:2505–2510, 1990.
53. Land H, Chen AC, Morgenstern JP, Parada LF, Weinberg RA. Behavior of *myc* and *ras* oncogenes in transformation of rat embryo fibroblasts. Mol Cell Biol 6:1917–1925, 1986.
54. Lee WM, Schwab M, Westaway D, Varmus H. Augmented expression of normal c-*myc* is sufficient for cotransformation of rat embryo cells with a mutant *ras* gene. Mol Cell Biol 5:3345–3356, 1985.
55. Kelly K, Cochran BH, Stiles CD, Leder P. Cell-specific regulation of the c-*myc* gene by lymphocyte mitogens and platelet-derived growth factor. Cell 35:603–610, 1983.
56. Yancopoulos GD, Nisen PD, Tesfaye A, Kohl NE, Goldfarb MP, Alt FW. N-*myc* can cooperate with *ras* to transform normal cells in culture. Proc Natl Acad Sci USA 82:5455–5459, 1985.
57. Ruley HE. Adenovirus early region 1A enables viral and cellular transforming genes to transform primary cells in culture. Nature 304:602–606, 1983.
58. Balmain A, Pragnell IB. Mouse skin carcinomas induced in vivo by chemical carcinogens have a transforming Harvey-*ras* oncogene. Nature 303:72–74, 1983.

59. Quintanilla M, Brown K, Ramsden M, Balmain A. Carcinogen-specific mutation and amplification of Ha-*ras* during mouse skin carcinogenesis. Nature 322:78–80, 1986.
60. Bizub D, Wood AW, Skalka AW. Mutagenesis of the Ha-*ras* oncogene in mouse skin tumors induced by polycyclic aromatic hydrocarbons. Proc Natl Acad Sci USA 83:6048–6052, 1986.
61. Barbacid M. *ras* genes. Annu Rev Biochem 56:779–827, 1987.
62. Leon J, Kamino H, Steinberg JJ, Pellicer A. H-*ras* activation in benign and self-regressing skin tumors (keratoacanthomas) in both human and animal model systems. Mol Cell Biol 8:786–793, 1988.
63. Bishop J. Cellular oncogenes and retroviruses. Annu Rev Biochem 52:301–354, 1983.
64. Brown K, Quintanilla M, Ramsden M, Kerr IB, Young S, Balmain A. V-*ras* genes from Harvey and BALB murine sarcoma viruses can act as inhibitors of two-stage mouse skin carcinogenesis. Cell 46:447–456, 1986.
65. Husain Z, Fei Y, Roy S, Solt DB, Polverini PJ, Biswas DK. Sequential expression and cooperative interaction of c-Ha-*ras* and c-*erb* B genes in in vivo chemical carcinogenesis. Proc Natl Acad Sci USA 86:1264–1268, 1989.
66. Wong DTW, Gertz R, Chow P, Chang ALC, McBride J, Chiang T et al. Detection of Ki-*ras* messenger RNA in normal and chemically transformed hamster oral keratinocytes. Cancer Res 49:4562–4567, 1989.
67. Campisi J, Gray HE, Pardee AB, Dean M, Soneshein G. Cell control of c-*myc* but not c-*ras* expression is lost following chemical transformation. Cell 36:241–247, 1984.
68. Solt DB. Localization of gamma-glutamyl transpeptidase in hamster buccal pouch epithelium treated with 7,12-dimethylbenz(*a*)anthracene. J Natl Cancer Inst 67:193–199, 1981.
69. Solt DB, Shklar G. Rapid induction of gamma-glutamyl transpeptidase-rich intraepithelial clones in DMBA-treated hamster buccal pouch. Cancer Res 42:285–291, 1982.
70. Odajima T, Solt DB, Solt LC. Persistence of gamma-glutamyl transpeptidase-positive foci during hamster buccal pouch carcinogenesis. Cancer Res 44:2062–2067, 1984.
71. Murase N, Fukui S, Mori M. Heterogeneity of keratin distribution in the oral mucosa and skin of mammals as determined using monoclonal antibodies. Histochem J 85:265–276, 1986.
72. Tatemoto Y, Fukui S, Oosumi H, Horike H, Mori M. Expression of keratins during experimentally induced carcinogenesis in hamster cheek pouch visualized polyclonal and monoclonal antibodies. Histochemistry 86:445–452, 1987.
73. Gimenez-Conti IB, Shin DM, Bianchi AB, Roop DR, Hong WK, Conti CJ, et al. Changes in keratin expression during 7,12-dimethylbenz(*a*)anthracene-induced hamster cheek pouch carcinogenesis. Cancer Res 50:4441–4445, 1990.
74. Fugita J, Yoshida O, Tusas Y, Rhim JS, Hatamaka M, Aaronson SA. Ha-*ras* oncogenes are activated by somatic alterations in human urinary tract tumors. Nature 309:464–466, 1984.
75. Eva A, Tronick SR, Gol RA, Pierce JH, Aaronson SA. Transforming genes of human hematopoietic tumors: Frequent detection of *ras*-related oncogenes whose activation appears to be independent of tumor phenotype. Proc Natl Acad Sci USA 80:4926–4930, 1983.
76. Santos E, Martin-Zanca D, Reddy EP, Pierotti MA, Della Porta G, Barbacid MJ. Malignant activation of K-*ras* oncogene in lung carcinoma, but not in normal tissue of the same patients. Science 223:661–668, 1984.
77. Shih C, Shelo BF, Goldfarb MP, Dannenberg A, Weinberg RA. Passage of phenotypes of chemically transformed cells via transfection of DNA and chromatin. Proc Natl Acad Sci USA 76:5714–5718, 1979.
78. Der CJ, Krontris TG, Cooper GM. Transforming genes of human bladder and lung carcinoma cell lines are homologous to the *ras* genes of Harvey and Kirsten sarcoma virus. Proc Natl Acad Sci USA 79:3637–3640, 1982.

79. Der CJ, Cooper GM. Altered gene products are associated with activation of cellular ABSK genes in human lung and colon carcinomas. Cell 32:201–208, 1983.
80. Goldfarb MP, Shimizn K, Perucho M, Wigler MH. Isolation and preliminary characterization of a human transforming gene from T24 bladder carcinoma cells. Nature 296:405–409, 1982.
81. Papageorge A, Lowy D, Scolnick E. Comparative biochemical properties of P^{21} ras molecules coded for by viral and cellular *ras* genes. J Virol 44:509–519, 1982.
82. Thor A, Ohuchi N, Horan Hand P, Callahan R, Weeks MO, Liderean R, et al. *ras* gene alterations and enhanced levels of P^{21}ras expression in a spectrum of benign and malignant human mammary tissue. J Lab Invest 55:603–615, 1986.
83. Bos JL. The *ras* gene family and human carcinogenesis. Mutat Res 195:255–271, 1988.
84. Reddy EP, Reynolds RK, Santos E, Barbacid M. A point mutation is responsible for the acquisition of transforming properties by T24 human bladder carcinoma oncogene. Nature 300:149–152, 1982.
85. Taparowsky E, Suard Y, Fasano O, Shimizu K, Goldfarb M, Wigler M. Activation of the T24 bladder carcinoma transforming gene is link to a single amino acid change. Nature 300:762–765, 1982.
86. Tabin CJ, Bradley SM, Bargmann CI, Weinberg RA, Papageorge AG, Scolnick EM, et al. Mechanism of activation of a human oncogene. Nature 300:143–148, 1982.
87. Spandidos DA, Wilkie NM. Malignant transformation of early passage rodent cells by a single mutated human oncogene. Nature 310:469–475, 1984.
88. Slamon DJ, DeKernion JB, Verma IM, Cline MJ. Expression of cellular oncogenes in human malignancies. Science 224:256–262, 1984.
89. Horan-Hand P, Thor A, Wunderlich D, Muraro R, Casruso A, Schlom J. Monoclonal antibodies of predefined specificity-detected carcinomas. Proc Natl Acad Sci USA 81:5227–5231, 1984.
90. Viola MV, Fromowitz F, Oravez S, Deb S, Schlom J. *ras* oncogene P^{21} expression is increased in premalignant lesions and high-grade bladder carcinoma. J Exp Med 161:1213–1218, 1985.
91. Gallick G, Kurzrock R, Kloetzer W, Arlinghaus R, Gutterman J. Expression of P^{21} ras in fresh primary and metastatic human colorectal tumors. Proc Natl Acad Sci USA 82:1795–1799, 1985.
92. Vousden KH, Marshall CJ. Three different activated *ras* genes in mouse tumors; evidence of oncogene activation during progression of a mouse lymphoma. EMBO J 3:913–917, 1984.
93. Collard JG, Schnijven JF, Roos E. Invasive and metastatic potential induced by *ras*-transfection into mouse BW5147 T-lymphoma cells. Cancer Res 47:754–759, 1987.
94. Riou G. Proto-oncogenes and prognosis in early carcinoma of the uterine cervix. Cancer Surv 7:441, 1988.
95. Riou G, Barrois M, Sheng FM. Somatic deletions and mutations of Ha-*ras* gene in human cervical cancers. Oncogene 3:329–333, 1988.
96. Capon DJ, Chen EY, Levinson AD, Seeburg PH, Goeddel et al. Complete nucleotide sequences of the T24 human bladder carcinoma oncogene and its normal homologue. Nature 302:33–37, 1983.
97. Nordenskjold M, Cavence WK. Genetics and the etiology of solid tumors. In: VT DeVita Jr, S Hellman, SA Rosenberg, eds. Important Advances in Oncology. Philadelphia: JB Lippincott, 1988, pp 83.
98. Jiang W, Kahn SM, Guillem JG, Lu SH, Weinstein IB. Rapid detection of *ras* oncogenes in human tumors: Application to colon, esophageal, and gastric cancer. Oncogene 4:923–928, 1989.
99. Azuma M, Furumoto N, Kawamata H, Yoshida H, Yanagawa T, Yura Y, et al. The relation of *ras* oncogene product P^{21} expression to clinicopathological status criteria and clinical outcome in squamous cell head and neck cancer. The Cancer J 1:375–380, 1987.
100. Furth ME, Davis LJ, Flenrdelys B, Scolnick EM. Monoclonal antibodies to the P^{21}

products of the transforming gene of Harvey murine sarcoma virus and of the cellular *ras* gene family. J Virol 43:294–304, 1982.

101. Sachs PG, Parnes SM, Gallick GE, Mansouri Z, Lichtner R, Satya-Prakash KL, et al. Establishment and characterization of two new squamous cell carcinoma cell lines derived from tumors of head and neck. Cancer Res 48:2858–2866, 1988.

102. Sheng ZM, Barrois M, Klijanienko J, Micheau C, Richard JM, Riou G. Analysis of the c-Ha-*ras*-1 gene for deletion, mutation, amplification, and expression in lymph node metastases of human head and neck carcinomas. Br J Cancer 62:398–404, 1990.

103. Rumsby G, Carter RL, Gusterson BA. Low incidence of *ras* oncogene activation in human squamous cell carcinomas. Br J Cancer 61:365–368, 1990.

104. Field JK, Lamothe A, Spandidos DA. Clinical relevance of oncogene expression in head and neck tumors. Anticancer Res 6:595–600, 1986.

105. Sakamoto H, Mori M, Taira M, Yoshida T, Matsukawa S, Shimizu K, et al. Transforming gene from human stomach cancers and a noncancerous portion of stomach mucosa. Proc Natl Acad Sci USA 83:3997–4001, 1986.

106. Yoshida MC, Wada M, Satoh H, Yoshida T, Sakamoto H, Myagawa K, et al. Human *HST2* (*HSTF1*) gene maps to chromosome band 11q13 and coamplifies with the *int*-2 gene in human cancer. Proc Natl Acad Sci USA 85:4861–4864, 1988.

107. Taira M, Yoshida T, Myagawa K, Sakamoto H, Terada M, Sugimura T. cDNA sequence of human transforming gene *hst* and identification of the coding squamous required for transforming activity. Proc Natl Acad Sci USA 84:2980–2984, 1987.

108. Yoshida T, Miyagawa K, Odagiri H, Sakamoto H, Little PFR, Terada M, et al. Genomic sequence of *hst*, a transforming gene encoding a protein homologous to fibroblast growth factor and the *int*-2-encoded protein. Proc Natl Acad Sci USA 84:7305–7309, 1987.

109. Miyagawa K, Sakamoto H, Yoshida T, Yamashita Y, Mitsui Y, Furusawa M, et al. *Hst*-1 transforming protein: Expression in silkworm cells and characterization as a novel heparin binding growth factor. Oncogene 3:383–389, 1988.

110. Casey G, Smith R, McGilliuray D, Peters G, Dickson C. Characterization and chromosome assignment of the human homolog of *int*-2, a potential protooncogene. Mol Cell Biol 6:502–510, 1986.

111. Tsutsumi M, Sakamoto H, Yoshida T, Kakizoe T, Koiso K, Sugimura T, et al. Coamplification of the *hst*-1 and *int*-2 genes in human cancer. Jpn J Cancer Res 79:428–432, 1988.

112. Tsuda Y, Tahara E, Kajiyama G, Sakamoto H, Terada M, Sugimora T. High incidence of coamplification of *hst*-1 and *int*-2 genes in human esophageal carcinomas. Cancer Res 49:5505–5508, 1989.

113. Adelaide J, Matter MG, Marics I, Raybaund F, Planche J, Lapeyriere OD, et al. Chromosomal localization of the *hst* oncogene and its coamplification with the *int*-2 oncogene in human melanoma. Oncogene 2:413–416, 1988.

114. Hatada I, Tokino T, Ochiya T, Matsubara K. Coamplification of integrated hepatitis B virus DNA and transforming gene *hst*-1 in a hepatocellular carcinoma. Oncogene 3:537–540, 1988.

115. Ali IU, Merlo G, Callahan R, Liderean R. The amplification unit of chromosome 11q13 in aggressive primary breast tumors entails the *bcl*-1, *int*-2 and *hst* loci. Oncogene 4:89–92, 1989.

116. Somers KD, Cartwright SL, Schechter GL. Amplification of the *int*-2 gene in human head and neck squamous carcinomas. Oncogene 5:915–920, 1990.

117. Zhou DJ, Casey G, Cline MJ. Amplification of human *int*-2 in breast cancers and squamous carcinomas. Oncogene 2:279–282, 1988.

118. Cole MD. The *myc* oncogene: Its role in transformation and differentiation. Annu Rev Genet 20:361–384, 1986.

119. Sheiness DK, Bishop JM. DNA and RNA from uninfected vertebrate cells containing nucleotide sequences related to the putative transforming gene of avian myelocytomatosis virus. J Virol 31:514–518, 1979.

120. Sheiness DK, Hughes SH, Varmus HE, Stubblefield E, Bishop JM. The vertebrate

homolog of the putative transforming gene of avian myelocytomatosis virus: Characteristics of the DNA locus and its RNA transcript. Virology 105:415–424, 1980.

121. Schwab M, Alitalo K, Klempnauer KH, Varmus HE, Bishop JM, Gilbert F, et al. Amplified DNA with limited homology to myc cellular oncogene is shared by human neuroblastoma cell lines and a neuroblastoma tumor. Nature 305:245–248, 1988.

122. Kohl NE, Gee CE, Alt FW. Activated expression of the N-myc gene in human neuroblastomas and related tumors. Science 226:1335–1337, 1984.

123. Nau MM, Brooks BJ, Battey J, Sausville E, Gazda AF, Kirsch IR, et al. L-myc, a new myc-related gene amplified and expressed in human small cell lung cancer. Nature 318:69–73, 1985.

124. Leder P, Battey J, Lenoir C, Moulding C, Murphy W, Potter H, et al. Translocations among antibody genes in human cancer. Science 222:765–771, 1983.

125. Croce CM, Nowell P. Molecular basis of human B-cell neoplasia. Blood 65:1–7, 1985.

126. Peschle C, Mavillo F, Sposi N, Giampaolo A, Care A, Bottero L, et al. Translocation and rearrangement of c-myc into immunoglobulin alpha heavy chain locus in primary cells from acute lymphocytic leukemia. Proc Natl Acad Sci USA 81:5514–5518, 1984.

127. Lee WH, Murphee AL, Benedict WF. Expression and amplification of the N-myc gene in primary retinoblastoma. Nature 309:458–460, 1984.

128. Seeger R, Brodeur G, Sather H, Dalton A, Siegel S, Wong K, et al. Association of multiple copies of the N-myc oncogene with rapid progression of neuroblastomas. N Engl J Med 313:1111–1119, 1985.

129. Brodeur G, Seeger R, Schwab M, Varmus H, Bishop JM. Amplification of N-myc in untreated human neuroblastomas correlates with advanced disease stage. Science 224:1121–1124, 1984.

130. Johnson BE, Ihde DC, Makuch RW, Gazdar AF, Carney DN, Oie H, et al. myc family oncogene amplification in tumor cell lines established from small cell lung cancer patients and its relationship to clinical status and course. J Clin Invest 79:1629–1634, 1987.

131. Field JK, Spandidos DA, Stell PM, Vaughan ED, Evan GI, Moore JP. Elevated expression of the c-myc oncoprotein correlates with poor prognosis in head and neck squamous cell carcinoma. Oncogene 4:1463–1468, 1989.

132. Sarnath D, Panchal R, Nair R, Mehta AR, Sanghavi V, Sumegi J, et al. Oncogene amplification in squamous cell cancer of the lung of the oral cavity. Jpn J Cancer Res 80:430–437, 1989.

133. Gusterson B, Cowley G, Smith JA, Ozanne B. Cellular localization of human epidermal growth factor receptor. Cell Biol Int Rep 8:659–667, 1984.

134. Filmus J, Pollak MN, Cailleau R, Buick RM. MDA-468, a human breast cancer cell line with a high number of epidermal growth factor (EGF) receptors, has an amplified EGF receptor gene and is growth inhibited by EGF. Biochem Biophys Res Commun 128:898–905, 1985.

135. Fitzpatrick SL, Brightwell J, Wittlift JL, Barrows GH, Shultz GS. Epidermal growth factor binding by breast biopsies and relationship to estrogen receptor and progestin receptor levels. Cancer Res 44:3448–3453, 1984.

136. Kamata N, Chida K, Rikimaru K, Horikoshi M, Enomoto S, Kuroki T. Growth inhibitory effects of epidermal growth factor and overexpression of its receptors on human squamous cell carcinomas in culture. Cancer Res 46:1648–1653, 1986.

137. Cohen S, Ushiro H, Stoscheck C, Gill GN. Regulation of the epidermal growth factor by phosphorylation. J Cell Biochem 29:195–208, 1985.

138. Cohen S, Carpenter G, King L. Epidermal growth factor receptor protein kinase interactions. J Biol Chem 255:4834–4842, 1980.

139. Ushiro H, Cohen S. Identification of phosphotyrosine as a product of epidermal growth factor-activated protein kinase in A431 cell membranes. J Biol Chem 255:8353–8365, 1980.

140. Yamamoto T, Nishida T, Miyajima M, Kawai S, Ooi T, Toyoshima K. The erb B gene of

avian erythoblastosis virus is a member of the *src* gene family. Cell 35:71–78, 1983.

141. Maxwell SA, Sacks PG, Gutterman JU, Gallick GE. Epidermal growth factor receptor protein-tyrosine kinase activity in human cell lines established from squamous carcinomas of the head and neck. Cancer Res 49:1130–1137, 1989.

142. Santini J, Formento JL, Francoual M, Milano G, Schneider M, Dassonville O, et al. Characterization, quantification, and potential clinical value of the epidermal growth factor receptor in head and neck squamous cell carcinomas. Head Neck 13:132–139, 1991.

143. Kearsley JH, Furlong KL, Cooke RA, Waters MJ. An immunohistochemical assessment of cellular proliferation markers in head and neck squamous cell cancers. Br J Cancer 61:821–827, 1990.

144. Weichselbaum RR, Dunphy EJ, Beckett MA, Tybor AG, Moran WJ, Goldman ME, et al. Epidermal growth factor receptor gene amplification and expression in head and neck cancer cell lines. Head Neck 11:437–442, 1989.

145. Lane DP, Crawford LV. T antigen is bound to a host protein in SV40-transformed cells. Nature 278:261–263, 1979.

146. Crawford LV, Pim DC, Gurney EG, Goodfellow P, Taylor-Papadimitriou J. Detection of a common feature in several human tumor cell lines — a 53,000-dalton protein. Proc Natl Acad Sci USA 78:41–45, 1981.

147. Miller C, Mohandas T, Wolf D, Prokocimer M, Rotter V, Koeffler HP. Human *p53* gene localized to the short arm of chromosome 17. Nature 319:783–784, 1986.

148. Isobe M, Emanuel BS, Givol D, Oren M, Croce CM. Localization of gene for human p53 tumor antigen to band 17p13. Nature 320:84–86, 1986.

149. Finlay CA, Hinds PW, Levine AJ. The *p53* proto-oncogene can act as a suppressor of transformation. Cell 57:1083–1093, 1989.

150. Eliyahu D, Michalovitz D, Eliyahu S, Pinhasi-Kimhi O, Oren M. Wild-type p53 can inhibit oncogene-mediated focus formation. Proc Natl Acad Sci USA 86:8763–8767, 1989.

151. Baker SJ, Fearon ER, Nigro JM, Hamilton SR, Preisinger AC, Jessup JM, et al. Chromosome 17 deletions and *p53* gene mutations in colorectal carcinomas. Science 244:217–221, 1989.

152. Soussi T, Caron DE, Fromentel C, Mechali M, Hay P, Kress M. Cloning and characterization of a cDNA from xenopus lavis coding for a protein homologous to human and murine *p53*. Oncogene 1:71–78, 1987.

153. Soussi T, Begue A, Kress M, Stehelin D, May P. Nucleotide sequence of a cDNA encoding the chicken p53 nuclear oncoprotein. Nucleic Acids Res 16:11383, 1988.

154. Wolf D, Laver-Rudich Z, Rotter V. In vitro expression of human *p53* cDNA clones and characterization of the cloned human *p53* gene. Mol Cell Biol 5:1887–1893, 1985.

155. Harlow E, Williamson NM, Ralston R, Halfman DM, Adams TE. Molecular cloning and in vitro expression of a cDNA clone for human cellular tumor antigen p53. Mol Cell Biol 5:1601–1610, 1985.

156. Mercer WE, Nelson D, DeLeo AB, Old IJ, Baserga R. Microinjection of monoclonal antibody to protein p53 inhibits serum-induced DNA synthesis in 3T3 cells. Proc Natl Acad Sci USA 79:6309–6312, 1982.

157. Reich NC, Levine AJ. Growth regulation of a cellular tumor antigen, p53, in nontransformed cells. Nature 308:199–201, 1984.

158. Shohat O, Greenberg M, Reisman D, Oren M, Rotter V. Inhibition of cell growth mediated by plasmids encoding p53 anti-sense. Oncogene 1:277–281, 1987.

159. Eliyahu D, Goldfinger N, Pinhasi-Kimhi O, Shaulsky G, Akurnik Y, Arai N, et al. Meth A fibrosarcoma cells express two transforming mutant p53 species. Oncogene 3:313–321, 1988.

160. Finlay CA, Hinds PW, Tan TH, Eliyahu D, Oren M, Levine AJ. Activating mutations for transformation by p53 produce a gene product that forms an *hsc* 70-p53 complex with an altered half-life. Mol Cell Biol 8:531–539, 1988.

161. Cavenee WK, Hastie ND, Stanbridge EJ, eds. Current Communications in Molecular

Biology: Recessive Oncogenes and Tumor Suppression. Cold Spring Harbor, NY: Cold Spring Harbor Laboratory Press, 1989.

162. Atkin NB, Baker MC. Chromosome 17p loss in carcinoma of the cervix uteri. Cancer Genet Cytogenet 37:229–233, 1989.

163. Yano T, Linehan M, Anglard P, Lerman MI, Daniel LN, Stein CA, et al. Genetic changes in human adrenocortical carcinomas. J Natl Cancer Inst 81:518–523, 1989.

164. Tsai CM, Gazdar AF, Venzon DJ, Steinberg SM, Dedrick RI, Mulshine JL, et al. Lack of in vitro synergy between etoposide and *cis*-diaminedichloroplatinum (II). Cancer Res 49:2390–2397, 1989.

165. Fearon ER, Hamilton SR, Vogelstein B. Clonal analysis of human colorectal tumors. Science 238:193–197, 1987.

166. Monpezat JPH, Delattre O, Bernard A, Grunwald D, Remvikos Y, Muleris M, et al. Loss of alleles on chromosome 18 and on the short arm of chromosome 17 in polyploid colorectal carcinomas. Int J Cancer 41:404–408, 1988.

167. Herskowitz I. Functional inactivation of genes by dominant negative mutations. Nature 329:219–222, 1987.

168. Eliyahu D, Michalovitz D, Eliyahu S, Pinhasi-Kimhi O, Oren M. Wild-type p53 can inhibit oncogene-mediated focus formation. Proc Natl Acad Sci USA 86:8763–8767, 1987.

169. Kraiss S, Quaiser A, Oren M, Montenarch M. Oligomerization of oncoprotein p53. J Virol 62:4737–4744, 1988.

170. Lane DP, Benchimol S. *p53*: Oncogene or anti-oncogene? Genes Dev 4:1–8, 1990.

171. Iggo R, Gatter K, Bartek J, Lane D, Harris AL. Increased expression of mutant forms of *p53* oncogene in primary lung cancer. Lancet 335:675–679, 1990.

172. Chiba I, Takehashi T, Nau M, D'Amico D, Curiel DT, Mitsudomi T, et al. Mutations in the *p53* gene are frequent in primary, resected non-small cell lung cancer. Oncogene 5:1603–1610, 1990.

173. Gusterson BA, Anbazhagan R, Warren W, Midgely C, Lane DP, Ohare M, et al. Expression of p53 in premalignant and malignant squamous epithelium. Oncogene 6:1785–1789, 1991.

174. Chiao PJ, Shin DM, Sacks PG, Hong WK, Tainsky MA. Elevated expression of the ribosomal protein *S2* gene in human tumors. Mol Carcinogen 5:219–231, 1992.

175. Chester KA, Robon L, Begent HJR, Talbot IC, Pringle HJ, Primrose L, et al. Identification of a human ribosomal protein mRNA with increased expression in colorectal tumors. Biochim Biophys Acta 1009:297–300, 1989.

176. Davies MS, Henney A, Ward HJW, Craig KR. Characterisation of an mRNA encoding a human ribosomal protein homologous to the yeast L44 ribosomal protein. Gene 45:183–191, 1984.

177. Pogue-Geile K, Geiser JR, Shu M, Miller C, Wool IG, Meisler AI, et al. Ribosomal protein genes are overexpressed in human colorectal cancer: Isolation of a cDNA clone encoding the human S3 ribosomal protein. Mol Cell Biol 11:3842–3849, 1991.

3. Squamous differentiation and retinoids

Reuben M. Lotan

Retinoids are structural or functional analogues of vitamin A, or retinol. They exert profound effects on the growth, maturation, and differentiation of many cells types, particularly epithelial cells, both in vivo and in vitro [1–8]. Vitamin A exerts a major effect on normal differentiation of epithelial cells, including those lining the oral cavity and upper aerodigestive tract [9]. The maintenance of the mucus-secreting function of these cells depends on the continuous presence of vitamin A. In its absence, squamous metaplasia develops that can be reversed by vitamin A replenishment [8–14]. β-all-*trans*-retinoic acid (tRA) can replace vitamin A in restoration of normal differentiation of epithelial tissues in vitamin A–deficient animals [14–19]. It is thought that squamous metaplasia in the upper aerodigestive epithelium is a precursor of certain cancers [20] and that agents like retinoids, which suppress keratinization and restore the normal nonkeratinizing phenotype to premalignant and malignant lesions, may also restore their responsiveness to normal growth control mechanisms. Consequently, such agents could suppress carcinogenesis and be useful in the prevention and treatment of squamous cell carcinomas [21–23]. This chapter describes the effects of retinoids on squamous differentiation in normal, premalignant, and malignant epithelial tissues.

Normal squamous cell differentiation

The skin is the major organ where epithelial cells undergo squamous cell differentiation and, not surprisingly, most of our basic knowledge on squamous cell differentiation has been derived from studies of this organ in vivo and from studies of cultured epidermal keratinocytes [24–26]. The keratinizing stratified squamous epithelium of the skin includes basal epithelial cells, which are separated from the dermis by a basal lamina. The basal

Hong, Waun Ki and Weber, Randal S., (eds.), Head and Neck Cancer. © *1995 Kluwer Academic Publishers.*
ISBN 0-7923-3015-3. All rights reserved.

cells are considered the stem cells of the skin in that they divide continuously and generate more basal cells as well as progeny that migrate from the basal layer outward. Cells in the suprabasal layers lose proliferating capacity and undergo a series of concerted changes in the expression of several genes, which result in terminally differentiated squames [24–27]. Epithelial cells covering the hard palate, the dorsal anterior part of the tongue, and the gingiva of the oral cavity resemble epidermis in that they are stratified and keratinizing cornified epithelium [28]. The epithelial cells of the esophagus and the uterine cervical mucosa are also keratinizing. In contrast, the majority of epithelial cells in the oral cavity and the tracheobronchial tree are normally nonkeratinizing.

Many of the genes expressed during squamous differentiation have been cloned and their products characterized extensively. Some of these markers are involved in the formation of the crosslinked envelope. They include the crosslinking enzyme transglutaminase type I (TGase-I), which is associated with the cytoplasmic face of the plasma membrane and catalyzes the formation of isopeptide linkages [ε-(γ-glutamyl)lysine] between protein-bound glutamine residues and primary amines such as protein-bound lysine that are present in various envelope protein precursors [29–36]. The TGase-I substrates that are abundant in the cytosol of cells in the upper spinous and granular layers are also differentiation markers. They include loricrin, a 25- to 30-kD protein found in the granular and lower cornified cell layers of epidermis [37,38]; cornifin, a 14-kD protein that is expressed in the suprabasal layer [39]; and involucrin, a 68-kD protein that is the major protein component of cornified envelopes in cultured keratinocytes [24,26, 29,34,40–46]. Because involucrin is also found in various stratified squamous epithelia, it is considered a general marker of squamous differentiation [47,48]. Additional TGase-I substrates found in the crosslinked envelope are keratolinin, a 16- to 26-kD protein [49–51]; annexin I, a 36-kD protein [52,53]; and sciellin, an 82-kD protein [54]. Another group of squamous differentiation markers is the intermediate filaments or keratins. Specifically, in human epidermis cells in the deep layers produce keratin molecules of 46- to 58-kD (keratins K5 and K14); however, as they move outward they begin to synthesize large keratins (e.g., keratin K1, 67 kD, and K10, 56.5 kD) that are characteristic of the suprabasal layers in cornifying stratified epithelia (e.g., epidermis) but not in simple or transitional stratified epithelia [55–62]. In the oral cavity, the cornified epithelium of the gingiva expresses K1 keratin, whereas the noncornifying stratified epithelia covering most of the oral cavity do not produce the K1 keratin but express other keratins [28,62]. The aggregation of keratin filaments is augmented by the protein filaggrin, which is a 37-kD protein derived from a higher molecular weight precursor in cornifying cells [63–67]. Other squamous differentiation markers are a 16–20 kD prorelaxin-like molecule [68,69], cholesterol sulfotransferase and cholesterol sulfate [70–75], acylceramides, and lanosterol lipid [76].

44

Aberrant squamous cell differentiation

Normal epithelial cells

The lining mucosa of the human oral epithelium that covers most of the oral cavity, including the soft palate, the tongue's ventral surface, the mouth's floor, the alveolar area, the lips, and the cheeks, is a nonkeratinizing epithelium [28]. Likewise, the epithelium of the tracheobronchial tree is noncornified [5]. Some columnar and transitional nonkeratinizing epithelial cells (e.g., lachrymal gland, trachea, bladder, and prostate) can undergo squamous metaplasia, indicating that they have the potential to differentiate along the squamous pathway [9,77]. This potential is expressed in vivo after mechanical injury [78], vitamin A deficiency [11,13,79,80], or exposure to carcinogens or tumor promoters [20,81–83]. The precursor cell type for the aberrant squamous cell may be the basal cell [84] or the secretory cell [85]. In rabbit tracheal epithelial cells, the squamous differentiation induced in vitro is accompanied by an increased expression of the K13 keratin [86]. In hamster trachea, squamous metaplasia induced by vitamin A deficiency is accompanied by increased expression of K5 keratin [8]. Squamous cell carcinomas (SCC), which account for over 90% of the tumors in the oral cavity, also undergo some degree of squamous differentiation [87]. Thus, squamous cell differentiation in the upper aerodigestive tract is usually an abnormal differentiation.

Premalignant and malignant lesions

The ability to form crosslinked envelopes is retained by many premalignant and malignant cells, which express transglutaminase and contain protein precursors for crosslinking [75,88–92]. For example, the exposure of buccal epithelial cells to the tumor-promoting agent 12-O-tetradecanoylphorbol-13-acetate increased the involucrin level and induced the formation of cross-linked envelopes [90]. Similarly, human keratinocytes immortalized by SV40 large T antigen continue to express involucrin and produce cornified envelopes [93]. Furthermore, involucrin is expressed in premalignant lesions and SCCs [46,88,89,94,95]. TGase-I was detected in benign and malignant neoplasms of the skin and oral cavity that show squamous differentiation but is not detected in severe oral epithelial dysplasia or undifferentiated invasive SCC [96,97]. TGase-I was expressed in the minority of several human lung SCCs grown in vitro or as xenografts in nude mice, whereas involucrin was expressed in all the cell lines, suggesting that control of the expression of these two markers is not tightly coordinated [98]. The expressions of TGase-I and involucrin are similarly uncoupled in lesions of severe oral epithelial dysplasia, in which TGase-I expression is suppressed but involucrin is present [97]. Studies with the hamster cheek pouch model of oral cancer have established that carcinogenesis is accompanied by increases in the expression of TGase-I during progression from normal cells through premalignant papilloma to carcinoma [82]. v-*ras*Ha-transduced mouse keratinocytes, which represent initiated cells, undergo a distinct reprogramming of the squamous differentiation program. The cells resist terminal differentiation induced by calcium (>0.1 mM), as evidenced by suppression of the level of loricrin. These v-*ras*Ha-transduced mouse keratinocytes also exhibit suppression of the level of the early suprabasal markers keratins K1 and K10. In contrast, the cells retain the ability to express filaggrin, albeit at higher calcium concentrations than normal cells [99]. Changes in the synthesis of keratins were noted during mouse skin carcinogenesis; the expression of keratins K6 and K16 increased in benign and malignant lesions, the expression of K13 increased after papilloma progressed to carcinoma, whereas the expression of K1 decreased in papilloma and diminished in carcinoma. These results suggest that the loss of K1 and the expression of K6, K13, and K16 could be considered as markers of progression to malignancy in skin lesions [60,100–103]. Similarly, studies with the hamster cheek pouch model of oral cancer have established that carcinogenesis is accompanied by increases in the expression of K1 keratin in hyperplastic lesions and decreases in dysplastic lesions and carcinomas during progression from normal through premalignant papilloma to carcinoma [83]. Thus, the expression of keratins 6/16 can serve as a marker for hyperplasia in premalignant lesions, and the expression of K1 can be a marker of squamous differentiation in premalignant lesions.

Although the K1 keratin is lost during carcinogenesis in mouse skin, there are reports on the presence of this keratin in squamous carcinomas in vivo and in vitro [59,91,92,104]. Some squamous cell carcinomas continue to produce the same keratins as the normal precursor cells [59,104,105]. However, neoplasms that arise in complex epithelia, such as stratified ones, often differ in the expression of keratin from the surrounding normal tissue, possibly because they represent an expanded subpopulation with a distinct keratin synthesis pattern [59,100]. For example, keratins K6 and K16 are usually present in very low amounts in normal epithelial tissues but are expressed in hyperproliferative states and in SCC [59,102].

Vitamin A and retinoids

β-carotene serves as the precursor for the in vivo biogenesis of retinol. β-all-*trans*-retinoic acid is a natural metabolite of retinol that can replace retinol in regulating epithelial differentiation and many other functions in vivo [15]. tRA is synthesized from retinol by various tissues and cultured cells, including keratinocytes [106–111]. Recently, it has been found that tRA can also be synthesized in various tissues and cultured epithelial cells from β-carotene without formation of retinol as an intermediate [107,108]. The production was at a rate that generated significant amounts of retinoic acid to make this pathway a potentially important one for retinoic acid generation in situ. Thus, tRA might be the active metabolite of both retinol and β-carotene. However, it should be noted the β-carotene and retinol may function without being metabolized to retinoic acid [112–117]. 13-*cis*-retinoic acid (13cRA) is an analogue of tRA that is also formed in vivo by isomerization [118]. It is present in human serum at concentrations similar to those of tRA [118]. 13cRA exhibits similar effects as tRA on cell growth, differentiation, and carcinogenesis but is less toxic and causes less side effects in vivo than the natural retinoic acid [119,120]. More recently 9-*cis*-retinoic acid has been shown to be a natural isomer of retinoic acid, and its presence in kidney and liver has been demonstrated [121,122].

Effects of retinoids on the growth of normal, premalignant, and malignant cells

Cell growth is tightly linked to squamous cell differentiation in that an irreversible growth arrest is a prerequisite for the expression of squamous cell differentiation markers and terminal differentiation [5,6]. Retinoids at physiological concentrations enhance the proliferation of cultured human epidermal cells [25,63,123–126] and are required in vivo for the maintenance of a normal architecture of the epithelia [8,63]. Pretreatment of growth factor–deprived human keratinocytes with retinoic acid enhanced the growth-stimulatory effects of a mixture of epidermal growth factor (EGF), bovine pituitary extract, and insulin [125]. Likewise, retinoic acid can enhance the growth of human buccal epithelial cells from explants maintained in a serum-free medium [90]. Recent studies have demonstrated that the targets for retinoid action in hamster trachea in vivo and in vitro are the columnar secretory (mucous) cells. Their proliferation is inhibited during vitamin A deficiency and enhanced upon restoration of vitamin A [126].

In contrast, several studies with SCCs reported that retinoids suppress cell proliferation in monolayer cultures [75,89,127–130], inhibit the formation of SCC colonies in semi-solid agarose [128], and decrease the growth of multicellular spheroids [131]. It is noteworthy that human keratinocytes immortalized by human papilloma virus type 16 show increased sensitivity to retinoids compared to the nonimmortalized precursor cells [132].

The growth of rabbit tracheal epithelial cells in serum-free medium was not affected by retinoids [5]. Furthermore, the responses of mouse keratinocytes were different from those of the human cells in that retinoic acid exhibited both stimulatory [125,133] and inhibitory [125,133,134] effects on the growth of the mouse skin keratinocytes. The dual effects of retinoids on mouse keratinocytes were attributed to different concentrations of calcium and growth factors in the medium. Thus, retinoids enhanced the proliferation of slow-growing cells maintained in low-calcium medium and inhibited DNA synthesis in hyperproliferative cells maintained in a high calcium with

47

a low level of growth factors [133]. In serum- and growth factor-free medium, retinoic acid enhanced the mitogenic effect of epidermal growth factor (EGF) and the growth-inhibitory effect of transforming growth factor-beta (TGF-β) [125]. The latter effect is important in view of the observation that retinoic acid also increased the level of active TGF-β2 in the murine cells [134]. The lack of inhibition of the growth of human keratinocytes by retinoids was attributed to the inability of retinoic acid to increase TGF-β in the human cells [25,127]. These findings have led to the conclusion that the effects of retinoids on epidermal growth and differentiation are complex, and this may be in part due to the ability of retinoids to enhance the responses of keratinocytes to both positive and negative peptide growth factors [125–127]. Our finding that retinoic acid suppressed the level of EGF receptor mRNA and the autophosphorylating activity of the receptor in human squamous carcinomas is compatible with this contention [135].

It is plausible to assume that the ability of retinoids to inhibit the growth of SCC cells and possibly also of premalignant epithelial cells is responsible, at least in part, for their ability to suppress oral premalignant lesion (e.g., leukoplakia) [136], and to prevent the development of second primary tumors in head and neck cancer patients [137], skin cancer in xeroderma pigmentosum patients [138], and other types of cancers [139–142].

Effects of retinoids on squamous cell differentiation in normal, premalignant, and malignant cells

Numerous reports have documented the ability of retinoids to suppress squamous differentiation in normal, premalignant (e.g., papillomas), and malignant keratinocytes [6,19,25,123]. Our studies with human head and neck SCC (HNSCC) have demonstrated that some of them exhibit characteristic markers of squamous differentiation and respond to retinoids under specific culture conditions.

Retinoids have been shown to reduce spontaneous and calcium ionophore-induced crosslinked envelope formation, especially when the cells were cultured in vitamin A–deficient medium [6,29,88,89,143]. This effect appeared to be the result of a combination of the suppression of TGase-I activity and the level of envelope precursor proteins. Thus, retinoids suppressed TGase-I expression [6,29,144,145] and decreased the level of involucrin [88,89,146], loricrin [147,148], and cornifin [39,149]. Human and rabbit tracheal epithelial cells cultured in a serum-free defined medium responded to very low retinoid concentrations and exhibited a suppression of TGase-I activity and inhibition of envelope formation [5,6]. In human ectocervical cells, retinoids suppressed envelope formation but did not alter the level of involucrin, suggesting that the mechanism of inhibition of envelope formation may be distinct for different epithelia [150]. Several studies with a variety of cultured cell lines established from human squamous cell carcinoma tumors of the oral mucosa or the facial epidermis have demonstrated that different retinoids inhibit TGase-I, decrease involucrin content, and suppress the formation of cornified envelopes [6,88,89,91,145, 151]. The suppression of TGase-I was presumably at the transcriptional level, and the effect was twofold in that retinoic acid inhibited the expression of TGase-I when it was present during the growth of tracheobronchial epithelial cells as well as when added to already squamous-differentiated cells [144,152]. Retinoic acid exerted two distinct effects on loricrin expression in that it not only blocked the calcium-induced loricrin mRNA synthesisis but also suppressed elevated loricrin mRNA levels in differentiated cells that had been pretreated with calcium [147]. The expression of another envelope precursor, cornifin, was similarly inhibited by retinoids in rabbit tracheal epithelial cells and human keratinocytes [39].

We studied the effects of RA on the expression of TGase-I in eight cell lines derived from human head and neck squamous carcinomas (HNSCCs) in the oral cavity and found that tRA suppressed the expression of this marker to different degrees in the different cell lines [6,128,130]. One of the cell lines, HNSCC 1483, was selected for investigation of the effects of retinoic acid on envelope formation, on the activity and amount of TGAse-I, and on the levels of involucrin. The cells' potential to crosslink proteins in the presence of the Ca^{2+} ionophore Ro2-2985 was suppressed by tRA [130]. A similar suppression of envelope competence by RA was reported for normal keratinocytes [153], a premalignant papilloma cell line [143], malignant SCC-13 cells from a tumor of the facial skin [88,151], and buccal SqCC/Y1 cells [89]. The tRA effect on envelope competence was the result of both a suppression of TGase-I and a decrease in involucrin expression at the mRNA and protein levels [91]; Zou and Lotan, unpublished].

A physiological role of vitamin A in the regulation of keratin synthesis was implied by examination of changes in keratin expression following vitamin A deficiency in experimental animals [154,155]. Vitamin A deficiency in rabbits was accompanied by increased keratinization of conjunctival and corneal epithelia, and by corresponding changes in keratins [155]. Whereas the normal corneal and conjunctival epithelial cells do not express significant amounts of the 56.5-kD (K10) and the 65- to 67-kD keratins (K1 and K2), the same epithelia express these keratins during vitamin A deficiency [155]. Similar changes in keratins were detected in esophageal epithelium, although this epithelium did not seem morphologically to undergo keratinization during vitamin A deficiency, and it was suggested that the biochemical changes may precede the morphological keratinization [155].

Further insight into the modulation of keratin expression by retinoids was derived from studies with cultured epithelial cells. Epidermal cells cultured in medium containing 10–20% serum do not synthesize the large keratins unless the serum is delipidized [156]. It has been found that the delipidation removes vitamin A and allows the cells to synthesize a 67-kD (K1) keratin while decreasing the synthesis of 52 (K13)- and 40-kD (K19) keratins [156].

When exogenous retinyl acetate was added to the delipidized serum in which the cells were cultured, the synthesis of the 67-kD keratin was inhibited and the synthesis of K13 and K19 keratins was stimulated [156]. Various synthetic retinoids can also modulate the synthesis of these specific keratins at the mRNA level [157–159]. Many cell lines established in culture from squamous carcinomas suffer from a defect in terminal differentiation and produce large amounts of a 40-kD keratin and very low amounts of the 67-kD keratin. These cells can be induced to produce more of the 67-kD keratin and less of the 40-kD keratin by reducing the level of vitamin A in the growth medium by delipidation of the serum supplement [104]. The level of 67-kD keratin produced under such conditions is still lower than that produced by normal keratinizing cells in culture, suggesting the existence of a defect in differentiation that is unrelated to the vitamin A effect [104].

A study with a cultured small cell lung cancer cell line (Lu-134-B-S) revealed that these cells maintained the small cell phenotype only when cultured in the presence of regular fetal calf serum. When cultured in delipidized serum, the cells became squamous, as indicated by synthesis of involucrin and high molecular weight keratins, as well as the appearance of desmosomes [160]. The squamous phenotype reversed to the small cell phenotype upon addition of retinoic acid to cells maintained in delipidized serum [160].

We observed that HNSCC 1483 cells grown in delipidized serum depleted of endogenous retinoids expressed keratins with molecular weights of 67 (K1), 56 (K10), 54, 52, 48, 46, and 40 (K19) kD [91]. In contrast, cells grown in medium with 10% fetal bovine serum, which contained about $0.06\,\mu M$ retinol, expressed much less K1; the levels of keratins of molecular weight 46 and 48 kD were lower; and the amounts of the 52- and 40-kD keratins were higher than those expressed in cells grown in delipidized serum. Cells treated with tRA in delipidized serum contained less keratins with molecular weights of 67, 56, 54, 48, and 46 kD and more of the 52-kD (probably K8) and the 40-kD (probably K19) keratins than cells grown in without retinoic acid. Thus, tRA modulated the expression of several keratins in addition to K1 in the 1483 cells [91].

These results are similar to previous findings that normal keratinocytes [156] and cells from SCCs of human tongue and skin produce keratins larger than 60 kD, including K1, when grown in delipidized serum or floating on collagen rafts [161] or on de-epidermized dermis [153] at the air-liquid interface. That laryngeal epithelial cells and papilloma cells respond to retinoids was demonstrated recently in a study of cells cultured in vitro at the air-liquid interface [162,163]. tRA was found to modulate the differentiation of these cells along two distinct pathways; at low concentrations($<10^{-8}$ M) the cells formed stratified squamous epithelium and expressed K13, whereas at higher concentrations of tRA ($>10^{-7}$M) the cells differentiated into a columnar epithelium with occasional ciliated cells, lacking squamous markers [162,163].

Retinoids also inhibited the synthesis of loricrin [147] and profilaggrin as well as its conversion into filaggrin in cultured human epidermal keratin-ocytes [63,123,164], and the production of cholesterol sulfate in rabbit tracheal epithelial cells, human bronchial epithelial cells, human keratin-ocytes [70–72] and in several HNSCC cell lines [75]. The mechanism of this effect of retinoids is suppression of the activity of cholesterol sulfotransferase [71,75]. Likewise, retinoids suppressed the level of lipids (acylceramide and lanosterol) that increase during late stages of epidermal differentiation [76] and the expression of a preprorelaxin-like gene in rabbit and human tracheobronchial epithelial cells and in human keratinocytes [68,69].

Recent histologic and immunocytochemical analyses of the effects of topically applied tRA on the expression of squamous differentiation markers in human skin in vivo revealed some differences from the findings with cultured epidermal keratinocytes in vitro [165]. tRA treatment (either an acute 4 day or a chronic 16 week treatment) caused epidermal thickening, stratum granulosum thickening, and increases in the number of cell layers expressing epidermal TGase, involucrin, and filaggrin, and focal expression of the keratins K6 and K13, which are not expressed in normal epidermis. The acute tRA treatment decreased the loricrin level, whereas the chron-ically treated skin showed increased numbers of cell layers expressing loricrin. The in vivo treatment did not alter the expression of keratins K1, K10, and K14 [165]. A direct comparison of acutely in vivo–treated skin and cultured keratinocytes exposed to tRA in vitro revealed that keratinocyte TGase activity increased 2.8-fold in the skin but decreased six-fold in the cultured cells [166]. These results demonstrate clearly that some of the results obtained with cultured normal cells in vitro may not represent the response of cells in vivo. It should be noted that the topical treatment used 0.1% tRA (1 mg/ml in cream), whereas the cultured cells were exposed to a much lower concentration of tRA (0.3 μg/ml; 1 μM).

Mechanisms involved in the actions of retinoids

Although the ability of retinoids to inhibit proliferation and clonogenicity of malignant cells and to modulate their differentiation in vitro is well documented [1–8], the mechanism(s) responsible for these effects is not fully understood. Likewise, it is not entirely clear how retinoids exert chemopreventive effects on carcinogenesis in experimental animal models and clinical trials in humans [120,121,136–142]. The ability of retinoids to modulate gene expression is the most plausible mechanism by which they can modulate the differentiation and growth of malignant cells or suppress the progression of premalignant cells to frank neoplastic lesions by re-directing their differentiation. The identity of the genes that control the expression of the premalignant or the malignant phenotype is not known; however, the restoration of normal differentiation by retinoids may repre-sent a part of a retinoid-dependent program of gene expression that includes activation of intrinsic anticancer activity (e.g., suppressor genes) or inhibition of genes that maintain the malignant phenotype in HNSCC cells. In the case of leukoplakia, retinoids could activate a program of resistance to progression to the neoplastic state.

To modulate gene expression, retinoids must transmit signals to the cell nucleus. The mechanism of this signal transduction is beginning to be unravelled as understanding of the roles of the major components of the pathway increases. Both cytoplasmic and nuclear retinoid-binding proteins appear to play important roles in the series of events that are initiated with the uptake of a retinoid by a target cell and culminate in the modulation of gene transcription in the cell's nucleus.

Cellular retinoid-binding proteins in squamous epithelial tissues and cells

Several intracellular proteins have been identified in the cell cytoplasm and in the nucleus that bind retinoids with different specificities [1,8,167–170]. These proteins have been implicated in morphogenesis during embryonal development, cell growth, differentiation, and the development of neoplasia [1,8,167–170]. Cellular (cytoplasmic) retinoid-binding proteins have also been detected in squamous epithelial tissues (e.g., skin) and in oral mucosa. A high-molecular-weight retinol-binding protein (HMWRBP) and retinoic acid-binding protein (HMWRABP) were found in human skin [171] and oral mucosa [172], and in undifferentiated and differentiated cultured keratinocytes [173]. Cellular retinol-binding protein (CRBP) and cellular retinoic acid-binding protein (CRABP) with a molecular weight of about 15,000 Da have been found in suprabasal cells in skin in vivo, and CRABP levels increased in psoriatic skin tissue and in retinoid-treated skin [173–177]. CRABP was found in confluent cultures of human keratinocytes [178,179]. The level of this protein was very low in undifferentiated keratinocytes, but it increased during squamous differentiation [173]. Two distinct CRABPs, designated CRABP-I and CRABP-II, have been isolated and cloned [168, 179,180]. CRABP-II was expressed at high levels in the skin during mouse embryogenesis and in adult skin [179]. Human CRABP-I and -II have been cloned, but only CRABP-II was found to be expressed in epidermal keratinocytes and to be modulated during squamous differentiation and retinoid treatment [180,181]. Topical treatment of human skin with tRA increased the level of CRABP-II mRNA 16-fold [180], consistent with the earlier reports on increased RA-binding activity in retinoid-treated skin [175,176]. CRABP-II mRNA levels increased in cultured keratinocytes under conditions that increase squamous differentiation, such as high Ca^{+2} concentration (2 mM) and growth to a high cell density [180]. Furthermore, tRA treatment of cultured keratinocytes, which suppressed squamous differentiation, also suppressed the expression of CRABP-II [180,181]. The apparent discrepancy between the effect of tRA on CRABP-II expression in vitro and in vivo may reflect the fact that tRA suppressed some markers of squamous differentiation in culture but not in vivo [166].

The presence of both CRBP and CRABP in normal tissue and HNSCC and lung SCCs has been described in several reports [1,167,168,182–187]. These studies have demonstrated that the levels of CRBP and CRABP were higher in the malignant than the normal tissues, and that the levels were higher in differentiated carcinomas than in less differentiated tumors. The levels of CRABP in squamous cell carcinoma cultured from tumors in the oral epithelium were found to be two to three times lower than in cultured normal keratinocytes. This observation has led to the proposal that the higher level of these proteins may be predictive of the responsiveness of the tumors to the antitumor action of retinoids. However, there is no experimental support for this suggestion.

We have compared the expression of CRABP-I and CRABP-II in four HNSCC cell lines and found that CRABP-I was not detectable in any of them, whereas CRABP-II was expressed by three of the four cell lines. One responsive HNSCC cell line (MDACC886Ln) had no detectable CRABP, whereas a nonrepsonsive cell line (183A) expressed as high a level of CRABP-II as did two responsive cell lines (1483 and SqCC/Y1) [188]. Thus, there was no correlation between the presence and level of CRABP and the response to the growth-inhibitory effects of RA.

In addition, uncertainties exist as to the precise function(s) of CRABP. A positive role in the retinoid signal transduction pathway was proposed after these binding proteins were shown to transport retinoids to the cell nucleus, where they can affect gene expression [189,190]. However, it has been shown that CRABP can function as a storage or sequestration function during embryonal development [191], and an overexpression of a transfected CRABP decreased the responsiveness of embryonal carcinoma cells to the differentiation-inducing effects of tRA, supporting the conclusion that CRABP may sequester retinoic acid and prevent it from reaching the cell nucleus [192]. Difficulties in reaching unambiguous conclusions on the role of CRABPs arise from various studies that have demonstrated a lack of correlation between the presence or level of the CRABPs and cells' sensitivity to various effects of retinoids. For example, some cell lines were responsive to the growth-inhibitory effects of tRA or retinyl acetate but did not possess detectable levels of either CRABP or CRBP [193], and, conversely, some retinoid-resistant cell lines did express these proteins [194]. Furthermore, a number of synthetic retinoids (e.g., Ch55 and CD271) that did not bind to CRABP were as active or more active than tRA in suppression of TGase in tracheobronchial epithelial cells [195] and control of keratinocyte differentiation, such as inhibition of the synthesis of suprabasal keratins, filaggrin, and TGase [196]. These findings suggest that CRABP may be not be necessary for the response of some cells to retinoids, but when it is present it may affect the response to retinoic acid by altering its effective concentration through sequestration in the cytoplasm or via increased catabolism [192,197].

Nuclear retinoic acid receptors

General properties of nuclear RA receptors. The understanding of the mechanism of retinoid action was enhanced following the discovery that some 'orphan' members of the large family of nuclear receptors for steroids, vitamin D, and thyroid hormones can bind retinoids. These nuclear retinoic acid receptors (RARs), like other members of the family, are ligand-activated, *trans*-acting, transcription-modulating factors. They bear strong DNA sequence homology to thyroid and steroid hormone receptors, especially in the DNA-binding domain [8,169,170,198,199]. Like other members of the steroid receptor superfamily, the RA receptors are constructed from six distinct domains, designated A–F [169,170,198,199]. The C domain, which is the most highly conserved domain among the different receptor family members, contains a zinc finger DNA-binding motif. Less well conserved is the E domain, which is responsible for ligand binding and dimerization function. Three RAR subtypes (RAR-α, RAR-β, and RAR-γ) encoding proteins of molecular weight of about 50,000 Da were cloned from human and mouse cell lines [200–206]. The RAR-α, RAR-β, and RAR-γ genes have been localized to the q21 band of chromosome 17 [207], the p24 band of chromosome 3 [208], and chromosome 12 [205], respectively. Each subtype had different tissue distributions. For example, in humans RAR-α mRNA was expressed in all tissues tested, with overexpression in hematopoietic cell lines, and RAR-β was expressed in a more variable and limited pattern in the tissues tested, with prevalence in neural tissues, whereas a third RA receptor, RAR-γ, was expressed predominantly in the skin, which is a tissue highly responsive to RA, and in precartilagenous and epithelial structures in the mouse embryo [206,209–211]. More recently, another subfamily of retinoic acid receptors, named RXR (-α, -β, and -γ), was discovered [212,213]. Although these receptors exhibit sequence homology with the steroid hormone receptors and with the retinoid receptors described above, they are substantially different in their primary structure and ligand specificity (e.g., they bind 9-*cis* RA much better than *trans* RA [121,122]) from the RARs and represent an alternative molecular pathway for gene regulation modulated by retinoids [212,213]. The tissue distribution of RXR mRNAs also differs from that of the RARs, with especially high levels of RXR-α in the adult in liver, muscle, lung, kidney, hearts, and spleen, all tissues in which there are very low levels of the RARs [212,213]. Whereas RXR-β was found in almost all tissues, the distribution of RXR-α and RXR-γ was more restricted [212,213]. The RXRs can form heterodimers with the RARs, and this dimerization is required for maximal transcriptional activation of retinoic acid response elements (e.g., RAREs and TREs) by RARs, whereas RAR homodimers may be inactive as transcription enhancers [214–217]. The response elements of the nuclear RARs are DNA sequences present in the promotor region of genes that are regulated transcriptionally by retinoids. The first RARE was identified in the promotor region of the RAR-β receptor. It is a direct repeat of the sequence GTTCAC separated by five nucleotides [218–220]. There are similar RAREs in the promotors found in both the RAR-α and RAR-γ genes [221,222]. Other genes for which RAREs have been discovered include laminin, *CRABP-II*, *CRBP-I*, alcohol dehydrogenase, complement factor H, oxytocin, *HOX3D*, and osteocalcin [223–229]. Response elements that appear to be specifically activated by RXRs were recently identified in several genes, including the *CRBP-II* gene, the apolipoprotein AI, and medium-chain acyl-CoA dehydrogenase genes [230–232]. In the *CRBP-II* gene the RXRE includes a 35-base pair sequence of five tandem repeats that responds to RXR-α but not to any of the RARs [231]. This response element has also been shown to bind RXR-α homodimers in the presence of 9-*cis* RA, which have a positive *trans*-activating function, as well as binding RAR-RXR heterodimers, which repress transcription [233].

RARs interact antagonistically with components of the AP-1 (*jun-fos*) transcription factor complex in stromelysin, collagenase, and osteocalcin promotors, possibly by direct protein-protein interactions [224,234,235]. Thus the regulation of a given gene by retinoids may depend on the relative concentrations of particular RARs, RXRs, the nature of the RAREs in that gene, as well as on the presence of a number of other transcription factors.

Nuclear RA receptors in normal keratinizing and nonkeratinizing epithelial cells. The expression of nuclear retinoic acid receptors in various embryonal tissues and in keratinizing and nonkeratinizing epithelial tissues and cells in skin and oral mucosa has been analyzed by northern blotting or in situ hybridization. RAR-γ was the predominant receptor in skin, RAR-α was expressed at much lower levels than RAR-γ, whereas *RAR-β* mRNA was undetectable [204,206,236–244]. A similar pattern of receptor expression was also found in RA-treated skin [239]. *RAR-γ1* mRNA was localized to all layers of the epidermis, including the basal cells [243]. Cultured epidermal keratinocytes also expressed primarily the RAR-γ receptor, and tRA treatment of these cells did not increase the RAR-γ level, nor did it induce the expression of RAR-β, although RAR-β was induced in cultured dermal fibroblasts [239–241].

Cultured undifferentiated tracheobronchial epithelial cells from human (HBE) and rabbit (RbTE) expressed both RAR-α and RAR-γ constitutively, and the expression of these receptors was not altered after the cells had undergone squamous cell differentiation or after RA treatment [245]. In contrast, the constitutive *RAR-β* mRNA level, which was low in HBE and RbTE, increased severalfold after RA treatment of both types [245]. All but one of nine surgical specimens of 'normal' lung tissue adjacent to lung carcinomas expressed RAR-β when analyzed by northern blotting, indicating that this receiver is constitutively expressed in vivo [246]. However, the method used was not appropriate to indicate whether the RAR-β is present in the epithelial cells, the stromal cells, or both.

The expression of mRNA for *RAR-α* and *RAR-γ* was detected in all cell strains derived from normal oral mucosa [244,247]. In contrast, *RAR-β* mRNA was detected only in cell strains derived from nonkeratinizing soft palate and the floor of the mouth, and was not detectable in nonkeratinizing buccal mucosa and in the keratinizing epithelial strains from the hard palate and gingiva [244,247]. RA treatment increased *RAR-β* mRNA levels in all three nonkeratinizing cell strains but not in the keratinizing ones. These results suggested that RAR-β expression is inversely related to keratinization [244,247].

Nuclear RA receptors in oral leukoplakias. Cell lines derived from oral leukoplakias in different regions of the oral cavity expressed RAR-α and RAR-γ constitutively, but the level of RAR-γ was about one half of that of the level in normal epithelial cells derived from the corresponding region of the oral cavity [244,247]. In contrast, only those cells derived from leukoplakia of the soft palate expressed RAR-β [244,247]. Treatment with RA increased RAR-β levels in the cells that expressed it constitutively but not in any of the cells that did not express it before treatment [244,247]. Our analysis by in situ hybridization of surgical specimens from oral leukoplakia lesions revealed that RAR-β was present in four of six tongue specimens but was not detectable in any of four buccal mucosa specimens [248]. The latter finding suggests that leukoplakia in buccal mucosa does not involve any change in RAR-β, since a normal cell strain from normal mucosa also failed to express RAR-β [244].

Nuclear RA receptors in squamous cell carcinomas of the skin. Two squamous cell carcinoma cell lines (SCC12 and SCC13) derived from facial skin cancers expressed RAR-α and RAR-γ constitutively, but failed to express RAR-β when cultured in the absence or presence of RA [241,247]. This pattern of expression was similar to that found in normal human epidermal keratinocytes [241,247]. In situ hybridization analysis of skin cancer specimens revealed that basal cell carcinoma and squamous cell carcinoma of the skin expressed RAR-γ; however, one of six SCCs showed a loss of RAR-γ expression [243].

Nuclear RA receptors in squamous cell carcinomas of the oral cavity. Squamous cell carcinoma cell lines derived from cancers of the oral cavity expressed RAR-α and RAR-γ, with RAR-γ being lower in six of nine SCCs relative to their normal counterparts [247]. RAR-β was expressed in only two of seven HNSCC cell lines, and a loss of expression relative to normal counterparts was evident two soft palate SCCs and one floor of the mouth tumor [247]. These results raised the suggestion that abnormally low level of RAR-β may contribute to neoplastic progression in stratified squamous epithelia [247].

We have analyzed the expression of six nuclear retinoic acid receptors (RAR-α, RAR-β, RAR-γ, RXR-α, RXR-β, and RXR-γ) in four HNSCC cell lines derived from tonsil (HNSCC183), larynx (HNSCC886Ln), retromolar trigon (HNSCC1483), and buccal mucosa (SqCC/Y1) grown in the absence or the presence of retinoic acid [188]. All four cell lines expressed mRNAs for *RAR-α*, *RAR-γ*, and *RXR-α*; three cell lines (183,886, and 1483) expressed *RAR-β*; and none expressed *RXR-β* or -γ. SqCC/Y1 did not express *RAR-β*, as was reported earlier [241], tRA treatment increased the level of *RAR-β* in the cell lines that expressed it constitutively but not in the one (SqCC/Y1) that did not express it. In contrast, the treatment had little or no effect on the expression of *RAR-α* or *RXR-α*.

To assess the expression of nuclear RA receptors in vivo, we used digoxigenin-labeled cRNA probes of *RAR-α*, *RAR-β*, and *RAR-γ* antisense for in situ hybridization to sections of head and neck surgical specimens, including normal tissue and hyperplastic, dysplastic, premalignant (e.g., leukoplakia), and malignant (squamous cell carcinomas) tissues. An analysis of 31 head and neck tissue specimens, including 14 cases from the oral cavity and 17 cases from the pharynx and larynx, revealed that *RAR-α* and *RAR-γ* mRNAs were present in most of the tissue specimens at similar levels. In contrast, *RAR-β*, which was detected in 70% of the normal and hyperplastic lesions, was detected in only in 56% of the dysplastic lesions and 35% of the carcinomas [248]. These results strongly indicate that the decreased expression of *RAR-β* may be associated with the development of head and neck cancer. The loss of expression of *RAR-β* in many HNSCC cell lines and SCC tumor specimens is intriguing in view of the recent report [249] that the commonly deleted region (distal to 3p14 and proximal to 3p25) of chromosome 3p in HNSCC cell lines derived from early stage tumors includes 3p24 where *RAR-β* is located [208]. The loss of heterozygosity suggests that tumor suppressor genes may be located in the deleted region; however, an analysis of DNA samples from five HNSCC cell lines that did not express *RAR-β* mRNA did not detect any gross rearrangements in the *RAR-β* gene [247], suggesting that the lack of RAR-β expression did not result from deletions of this gene.

Nuclear RA receptors in squamous cell carcinomas of the lung. The expression of nuclear RA receptors in human lung squamous carcinomas was reported independently by three laboratories [246,246,250,251]. Their results were based on northern blotting and showed that most squamous and adenosquamous carcinomas expressed *RAR-α* and *RAR-γ* mRNAs. The level of *RAR-γ* was higher in three of seven squamous carcinomas than in other cell lines and normal lung [246]. The expression of *RAR-β* was variable. It was expressed by three of eight squamous cell carcinomas and was induced by RA in four of eight cell lines. *RAR-β* mRNA was expressed in 5 out of 7 adenosquamous carcinomas and was increased by RA treatment in two of seven of these cell lines [245,246,250]. Interestingly, *RAR-β* abnormalities were also observed in small cell lung carcinomas, as three of eleven cell lines failed to express *RAR-β* mRNA [246]. *RAR-β* DNA showed rearrangements in one SCC that did not express RAR-β and in an adenocarcinoma and a small cell carcinoma that did express RAR-β [246]. Northern blotting analyses of *RAR-β* mRNA in surgical specimens of adjacent 'normal' and lung carcinomas showed that three of nine tumor samples contained no or low transcript levels relative to the normal tissue [246]. The abnormalities in RAR-β expression suggested that this receptor may be involved in the pathogenesis of lung cancer, possibly as a suppressor gene [246,250]. The *RAR-β* gene is located on chromosome 3p24 close to a region that is often deleted in lung cancer (from 3p14 to the telomer) [251–253]. However, no rearrangements of the *RAR-β* gene were detected in several surgical specimens of lung cancer [246], and the expression of thyroid hormone receptor, which is located close to *RAR-β* on chromosome 3p24 [208] in cell lines that did not express RAR-β, indicated that the *RAR-β* gene was not deleted in the lung carcinoma cells [250]. Thus the molecular mechanism underlying the relationship between aberrant expression of RAR-β and the development of lung cancer is still unknown.

Implication of nuclear RA receptors in the response of squamous epithelial cells to retinoids. Several lines of evidence indicate that RARs are the ultimate mediators of RA action on gene expression and the subsequent differentiation. For example, overexpression of a modified RAR-α in embryonal carcinoma cells inhibited in a dominant negative fashion the induction by retinoic acid of some markers of endodermal differentiation, and it was suggested that the truncated RAR-α formed inactive heterodimers with endogenous wild-type receptor(s) [254]. More related to the subject of this chapter is the report that *RAR-α* antisense oligonucleotides inhibited in malignant keratinocytes (SCC) both alkaline phosphatase induction and clonogenicity suppression by retinoids [255]. More direct evidence for the role of nuclear receptors in mediating the effects of retinoids on cell growth and differentiation was provided by the studies of a RA-resistant mutant subclone of HL-60 promyelocytic leukemia cells, designated HL-60R, which has a defective RAR-a, and K562, an erythroleukemia cell line that expresses a very low level of this receptor and is also resistant to RA [256–258]. By transducing normal *RAR-α* via a retroviral vector it was possible to restore sensitivity to retinoic acid in the mutant cells [256]. Furthermore, transduction of *RAR-β*, *RAR-γ*, or *RXR-α* also restored sensitivity to RA in these mutant cells [257].

Gene expression in keratinocytes is thought to be regulated by retinoids at the transcriptional level [259–261]. Nuclear RARs have been implicated in the regulation of epidermal keratinocyte differentiation based on the correlation between the ability of several synthetic retinoids to bind to RARs and transactivate transcription from RARE, and to suppress the expression of squamous differentiation markers such as involucrin, type I TGase, and cornifin (SQ37) in transfected normal human epidermal keratinocytes [241]. A role for nuclear RA receptors in the regulation of squamous differentiation has been demonstrated more directly for the regulation of keratin genes [260]. The three RAR receptor subtypes were able to suppress transcription from the 5' regulatory regions of keratins K5, K6, K10, and K14 in cotransfection experiments [260]. Although direct binding of the RARs to DNA was not demonstrated, it was proposed that the RARs bind to a putative negative recognition element in the upstream DNAs of keratin genes [260]. Roles for nuclear RA receptors in both positive and negative regulation of epidermal differentiation have been implied by the effects of a truncated RAR-γ receptor [261]. Transfection of *RAR-γ* truncated in the ligand-binding domain enhanced the growth and inhibited the squamous differentiation (e.g., production of keratins K1/10 and K6/16, involucrin, and filaggrin) of human squamous carcinoma cells SCC13. In addition, the transfected cells expressed low levels of K13 and K19, which are positively regulated by retinoids in the parental SCC13 cells. Thus it appears that RARs may be required for induction of terminal differentiation of keratinocytes [261]. *RAR-β* mRNA expression in cultured normal oral epithelial cell strains was correlated with the expression of keratin 19, and it was suggested that RAR-β plays a role in keratin expression and suprabasal differentiation of stratified squamous epithelia [244]. This correlation was abrogated in head and neck squamous cell carcinomas, in which the expression of K19 was independent of the expression of RAR-β [247]. Likewise, there was no apparent correlation between the expression of the nuclear receptors and the status of squamous cell differentiation of the HNSCC cell lines (two well differentiated and two poorly differentiated), and there was no correlation between the expression of RAR-β and the response of HNSCC cells to the growth-inhibitory or differentiation-suppressing effects of tRA [188].

Acknowledgments

I thank members of my group (Drs. X-C Xu, C-P Zou, S. Poddar, and J. Kim) and collaborators in the studies described in this chapter (Drs. P. Sacks, A. Jetten, and Waun Hong). The work from our laboratory, described in this chapter, was supported in part by Public Health Service NCI grant PO1-CA 52051.

References

1. Lotan R. Effects of vitamin A and its analogs (retinoids) on normal and neoplastic cells. Biochim Biophys Acta 605:33–91, 1980.

2. Roberts AB, Sporn MB. Cellular biology and biochemistry of the retinoids. In: MB Sporn, AB Roberts, DS Goodman, eds. The Retinoids. Orlando: Academic Press, pp 209–286, 1986.
3. Sherman MI (ed), Retinoids and Cell Differentiation. Boca Raton, FL: CRC Press.
4. Gudas LJ. Molecular mechanisms of retinoid action. Am J Respir Cell Mol Biol 2:319–320, 1989.
5. Jetten AM. Multistep process of squamous differentiation in tracheobronchial epithelial cells in vitro: Analogy with epidermal differentiation. Environ Health Perspect 80: 149–160, 1989.
6. Jetten AM. Multi-stage program of differentiation in human epidermal keratinocytes: Regulation by retinoids. J Invest Dermatol 95:44–46, 1990.
7. Amos B, Lotan R. Retinoid-sensitive cells and cell lines. Methods Enzymol 190:217–225, 1991.
8. DeLuca LM. Retinoids and their receptors in differentiation, embryogenesis and neoplasia. FASEB J 5:2924–2933, 1991.
9. Wolbach SB, Howe PR. Tissue changes following deprivation of fat soluble vitamin A. J Exp Med 42:753–777, 1925.
10. Wolbach SB. Effects of vitamin A deficiency and hypervitaminosis in animals. In: WH Sebrell, RS Harris, eds. The Vitamins, vol 1. New York: Academic Press, 1956, pp 106–137.
11. Wong YC, Buck RC. An electron microscopic study of metaplasia of the rat tracheal epithelium in vitamin A-deficiency. Lab Invest 24:55–66, 1971.
12. Harris CC, Silverman T, Smith JM, Jackson F, Boren HG. Proliferation of tracheal epithelial cells in normal and vitamin A-deficient Syrian golden hamsters. J Natl Cancer Inst 51:1059–1062, 1973.
13. Chopra DP. Squamous metaplasia in organ culture of vitamin A-deficient hamster trachea. Cytokinetic and ultrastructural alterations. J Natl Cancer Inst 69:895–905, 1982.
14. Chopra DP. Retinoid reversal of squamous metaplasia in organ cultures of tracheas derived from hamsters fed an vitamin A-deficient diet. Eur J Cancer Clin Oncol 9: 847–857, 1983.
15. Dowling JE, Wald G. The role of vitamin A acid. Vitam Horm 18:515–541, 1960.
16. Sporn MB, Clamon GH, Dunlop NM, Newton DL, Smith JM, Saffiotti U. Activity of vitamin A analogues in cell cultures of mouse epidermis and organ cultures of hamster trachea. Nature 253:47–50, 1975.
17. Sporn MB, Dunlop NM, Newton DL, Henderson WR. Relationships between structure and activity of retinoids. Nature 263:110–113, 1976.
18. Chytil F. Retinoic acid: Biochemistry and metabolism. J Am Acad Dermatol 15:741–747, 1986.
19. Darmon M. Retinoic acid in skin and epithelia. Semin Dev Biol 2:219–228, 1991.
20. Auerbach O, Stout AP, Hammond EC, Garfinkel L. Changes in bronchial epithelium in relation to cigarette smoking and in relation to lung cancer. N Engl J Med 265:253–267, 1961.
21. Saffioti U, Montesano R, Sellakumar AR, Bork SA. Experimental cancer of the lung. Inhibition by vitamin A of the induction of tracheobronchial metaplasia and squamous cell tumor. Cancer 20:857–864, 1967.
22. Sporn MB, Newton DL. Chemoprevention of cancer with retinoids. Fed Proc 38:2528–2534, 1979.
23. Lotan R, Lippman SM, Hong WK. Retinoid modulation of squamous cell differentiation and carcinogenesis. Cancer Bull 43:490–498, 1991.
24. Eckert RL. Structure, function, and differentiation of the keratinocyte. Physiol Rev 69:1316–1346, 1989.
25. Fuchs E. Epidermal differentiation: The bare essentials. J Cell Biol 111:2807–2814, 1990.
26. Hohl D. Cornified cell envelope. Dermatologica 180:201–211, 1990.

27. Darmon M, Rocher M, Cavey MT, Martin B, Ribald T, Delescluse C, Shroot B. Biological activity of retinoids correlates with affinity for nuclear receptors but not for cytosolic binding protein. Skin Pharm 1:161–175, 1988.
28. Ohayoun J-P, Gosselin F, Forest N, Winter S, Franke WW. Cytokeratin patterns of human oral epithelia: Differences in cytokeratin synthesis in gingival epithelium and the adjacent alveolar mucosa. Differentiation 30:123–129, 1985.
29. Thacher SM, Rice RH. Keratinocyte-specific transglutaminase of cultured human epidermal cells: Relation to cross-linked envelope formation and terminal differentiation. Cell 40:685–695, 1985.
30. Thacher SM. Purification of keratinocyte transglutaminase and its expression during squamous differentiation. J Invest Dermatol 89:578–584, 1989.
31. Folk JE. Mechanisms and basis for specificity of transglutaminase-catalyzed ε-(γ-glutamyl) lysine bond formation. Adv Enzymol 54:1–54, 1983.
32. Chakravarty R, Rice RH. Acylation of keratinocyte transglutaminase by palmitic and myristic acids in the membrane anchorage region. J Biol Chem 264:625–629, 1989.
33. Rice RH, Green H. Relationship of protein synthesis and transglutaminase activity to formation of the cross-linked envelope during terminal differentiation of the cultured human epidermal keratinocyte. J Cell Biol 76:705–711, 1978.
34. Simon M, Green H. Enzymatic crosslinking of involucrin and other proteins by keratinocyte particulates in vitro. Cell 40:677–683, 1985.
35. Lichti U, Ben T, Yuspa SH. Retinoic acid-induced transglutaminase in mouse epidermal cells is distinct from epidermal transglutaminase. J Biol Chem 260:1422–1426, 1985.
36. Rice RH, Thacher SM. In: J Breiter-Hahn, AG Matoltsky, KS Richards, eds. Biology of the Integument, vol 2. Heidelberg: Springer-Verlag, 1986, pp 752–761.
37. Hohl D, Mehrel T, Lichti U, Turnerm ML, Roop D, Steinert PM. Characterization of human loricrin structure and function of a new class of epidermal cell envelope proteins. J Biol Chem 266:6626–6636, 1991.
38. Magnaldo T, Bernerd F, Asselineau D, Darmon M. Expression of loricrin is negatively controlled by retinoic acid in human epidermis reconstructed in vitro. Differentiation 49:39–46, 1982.
39. Marvin KW, George MD, Fujimoto W, Saunders N, Bernacki SH, Jetten AM. Cornifin: A new cross-linked envelope precursor in keratinocytes. Down regulation by retinoids. Proc Natl Acad Sci USA, 89:11026–11030, 1992.
40. Simon M, Green H. Participation of membrane-associated proteins in the cross-linked envelope of the keratinocyte. Cell 36:827–834, 1984.
41. Rice RH, Green H. The cornified envelope of terminally differentiated human epidermal keratinocytes consists of cross-linked protein. Cell 11:417–422, 1977.
42. Rice RH, Green H. Presence in human epidermal cells of a soluble protein precursor of the cross-linked envelope: Activation of cross-linking by calcium ions. Cell 18:681–694, 1979.
43. Eckert RL, Green H. Structure and evolution of the human involucrin gene. Cell 46:583–589, 1986.
44. Simon M, Green H. The glutamine residues reactive in transglutaminase-catalyzed cross-linking of involucrin. J Biol Chem 263:18093–18098, 1988.
45. Green H, Watt FM. Regulation by vitamin A of envelope cross-linking in cultured keratinocytes derived from different human epithelia. Mol Cell Biol 2:1115–1117, 1982.
46. Murphy GM, Flynn TC, Rice RH, Pinkus GS. Involucrin expression in normal and neoplastic human skin: A marker for keratinocyte differentiation. J Invest Dermatol 82:453–457, 1984.
47. Banks-Schlegl S, Green H. Involucrin synthesis and tissue assembly by keratinocytes in natural and cultured human epithelia. J Cell Biol 90:732–737, 1981.
48. Klein-Szanto AJP, Boysen M, Reith A. Keratin and involucrin in preneoplastic and neoplastic lesions. Arch Pathol Lab Med 111:1057–1061, 1987.
49. Zettergren JG, Peterson LL, Wuepper KD. Keratolinin: The soluble substrate of epider-

mal transglutaminase from human and bovine tissue. Proc Natl Acad Sci USA 81:238–242, 1984.

50. Lobitz CJ, Buxman MM. Characterization and localization of bovine epidermal transglutaminase substrate. J Invest Dermatol 78:150–154, 1982.

51. Passavant CW, Coulter SN, Wuepper KD. The identification of cDNA clones coding for a protein which reacts with anti-keratolinin. J Invest Dermatol 92:497, 1989.

52. Moore KG, Sartorelli AC. Annexin I and involucrin are cross-linked by particulate transglutaminase into the cornified cell envelope of squamous cell carcinoma Y1. Exp Cell Res 200:186–195, 1992.

53. Ando Y, Imamura S, Owada MK, Kannagi R. Calcium-induced intracellular cross-linking of lipocortin I by tissue transglutaminase in A431 cells. J Biol Chem 266:1101–1108, 1991.

54. Kvedar JC, Manabe M, Phillips SB, Ross BS, Baden HP. Characterization of sciellin, a precursor to the cornified envelope of human keratinocytes. Differentiation 49:195–204, 1992.

55. Roop DR, Huitfeldt H, Kilkenny A, Yuspa SH. Regulated expression of differentiation-associated keratins in cultured epidermal cells detected by monospecific antibodies derived from different human epithelia. Differentiation 35:143–150, 1987.

56. Fuchs E, Green H. Changes in keratin gene expression during terminal differentiation of the keratinocyte. Cell 19:1033–1042, 1980.

57. Sun TT, Tseng SCG, Huang AJ-W, Cooper D, Schermer A, Lynch MH, Weiss R, Eichner R. Monoclonal antibody studies of mammalian epithelial keratins: A review. Ann NY Acad Sci 455:307–329, 1985.

58. Franke WW, Schiller DL, Moll R, Winter S, Schmidt E, Engelbrecht I, Denk H, Krepler R, Platzer B. Diversity of cytokeratin polypeptides in epithelial cells and tissues. J Mol Biol 153:933–959, 1981.

59. Moll R, Franke WW, Schiller DL, Geiger B, Krepler R. The catalog of human cytokeratins: Patterns of expression in normal epithelia, tumors and cultured cells. Cell 31:11–24, 1982.

60. Moll R, Krepler R, Franke WW. Complex cytokeratin polypeptide patterns observed in certain human carcinomas. Differentiation 23:256–269, 1983.

61. Roop DR, Krieg TM, Mehrel T, Chung CK, Yuspa SH. Transcriptional control of high molecular weight keratin gene expression in multistage mouse skin carcinogenesis. Cancer Res 48:3245–3252, 1988.

62. Nagle RB, Moll R, Weidauer H, Nemetschek H, Franke WW. Different patterns of cytokeratin expression in the normal epithelia of the upper respiratory tract. Differentiation 30:130–140, 1985.

63. Fleckman P, Dale BA, Holbrook KA. Profilaggrin, a high molecular weight precursor of filaggrin in human epidermis and cultured keratinocytes. J Invest Dermatol 85:507–512, 1985.

64. Asselineau D, Bernard BA, Bailly C, Darmon M. Retinoic acid improves epidermal morphogenesis. Dev Biol 133:322–335, 1989.

65. Rothnagel JA, Steinert PM. The structure of the gene for mouse filaggrin and a comparison of the repeating units. J Biol Chem 265:1862–1865, 1990.

66. Manabe M, Sanchez M, Sun T-T, Dale BA. Interaction of filaggrin with keratin filaments during advanced stages of normal human epidermal differentiation and in ichtiosis vulgaris. Differentiation 48:43–50, 1991.

67. Korge B, Gan S-O, Yoneda K, Compton JG, Volz A, Steinert PM, Ziegler A, Mischke D. Physical mapping of the epidermal differentiation markers loricrin, profilaggrin, and involucrin on chromosome 1q21 by pulsed field electrophoresis. Clin Res 40:490A, 1992.

68. Lotan R, Pieniazek J, George MD, Jetten AM. Identification of a new squamous cell differentiation marker and its suppression by retinoids. J Cell Physiol 151:94–102, 1992.

69. Jetten AM, Bernacki SH, Floyd EE, Saunders NA, Pieniazek J, Lotan R. Expression of a preprorelaxin-like gene during squamous differentiation of rabbit tracheobronchial epithelial cells and its suppression by retinoic acid. Cell Growth Differ 3:549–556, 1992.

70. Rearick JI, Jetten AM. Accumulation of cholesterol 3-sulfate during in vitro squamous differentiation of rabbit tracheal epithelial cells and its regulation by retinoids. J Biol Chem 261:13898–13904, 1986.

71. Rearick JI, Albro PW, Jetten AM. Increase in cholesterol sulfotransferase activity during in vitro squamous differentiation of rabbit tracheal epithelial cells and its inhibition by retinoic acid. J Biol Chem 262:13069–13074, 1987.

72. Rearick JI, Hesterberg TW, Jetten AM. Human bronchial epithelial cells synthesize cholesterol sulfate during squamous differentiation in vitro. J Cell Physiol 133:573–578, 1987.

73. Jetten AM, George MA, Nervi C, Boone LR, Rearick JI. Increased cholesterol sulfate and cholesterol sulfotransferase activity in relation to multistep process of differentiation in human epidermal keratinocytes. J Invest Dermatol 92:203–209, 1989.

74. Jetten AM, George MA, Pettit GR, Rearick JI. Effects of bryostatins and retinoic acid on phorbol ester- and diacylglycerol-induced squamous differentiation in human tracheo-bronchial epithelial cells. Cancer Res 49:3990–3995, 1989.

75. Jetten AM, Kim JS, Sacks PG, Rearick JI, Lotan D, Hong WK, Lotan R. Suppression of growth and squamous cell differentiation markers in cultured human head and neck squamous carcinoma cells by β-all *trans* retinoic acid. Int J Cancer 45:195–202, 1990.

76. Brod J, Bavelier E, Justine P, Weerheim A, Ponec M. Acylceramides and lanosterol-lipid markers of terminal differentiation in cultured human keratinocytes: Modulating effects of retinoic acid. In Vitro 27:163–168, 1991.

77. Lasnitzki I. Hypovitaminosis A in the mouse prostate gland cultured in chemically defined medium. Exp Cell Res 28:40–51, 1962.

78. Keenan KP, Combs JW, McDowell EM. Regeneration of hamster tracheal epithelium after mechanical injury. IV. Histochemical, immunocytochemical studies. Virchows Arch Cell Pathol 41:213–240, 1983.

79. Marchok AC, Cone V, Nettesheim P. Induction of squamous metaplasia (vitamin A deficiency) and hypersecretory activity in tracheal organ culture. Lab Invest 33:451–460, 1975.

80. McDowell EM, Keenan KP, Huang M. Effects of vitamin A deprivation on hamster tracheal epithelium. A quantitative morphologic study. Virchows Arch [Cell Pathol] 45:197–219, 1984.

81. Harris CC, Sporn MB, Kaufman DG, Smith JM, Jackson FE, Saffiotti U. Histogenesis of squamous metaplasia in the hamster tracheal epithelium caused by vitamin A deficiency or benzo[a]pyrene ferric oxide. J Natl Cancer Inst 48:743–761, 1973.

82. Shin DM, Gimenez IB, Lee JS, Nishioka K, Wargovich MJ, Thacher S, Lotan R, Slaga TJ, Hong WK. Expression of epidermal growth factor receptor, polyamine levels, ornithine decarboxylase activity, micronuclei, and transglutaminase I in DMBA-induced hamster buccal pouch carcinogenesis model. Cancer Res 50:2505–2510, 1990.

83. Gimenez IB, Shin DM, Bianchi AB, Roop DR, Hong WK, Conti CJ, Slaga TJ. Changes in keratin expression during 7,12-dimethylbenz[a]anthracene-induced hamster cheek pouch carcinogenesis. Cancer Res 50:4441–4445, 1990.

84. Ford JR, Howe-Terzaghi M. Basal cells are the progenitors of primary tracheal epithelial cell cultures. Exp Cell Res 198:69–77, 1992.

85. Sigler RE, Newkirk C, McDowell EM. Histogenesis and morphogenesis in epidermoid metaplasia in hamster tracheal organ explant culture. Virchows Arch [B] 55:47–55, 1988.

86. Jetten AM, George MA, Smits HL, Vollberg TM. Keratin 13 expression is linked to squamous differentiation in rabbit tracheal epithelial cells and down-regulated by retinoic acid. Exp Cell Res 182:622–634, 1989.

87. Shafer WG, Hine MA, Levy BM. A Textbook of Oral Pathology. Philadelphia: WB Saunders, 1974, pp 81–211.

88. Cline PR, Rice RH. Modulation of involucrin and envelope competence in human keratinocytes by hydrocortisone, retinyl acetate, and growth arrest. Cancer Res 43:3203–3207, 1983.

89. Reiss M, Pitman SW, Sartorelli AC. Modulation of the terminal differentiation of human squamous carcinoma cells in vitro by all-*trans*-retinoic acid. J Natl Cancer Inst 74:1015–1023, 1985.

90. Sundqvist K, Liu Y, Arvidson K, Ormstad K, Nilsson L, Toftgard R, Grafstrom RC. Growth regulation of serum-free cultures of epithelial cells from normal human buccal mucosa. In Vitro Cell Dev Biol 27:562–568, 1991.

91. Poddar S, Hong WK, Thacher SM, Lotan R. Suppression of type I transglutaminase, involucrin, and keratin K1 in cultured human head and neck squamous carcinoma 1483 cells by retinoic acid. Int J Cancer 48:239–247, 1991.

92. Breitkreutz D, Boukamp P, Ryle CM, Stark HJ, Roop DR, Fusenig NE. Epidermal morphogenesis and keratin expression in c-Ha-*ras*-transfected tumorigenic clones of the human HaCaT cell line. Cancer Res 51:4402–4409, 1991.

93. Agarwal C, Eckert RL. Immortalization of human keratinocytes by simian virus 40 large T antigen alters keratin gene response to retinoids. Cancer Res 50:5947–5953, 1990.

94. Kaplan MJ, Mills SE, Rice RH, Johns ME. Involucrin in laryngeal dysplasia. Arch Otolaryngol 110:713–716, 1984.

95. Said JW, Sassoon AF, Shintaku P, Banks-Schlegel S. Involucrin in squamous and basal cell carcinomas of the skin: An immunohistochemical study. J Invest Dermatol 82:449–552, 1984.

96. Thacher SM, Coe EL, Rice RH. Retinoid suppression of transglutaminase activity and envelope competence in cultured human epidermal carcinoma cells. Differentiation 29:82–87, 1985.

97. Ta BM, Gallagher GT, Chakravarty R, Rice RH. Keratinocyte transglutaminase in human skin and oral mucosa: Cytoplasmic localization and uncoupling of differentiation markers. J Cell Sci 95:631–638, 1990.

98. Levitt ML, Gazdar AF, Oie HK, Schuller H, Thacher SM. Cross-linked envelope-related markers for squamous differentiation in human hung cancer cell lines. Cancer Res 50:120–128, 1990.

99. Cheng C, Kilkenny AE, Roop D, Yuspa SH. The v-Ha-*ras* oncogene inhibits the expression of differentiation markers and facilitates expression of cytokeratins 8 and 18 in mouse keratinocytes. Mol Carcinog 3:363–373, 1990.

100. Nelson KG, Slaga TJ. Keratin modifications in epidermis, papillomas, and carcinomas during two-stage carcinogenesis in the SENCAR mouse. Cancer Res 43:4176–4181, 1982.

101. Weiss RA, Eichnerm R, Sun T-T. Monoclonal antibody analysis of keratin expression in epidermal diseases: 48- and 56-keratins as molecular markers for hyperproliferative keratinocytes. J Cell Biol 98:1397–1406, 1984.

102. Toftgard R, Yuspa SH, Roop DR. Keratin gene expression in mouse skin tumors and in mouse skin treated with 12-O-tetradecanoylphorbol-13-acetate. Cancer Res 45:5845–5850, 1985.

103. Gimenez-Conti IB, Aldaz CM, Bianchi AB, Roop DR, Slaga TJ, Conti CJ. Early expression of type I K13 in the progression of mouse skin papillomas. Carcinogenesis 11:1995–1999, 1990.

104. Kim KH, Schwartz F, Fuchs E. Differences in keratin synthesis between normal epithelial cells and squamous cell carcinomas are mediated by vitamin A. Proc Natl Acad Sci USA 81:4280–4284, 1984.

105. Stoler A, Kopan R, Duvic M, Fuchs E. Use of monospecific antisera and cDNA probes to localize the major changes in keratin expression during normal and abnormal epidermal differentiation. J Cell Biol 107:427–446, 1988.

106. Napoli JL, Race KR. The biosynthesis of retinoic acid from retinol by rat tissues in vitro. Arch Biochem Biophys 255:95–101, 1987.

107. Napoli JL, Race KR. Biogenesis of retinoic acid from β-carotene: Differences between the metabolism of β-carotene and retinol. J Biol Chem 263:17372–17377, 1988.

108. Napoli JL. The biogenesis of retinoic acid: A physiologically significant promoter of differentiation. In: MI Dawson, WH Nakamura, eds. Chemistry and Biology of Synthetic

Retinoids. Boca Raton, FL: CRC Press, 1990, pp 229–249.

109. Siegenthaler G, Saurat J-H, Ponec M. The formation of retinoic acid from retinol in relation to the differentiation state of cultured human keratinocytes. Pharmacol Skin 3:52–55, 1989.

110. Connor MJ, Smith MH. The formation of all-*trans*-retinoic acid from all-*trans* retinol in hairless mouse skin. Biochem Pharmacol 36:919–924, 1987.

111. Bhat PV, Jetten AM. Metabolism of all-*trans*-retinol and all-*trans*-retinoic acid in rabbit tracheal epithelial cells in culture. Biochim Biophys Acta 922:18–27, 1987.

112. Seifter E, Rettura G, Padawer J, Levenson SM. Moloney murine sarcoma virus tumors in CBA/J mice: Chemopreventive and chemotherapeutic actions of supplemental β-carotene. J Natl Cancer Inst 68:835–840, 1982.

113. Som S, Chatterjee MM, Banerjee MR. β-carotene inhibition of 7,12-dimethylbenz[*a*] anthracene-induced transformation of murine mammary cells in vitro. Carcinogenesis 5:937–940, 1984.

114. Burton GW, Ingold KU. β-carotene: An unusual type of lipid antioxidant. Science 224:569–573, 1984.

115. Krinsky NI. Mechanism of inactivation of oxygen species by carotenoids. In: MG Simic, O Nygaard, eds. Anticarcinogenesis and Radiation Protection. New York: Plenum Press, 1988, pp 41–46.

116. Peto R, Doll R, Buckley JD, Sporn MB. Can dietary β-carotene materially reduce human cancer rates? Nature 290:201–208, 1981.

117. Krinsky NI. Evidence for the role of carotenoids in preventive health. Clin Nutr 7: 107–114, 1988.

118. Pung A, Rundhaug JE, Yoshizawa CN, Bertram JS. β-carotene and canthaxanthine inhibit chemically- and physically-induced neoplastic transformation in 10T1/2 cells. Carcinogenesis 9:1533–1539, 1988.

119. Tang G, Russell RM. 13-*cis*-retinoic acid is an endogenous compound in human serum. J Lipid Res 31:175–182, 1990.

120. Moon RC, Mehta RC. Retinoid inhibition of experimental carcinogenesis. In: MI Dawson, WH Okamura, eds. Chemistry and Biology of Synthetic Retinoids. Boca Raton, FL: CRC Press, 1990, pp 501–518.

121. Levin AA, Sturzenbecker LJ, Kazmer S, Bosakowski T, Huselton C, Allenby G, Speck J, Kratzeisen C, Rosenberger M, Lovey A, Grippo JF. 9-*cis* retinoic acid stereoisomer binds and activates the nuclear receptor RXRα. Nature 335: 359, 1992.

122. Heyman RA, Mangelsdorf DJ, Dyck JA, Stein RB, Eichele G, Evans RM, Thaller C. 9-*cis* retinoic acid is a high-affinity ligand for the retinoid X receptor. Cell 68:397–406, 1992.

123. Eichner R. Epidermal effects of retinoids: In vitro studies. J Am Acad Dermatol 15:789–797, 1986.

124. Varani J, Nockoloff BJ, Dixit VM, Mitra RS, Voorhees JJ. All-*trans*-retinoic acid stimulates growth of adult keratinocytes cultured in growth factor-deficient medium, inhibits production of thrombospondin and fibronectin, and reduces adhesion. J Invest Dermatol 93:449–454, 1989.

125. Tong PS, Horowitz NN, Wheeler LA. *Trans* retinoic acid enhances the growth response of epidermal keratinocytes to epidermal growth factor and transforming growth factor beta. J Invest Dermatol 94:126–131, 1990.

126. McDowell EM, Ben T, Colemen B, Chang S, Newkirk C, De Luca LM. Effects of retinoic acid on the growth and morphology of hamster tracheal epithelial cells in primary culture. Virchows Arch [Cell Pathol] 54:38–51, 1987.

127. Choi Y, Fuchs E. TGF-β and retinoic acid: Regulators of growth and modifiers of differentiation in human epidermis. Cell Regul 1:791–809, 1990.

128. Lotan R, Lotan D, Sacks PG. Inhibition of tumor cell growth by retinoids. Methods Enzymol 190:100–110, 1990.

129. Frey JR, Peck R, Bollag W. Antiproliferative activity of retinoids, interferon α and their

65

combination in five human transformed cell lines. Cancer Lett 57:223–227, 1991.

130. Lotan R, Sacks PG, Lotan D, Hong WK. Differential effects of retinoic acid on the in vitro growth and cell-surface glycoconjugates of two human head and neck squamous-cell carcinomas. Int J Cancer 40:224–229, 1987.

131. Sacks PG, Oke V, Vasey T, Lotan R. Modulation of growth, differentiation, and glycoprotein synthesis by β-all-*trans* retinoic acid in a multicellular tumor spheroid model for squamous carcinoma of the head and neck. Int J Cancer 44:926–933, 1989.

132. Pirisi L, Batova A, Jenkins GR, Hodam JR, Creek KE. Increased sensitivity of human keratinocytes immortalized by human papillomavirus type 16 DNA to growth control by retinoids. Cancer Res 52:187–193, 1992.

133. Tong PS, Mayes DM, Wheeler LA. Differential effects of retinoids on DNA synthesis in calcium-regulated murine epidermal keratinocyte cultures. J Invest Dermatol 90:861–868, 1988.

134. Glick AB, Flanders KC, Danielpour D, Yuspa SH, Sporn MB. Retinoic acid induces transforming growth factor-beta2 in cultured keratinocytes and mouse epidermis. Cell Regul 1:87–97, 1989.

135. Kim JS, Steck PA, Gallick GE, Lee JS, Blick M, Hong WK, Lotan R. Suppression by retinoic acid of epidermal growth factor receptor autophosphorylation and glycosylation in cultured human head and neck squamous carcinoma cells. Monogr Natl Cancer Inst 13:101–110, 1992.

136. Hong WK, Endicott J, Itri LM, Doos W, Batsakis JG, Bell R, Fofonoff S, Byers R, Atkinson EN, Vaughan C, Toth BB, Kramer A, Dimery IW, Skipper P, Strong S. The efficacy of 13-*cis* retinoic acid in the treatment of oral leukoplakia. N Engl J Med 315:1501–1505, 1986.

137. Hong WK, Lippman SM, Itri LM, Karp DD, Lee JS, Byers RM, Schantz SS. Kramer AM, Lotan R, Peters LL Dimery IW, Brown BW, Goepfert H. Prevention of second primary tumors with isotretinoin in squamous-cell carcinoma of the head and neck. N Engl J Med 323:795–801, 1990.

138. Kraemer KH, DiGiovanna JJ, Moshell AN, Tarone RE, Peck GL. Prevention of skin cancer in xeroderma pigmentosum with the use of oral isotretinoin. N Engl J Med 318:1633–1637, 1988.

139. Lippman S, Kessler JF, Meyskens F Jr. Retinoids as preventive and therapeutic anticancer agents. Cancer Treat Rep 71:391–405 (Part 1); 493–515 (Part 2), 1987.

140. Lippman SM, Hong WK. Prevention of aerodigestive cancers with retinoids. Cancer Bull 43:525–533, 1991.

141. Lippman SM, Meyskens FL. Results of the use of vitamin A and retinoids in cutaneous malignancies. Pharmacol Ther 40:107–122, 1989.

142. Smith MA, Parkinson DR, Cheson BD, Friedman MA. Retinoids in cancer therapy. J Clin Oncol 10:839–864, 1992.

143. Nagae S, Lichti U, DeLuca LM, Yuspa SH. Effect of retinoic acid on cornified envelope formation: Difference between spontaneous envelope formation in vivo or in vitro. J Invest Dermatol 89:51–58, 1987.

144. Floyd EE, Jetten AM. Regulation of type I (epidermal) transglutaminase mRNA levels during squamous differentiation: Down regulation by retinoids. Mol Cell Biol 9:4846–4851, 1989.

145. Rubin AL, Rice RH. Differential regulation by retinoic acid and calcium of transglutaminases in cultured neoplastic and normal human keratinocytes. Cancer Res 46:2356–2361, 1986.

146. Rubin AL, Parenteau NL, Rice RH. Coordination of keratinocyte programming in human SCC-13 squamous carcinoma and normal epidermal cells. J Cell Physiol 138:208–214, 1989.

147. Hohl D, Lichti U, Breitkreutz D, Steinert PM, Roop D. Transcription of the human loricrin gene in vitro is induced by calcium and cell density and suppressed by retinoic

acid. J Invest Dermatol 96:414–418, 1991.

148. Magnaldo T, Pommes L, Asselineau D, Darmon M. Isolation of a GC-rich cDNA identifying mRNA present in human epidermis and modulated by calcium and retinoic acid in cultured keratinocytes. Mol Biol Rep 14:237–246, 1990.

149. Smits HL, Floyd EE, Jetten AM. Molecular cloning of gene sequences regulated during squamous differentiation of tracheal epithelial cells and controlled by retinoic acid. Mol Cell Biol 7:4017–4023, 1987.

150. Gorodeski GI, Eckert RL, Utian WH, Sheean L, Rorke EA. Retinoids, sex steroids, and glucocorticoids regulate ectocervical cell envelope formation but not the level of the envelope precursor, involucrin. Differentiation 42:75–80, 1989.

151. Rice RH, Cline PR, Coe EL. Mutually antagonistic effects of hydrocortisone and retinyl acetate on envelope competence in cultured malignant human keratinocytes. J Invest Dermatol 81:176s–178s, 1983.

152. Michel S, Reichert U, Isnard JL, Shroot B, Schmidt R. Retinoic acid controls expression of epidermal transglutaminase at the pre-translational level. FEBS Lett 258:35–38, 1989.

153. Regnier M, Darmon M. Human epidermis reconstructed in vitro: A model to study keratinocyte differentiation and its modulation by retinoic acid. In Vitro 25:1000–1008, 1989.

154. Tseng SCG, Hatchell D, Tierney N, Huang AJ-W, Sun T-T. Expression of specific keratin markers by rabbit corneal, conjunctival, and esophageal epithelia during vitamin A deficiency. J Cell Biol 99:2279–2286, 1984.

155. Huang FL, Roop DR, DeLuca LM. Vitamin A deficiency and keratin biosynthesis in cultured hamster trachea. In Vitro Cell Dev Biol 22:223–230, 1986.

156. Fuchs E, Green H. Regulation of terminal differentiation of cultured human keratinocytes by vitamin A. Cell 25:617–625, 1981.

157. Gilfix BM, Green H. Bioassay of retinoids using cultured human conjunctival keratinocytes. J Cell Physiol 119:172–174, 1984.

158. Gilfix BM, Eckert RL. Coordinate control by vitamin A of keratin gene expression in human keratinocytes. J Biol Chem 260:14026–14029, 1985.

159. Eckert RL, Green H. Cloning of cDNAs specifying vitamin A-responsive human keratins. Proc Natl Acad Sci USA 81:4321–4325, 1984.

160. Terasaki T, Shimosato Y, Nakajima T, Tsumuraya M, Ichinose H, Nagatsu T, Kato K. Reversible squamous cell characteristics induced by vitamin A deficiency in a small cell lung cancer cell line. Cancer Res 47:3533–3537, 1987.

161. Kopan R, Traska G, Fuchs E. Retinoids as important regulators of terminal differentiation: Examining keratin expression in individual epidermal cells at various stages of keratinization. J Cell Biol 105:427–440, 1987.

162. Mendelsohn MG, DiLorenzo TP, Abramson AL, Steinberg BM. Retinoic acid regulates, in vitro, the two normal pathways of differentiation of human laryngeal keratinocytes. In Vitro Cell Dev Biol 27A:137–141, 1991.

163. Reppucci AD, DiLorenzo TP, Abramson AL, Steinberg BM. In vitro modulation of human laryngeal papilloma cell differentiation by retinoic acid. Otolaryngol Head Neck Surg 105:528–532, 1991.

164. Asselineau D, Dale BA, Bernard BA. Filaggrin production by cultured human epidermal keratinocytes and its regulation by retinoic acid. Differentiation 45:221–229, 1990.

165. Rosenthal DS, Griffiths CE, Yuspa SH, Roop DR, Voorhees JJ. Acute or chronic topical retinoic acid treatment of human skin in vivo alters the expression of epidermal transglutaminase, loricrin, involucrin, filaggrin, and keratins 6 and 13 but not keratins 1, 10, and 14. J Invest Dermatol 98:343–350, 1992.

166. Griffiths CE, Rosenthal DS, Reddy AP, Elder JT, Astrom A, Leach K, Wang TS, Finkel LJ, Yuspa SH, Voorhees JJ, Fisher GJ. Short-term retinoic acid treatment increases in vivo, but decreases in vitro, epidermal transglutaminase-K enzyme activity and imunoreactivity. J Invest Dermatol 99:283–288, 1992.

167. Chytil F, Ong D. Cellular retinoid-binding proteins. In: MB Sporn, AB Roberts, DS Goodman, eds. The Retinoids. New York: Academic Press, 1984, pp 90–123.
168. Wolf G. The intracellular vitamin A-binding proteins: An overview of their functions. Nutr Rev 49:1–12, 1991.
169. Mangelsdorf DJ, Evans RM. Vitamin A receptors: New insights on retinoid control of transcription. In: G Morriss-Kay, ed. Retinoids in Normal Development and Teratogenesis. New York: Oxford University Press, 1992, pp 27–50.
170. Lotan R, Clifford JL. Nuclear receptors for retinoids: Mediators of retinoid effects on normal and malignant cells. Biomed Pharmocother 45:145–156, 1990.
171. Siegenthaler G, Saurat J-H, Morin C, Hotz R. Cellular retinol and retinoic acid-binding proteins in the epidermis and dermis of normal human skin. Br J Dermatol 111:647–654, 1984.
172. Siegenthaler G, Samson J, Bernard JP, Fiore-Donno G, Saurat JH. Retinoid-binding proteins in human oral mucosa. J Oral Pathol 17:106–112, 1988.
173. Siegenthaler G, Saurat J-H, Ponec M. Terminal differentiation in cultured human keratinocytes is associated with increased levels of cellular retinoic acid-binding protein. Exp Cell Res 178:114–126, 1988.
174. Siegenthaler G, Saurat J-H, Hotz R, Camenzind M, Merot Y. Cellular retinoic acid, but not cellular retinol-binding protein, is elevated in psoriatic plaques. J Invest Dermatol 86:42–45, 1984.
175. Siegenthaler G, Saurat J-H. Plasma and skin carriers for natural and synthetic retinoids. Arch Dermatol 123:1690–1692, 1987.
176. Hirschel-Scholz S, Siegenthaler G, Saurat J-H. Ligand-specific and nonspecific in vivo modulation of human epidermal cellular retinoic acid binding protein (CRABP). Eur J Clin Invest 19:220–227, 1989.
177. Gates RE, Maytield C, Allred LE. Human neonatal keratinocytes have very high levels of cellular vitamin A-binding proteins. J Invest Dermatol 88:37–41, 1987.
178. Bailey JS, Siu CH. Purification and partial characterization of a novel binding protein from the neonatal rat. J Biol Chem 263:9326–9332, 1988.
179. Giguere V, Lyn S, Yip P, Siu C-H, Amin S. Molecular cloning of cDNA encoding a second cellular retinoic acid-binding protein. Proc Natl Acad Sci USA 87:6233–6237, 1990.
180. Astrom A, Tavakkol A, Pettersson U, Cromie M, Elder JT, Voorhees JJ. Molecular cloning of two human cellular retinoic acid-binding proteins (CRABP). J Biol Chem 266:17662–17666, 1991.
181. Eller MS, Oleksiak MF, McQuaid TJ, McAfee SG, Gilchrest BA. The molecular cloning and expression of two CRABP cDNAs from human skin. Exp Cell Res 199:328–336, 1992.
182. Ong DE, Goodwin WJ, Jesse RH, Griffin AC. Presence of cellular retinol and retinoic acid-binding proteins in epidermoid carcinoma of the oral cavity and oropharynx. Cancer 49:1409–1412, 1982.
183. Gates RE, Rees RS. Altered vitamin A-binding proteins in carcinoma of the head and neck. Cancer 56:2598–2604, 1985.
184. Rallet A, Jardillier JC. Cellular binding proteins for retinol and retinoic acid in head and neck carcinomas and in human breast cancer cell lines. Steroids 52:397–398, 1988.
185. Fex G, Wahlberg P, Biorklund A, Wennerberg J, Willen R. Studies of cellular retinol-binding protein (CRBP) in squamous-cell carcinomas of the head and neck region. Int J Cancer 37:217–221, 1986.
186. Yanagita T, Komiyama S, Kuwano M. Cellular retinol-binding proteins in head and neck tumors and their adjacent tissues. Cancer 58:2251–2255, 1986.
187. Wahlberg P, Fex G, Biorklund A, Trope C, Willen R. Quantitation and localization of cellular retinol-binding protein in squamous cell carcinomas of the cervix uteri and of the oral cavity. Int J Cancer 41:771–776, 1988.
188. Zou C-P, Clifford J, Xu X-C, Sacks P, Jetten A, Eckert R, Roop D, Chambon P, Hong

K, Lotan R. Expression of differentiation markers, retinoic acid-binding proteins and nuclear receptors in human head and neck carcinoma cells and their modulation by retinoic acid. Proc Am Assoc Cancer Res 1993, in press.

189. Takase S, Ong DE, Chytil F. Cellular retinol-binding protein allows specific interaction of retinol with the nucleus in vitro. Proc Natl Acad Sci USA 76:2204–2208, 1979.

190. Takase S, Ong DE, Chytil F. Transfer of retinoic acid from its complex with cellular retinoic acid-binding protein to the nucleus. Arch Biochem Biophys 247:328–334, 1986.

191. Maden M, Ong DE, Summerbell D, Chytil F. Spatial distribution of cellular protein binding to retinoic acid in the chick limb bud. Nature 335:733–735, 1988.

192. Boylan JF, Gudas JI. Overexpression of the cellular retinoic acid binding protein-I (CRABP-I) results in reduction in differentiation-specific gene expression in F9 teratocarcinoma cells. J Cell Biol 112:965–979, 1991.

193. Lotan R, Ong DE, Chytil F. Comparison of the level of cellular retinoid-binding proteins and susceptibility to retinoid-induced growth inhibition of various neoplastic cell lines. J Natl Cancer Inst 64:1259–1262, 1980.

194. Lotan R, Stolarsky T, Lotan D. Isolation and analysis of melanoma cell mutants resistant to the antiproliferative action of retinoic acid. Cancer Res 43:2868–2875, 1983.

195. Jetten AM, Anderson K, Deas MA, Kagechika H, Lotan R, Rearick JI, Shudo K. New benzoic acid derivatives with retinoid activity: Lack of direct correlation between biological activity and binding to CRABP. Cancer Res 47:3523–3527, 1987.

196. Asselineau D, Cavey M-T, Shroot B, Darmon M. Control of epidermal differentiation by a retinoid analogue unable to bind to cytosolic retinoic acid-binding proteins (CRABP). J Invest Dermatol 98:128–134, 1992.

197. Boylan JF, Gudas JL. The level of CRABP-I expression influences the amounts and types of all-*trans*-retinoic acid metabolites in F9 teratocarcinoma cells. J Biol Chem 267:21486–21491, 1992.

198. Glass CK, DiRenzo J, Kurokawa R, Han Z. Regulation of gene expression by retinoic acid receptors. DNA Cell Biol 10:623–638, 1991.

199. Leid M, Kastner P, Chambon P. Multiplicity generates diversity in the retinoic acid signalling pathways. Trends Biochem Sci 17:427–433, 1992.

200. Petkovich M, Brand NJ, Krust A, Chambon P. A human retinoic acid receptor which belongs to the family of nuclear receptors. Nature 330:444–450, 1987.

201. Giguere V, Ong ES, Segui P, Evans RM. Identification of a receptor for the morphogen retinoic acid. Nature 330:624–629, 1987.

202. Brand N, Petkovich M, Krust A, Chambon P, de The H, Marchio A, Tiollas P, Dejean A. Identification of a second human retinoic acid receptor. Nature 332:850–853, 1988.

203. Benbrook D, Lernhardt E, Pfahl M. A new retinoic acid receptor identified from a hepatocellular carcinoma. Nature 33:669–672, 1988.

204. Krust A, Kastner P, Petkovich M, Zelent A, Chambon P. A third human retinoic acid receptor, hRAR-g. Proc Natl Acad Sci USA 86:5310–5314, 1989.

205. Ishikawa T, Umesono K, Mangelsdorf DJ, Aburatani H, Stanger BZ, Shibasaki Y, Imawari M, Evans RM, Takaku F. A functional retinoic acid receptor encoded by the gene on human chromosome 12. Mol Endocrinol 4:837–844, 1990.

206. Kastner P, Krust A, Mendelsohn C, Garnier JM, Zelent A, Leroy P, Staub A, Chambon P. Murine forms of retinoic acid receptor γ with specific patterns of expression. Proc Natl Acad Sci USA 87:2700–2704, 1990.

207. Mattei MG, Petkovich M, Mattei JF, Brand N, Chambon P. Mapping of the human retinoic acid receptor to the q21 band of chromosome 17. Hum Genet 80:186–188, 1988.

208. Mattei MG, de The H, Mattei JF, Marchio A, Tiollais P, Dejean A. Assignment of the human hap retinoic acid receptor RAR-beta gene to the p24 band of chromosome 3. Hum Genet 80:189–190, 1988.

209. Brockes JP. Retinoids, homeobox genes, and limb morphogenesis. Neuron 2:1285–1294, 1989.

210. Ruberte E, Dolle P, Krust A, Zelent A, Morris-Kay G, Chambon P. Spacial and

temporal distribution of retinoic acid receptor gamma transcripts during mouse embryogenesis. Development 108: 213–222, 1990.

211. Dolle P, Ruberte E, Kastner P, Petkovich M, Stoner CM, Gudas LJ, Chambon P. Differential expression of genes encoding α, β, and γ retinoic acid receptors and CRABP in the developing limbs of the mouse. Nature 342:702–705, 1989.

212. Mangelsdorf DJ, Ong ES, Dyck JA, Evans RM. Nuclear receptor that identifies a novel retinoic acid response pathway. Nature 345:224–229, 1990.

213. Mangelsdorf DJ, Borgmeyer U, Heyman RA, Zhou JY, Ong ES, Oro AE, Kakizuka A, Evans RM. Characterization of three RXR genes that mediate the action of 9-*cis* retinoic acid. Genes Dev 6:329–344, 1992.

214. Yu VC, Delsert C, Andersen B, Holloway JW, Devary OV, Naar AM, Kim SY, Boutin J-M, Glass CK, Rosenfeld MG. RXRβ: A coregulator that enhances binding of retinoic acid, thyroid hormone, and vitamin D receptors to their cognate response elements. Cell 67:1251–1266, 1991.

215. Kliewer SA, Umesono K, Mangelsdorf DJ, Evans RM. Retinoid X receptor interacts with nuclear receptors in retinoic acid, thyroid hormone and vitamin D3 signalling. Nature 355:446–449, 1992.

216. Leid M, Kastner P, Lyons R, Nakshatri H, Saunders M, Zacharewski T, Chen J-Y, Staub A, Garnier J-M, Mader S, Chambon P. Purification, cloning, and RXR identity of the HeLa cell factor with which RAR or TR heterodimerizes to bind target sequences efficiently. Cell 68:377–395, 1992.

217. Zhang X-K, Hoffmann B, Tran PB-V, Graupner G, Pfahl M. Retinoid X receptor is an auxillary protein for thyroid hormone and retinoic acid receptors. Nature 355:441–446, 1992.

218. de The H, Vivanco-Ruiz MdM, Tiollais P, Stunnenberg H, Dejean A. Identification of a retinoic acid responsive element in the retinoic acid receptor β gene. Nature 343:177–180, 1990.

219. Sucov HM, Murakami KK, Evans RM. Characterization of an autoregulated response element in the mouse retinoic acid receptor type β gene. Proc Natl Acad Sci USA 87:5392–5396, 1990.

220. Umesono K, Murakami KK, Thompson CC, Evans RM. Direct repeats as selective response elements for the thyroid hormone, retinoic acid, and vitamin D3 receptors. Cell 65:1255–1266, 1991.

221. Leroy P, Krust A, Zelent A, Mendelsohn C, Garnier J-M, Kastner P, Dierich A, Chambon P. Multiple isoforms of the mouse retinoic acid receptor α are generated by alternative splicing and differential induction by retinoic acid. EMBO J 10:59–69, 1991.

222. Lehmann JM, Zhang X-K, Pfahl M. RARγ2 expression is regulated through a retinoic acid response element embedded in Sp1 sites. Mol Cell Biol 12:2976–2985, 1992.

223. Vasios GW, Gold JD, Petkovich M, Chambon P, Gudas LJ. A retinoic acid-responsive element is present in the 5' flanking region of the laminin B1 gene. Proc Natl Acad Sci USA 86:9099–9103, 1989.

224. Schule R, Umesono K, Mangelsdorf DJ, Bolado J, Pike W, Evans RM. Jun-fos and receptors for vitamins A and D recognize a common response element in the human osteocalcin gene. Cell 61:497–504, 1990.

225. Munoz-Canoves P, Vik D, Tack B. Mapping of a retinoic acid-responsive element in the promotor region of the complement factor H gene. J Biol Chem 265:20065–20068, 1990.

226. Duester G, Shean M, McBride MS, Stewart MJ. Retinoic acid response element in the human alcohol dehydrogenase gene ADH3: Implications for regulation of retinoic acid synthesis. Mol Cell Biol 11:1638–1646, 1991.

227. Richard S, Zingg HH. Identification of a retinoic acid response element in the human oxytocin promotor. J Biol Chem 266:21428–21433, 1991.

228. Arcioni L, Simeone A, Guazzi S, Zappavigna V, Boncinelli E, Mavilio F. The upstream

region of the human homeobox gene *HOX3D* is a target for regulation by retinoic acid and HOX homeoproteins. EMBO J 11:265–277, 1992.

229. Durand B, Saunders M, Leroy P, Leid M, Chambon P. All-*trans* and 9-*cis* retinoic acid induction of mouse CRABP-II gene transcription is mediated by RAR/RXR heterodimers bound to DR1 and DR2 directly repeated motifs. Cell 71:73–85, 1992.

230. Rottman JN, Widom RL, Nadal-Ginard B, Mahdavi V, Karathanasis SK. A retinoic acid-responsive element in the apolipoprotein AI gene distinguishes between two different retinoic acid response pathways. Mol Cell Biol 11:3814–3820, 1991.

231. Mangelsdorf DJ, Umesono K, Kliewer SA, Borgmeyer U, Ong ES, Evans RM. A direct repeat in the cellular retinol-binding protein type II gene confers differential regulation by RXR and RAR. Cell 66:555–561, 1991.

232. Raisher BD, Gulick T, Zhang Z, Strauss AW, Moore DD, Kelly DP. Identification of a novel retinoid-responsive element in the promoter region of the medium chain acyl-coenzyme A dehydrogenase gene. J Biol Chem 267:20264–20269, 1992.

233. Zhang X-K, Hoffmann B, Tran PB-V, Graupner G, Pfahl M. Retinoid X receptor is an auxillary protein for thyroid hormone and retinoic acid receptors. Nature 355:441–446, 1992.

234. Nicholson RC, Mader S, Nagpal S, Leid M, Rochette-Egly C, Chambon P. Negative regulation of the rat stromelysin gene promoter by retinoic acid is mediated by an AP1 binding site. EMBO J 9:4443–4454, 1990.

235. Schule R, Rangarajan P, Yang N, Kliewer S, Ransone L, Bolado J, Verma IM, Evans RM. Retinoic acid is a negative regulator of AP-1 responsive genes. Proc Natl Acad Sci USA 88:6092–6096, 1991.

236. Zelent A, Krust A, Petkovich M, Kastner P, Chambon P. Cloning of murine α and β retinoic acid receptors and a novel receptor γ predominantly expressed in skin. Nature 339:714–717, 1989.

237. Rees JL, Redfern CPE. Expression of the α and β retinoic acid receptors in skin. J Invest Dermatol 93:818–820, 1989.

238. Dolle P, Ruberte E, Laroy P, Morris-Kay G, Chambon P. Retinoic acid receptors and cellular binding proteins. I. A systematic study of their differential pattern of transcription during mouse organogenesis. Development 110:1133–1151, 1990.

239. Elder JT, Fisher GJ, Zhang Q-Y, Eisen D, Krust A, Kastner P, Chambon P, Voorhees JJ. Retinoic acid receptor gene expression in human skin. J Invest Dermatol 96:425–433, 1991.

240. Redfern CPF, Todd C. Retinoic acid receptor expression in human skin keratinocytes and dermal fibroblasts in vitro. J Cell Sci 102:113–121, 1992.

241. Vollberg TM, Nervi C, George MD, Fujimoto W, Krust A, Jetten AM. Retinoic acid receptors as regulators of human epidermal keratinocyte differentiation. Mol Endocrinol 6:667–676, 1992.

242. Fujimoto W. Expression pattern of retinoic acid receptor genes in normal human skin. Jpn J Dermatol 100:1227–1233, 1990.

243. Finzi E, Blake MJ, Celano P, Skouge J, Diwan R. Cellular localization of retinoic acid receptor-gamma expression in normal and neoplastic skin. Am J Pathol 140:1463–1471, 1992.

244. Crowe DL, Hu L, Gudas LJ, Rheinwald JG. Variable expression of retinoic acid receptor (RAR beta) mRNA in human oral and epidermal keratinocytes; relation to keratin 19 expression and keratinization potential. Differentiation 48:199–208, 1991.

245. Nervi C, Vollberg TM, George MD, Zelent A, Chambon P, Jetten AM. Expression of nuclear retinoic acid receptors in normal tracheobronchial cells and in lung carcinoma cells. Exp Cell Res 195:163–70, 1991.

246. Gebert JF, Moghal N, Frangioni JV, Sugarbaker DJ, Neel BG. High frequency of retinoic acid receptor beta abnormalities in human lung cancer. Oncogene 6:1859–1868, 1991.

71

247. Hu L, Crowe DL, Rheinwald JG, Chambon P, Gudas LJ. Abnormal expression of retinoic acid receptors and keratin 19 by human oral and epidermal squamous cell carcinoma cell lines. Cancer Res 51:3972–3981, 1991.

248. Xu X-C, Ro JY, Lee JS, Shin DM, Hittelman WN, Lippman SM, Toth BB, Martin JW, Hong WK, Lotan R. Differential expression of nuclear retinoic acid receptors in surgical specimens from head and neck 'normal', hyperplastic, premalignant and malignant tissues. Proc Am Assoc Cancer Res 34:3285, 1993.

249. Latif F, Fivash M, Glenn G, Tory K, Orcutt ML, Hampsch K, Delisio J, Lerman M, Cowan J, Beckett M, Weichselbaum R. Chromosome 3p deletions in head and neck carcinomas: Statistical ascertainment of allelic loss. Cancer Res 52:1451–1456, 1992.

250. Houle B, Leduc F, Bradley WEC. Implication of RARB in epidermoid (squamous) lung cancer. Genes Chromosom Cancer 3:358–366, 1991.

251. Brauch H, Johnson B, Hovis J, Yano T, Gazdar Y, Fettengill OS, Graziano S, Sorensen OD, Poiesz BJ, Minna J, Linehan WM, Zbar B. Molecular analysis of the short arm of chromosome 3 in small cell and non-small cell carcinomas of the lung. N Engl J Med 317:1109–1113, 1987.

252. Naylor SL, Bishop DT. Report of the Committee on the Genetic Constitution of Chromosome 3 (HGM 10). Cytogenet Cell Genet 51:106–120, 1989.

253. Albertson DG, Sherrington PD, Rabbits PH. Localization of polymorphic DNA probes frequently deleted in lung carcinoma. Hum Genet 83:127–132, 1989.

254. Espeseth AS, Murphy SP, Linney E. Retinoic acid receptor expression vector inhibits differentiation of F9 embryonal carcinoma cells. Genes Dev 3:1647–1656, 1989.

255. Cope FO, Wille JJ. Retinoid receptor antisense DNAs inhibit alkaline phosphatase induction and clonogenicity in malignant keratinocytes. Proc Natl Acad Sci USA 86:5590–5594, 1989.

256. Collins SJ, Robertson KA, Mueller L. Retinoic acid-induced granulocytic differentiation of HL-60 myeloid leukemia cells is mediated directly through the retinoic acid receptor (RAR-α). Mol Cell Biol 10:2154–2163, 1990.

257. Robertson KA, Emami B, Mueller L, Collins SJ. Multiple members of the retinoic acid receptor family are capable of mediating the granulocytic differentiation of HL-60 cells. Mol Cell Biol 12:3743–3749, 1992.

258. Robertson KA, Mueller L, Collins SJ. Retinoic acid receptors in myeloid leukemia: Characterization of receptors in retinoic acid-resistant K-562 cells. Blood 77:340–347, 1991.

259. Stellmach V, Leask A, Fuchs E. Retinoid-mediated transcriptional regulation of keratin genes in human epidermal and squamous cell carcinoma cells. Proc Natl Acad Sci USA 88:4582–4596, 1991.

260. Tomic M, Jiang CK, Epstein HS, Freedberg IM, Samuels HH, Blumenberg M. Nuclear receptors for retinoic acid and thyroid hormone regulate transcription of keratins. Cell Regul 1:965–973, 1990.

261. Aneskievich BJ, Fuchs E. Teminal differentiation in keratinocytes involves positive as well as negative regulation by retinoic acid receptors and retinoid X receptors at retinoid response elements. Mol Cell Biol 12:4862–4871, 1992.

262. Leroy P, Krust A, Kastner P, Mendelsohn C, Zelent A, Chambon P. Retinoic acid receptors. In: G Morriss-Kay, ed. Retinoids in Normal Development and Teratogenesis. New York: Oxford University Press, 1992, pp 7–25.

4. Risk factors and genetic susceptibility

Margaret R. Spitz

Upper aerodigestive tract (oral cavity, pharyngeal, and laryngeal) cancers are sentinel diseases of exposure to tobacco and alcohol, and thus can be considered the paradigm of environmentally induced disease. The fact that only a fraction of exposed individuals develop these cancers suggests inter-individual differences in susceptibility to these environmental insults. In fact, heritable differences in susceptibility may be identified at almost every phase of carcinogenesis, for example, in the ability to metabolize carcinogens, DNA repair capability, genomic instability, and altered proto-oncogene and tumor suppressor gene expression [1]. This chapter will review briefly the environmental contribution to the incidence of upper aerodigestive tract cancers and will explore some of the host factors that modify genetic damage from these and other carcinogenic exposures.

Descriptive epidemiology

In 1994, it is estimated that there will be 42,100 incident cases of upper aerodigestive tract cancer and 11,725 deaths from these diseases [2]. From 1973 to 1989, the incidence of oral and pharyngeal cancers decreased in white men of all ages and white women under 65 years, and concomitantly, there has been an average 2% annual decline in mortality [3]. In contrast, there have been significant increases in incidence and mortality in black men and nonsignificant increases in black women. Incidence rates in black men under 65 years are now twice as high as in white men [3]. The secular pattern of incidence of laryngeal cancers resembles that of lung cancer: a small decline in white men under 65 years age but continuing increases in white and black men above 65 years and in all women, especially those above 65 years [3].

Hong, Waun Ki and Weber, Randal S., (eds.), Head and Neck Cancer. © 1995 Kluwer Academic Publishers.
ISBN 0-7923-3015-3. All rights reserved.

Cigarette smoking

The contribution of tobacco to risk of oral and laryngeal cancers is without question. Both prospective and retrospective studies worldwide have consistently demonstrated linear dose-response effects. A review of the relevant studies documents cancer risks of 5- to 25-fold higher for heavy smokers relative to nonsmokers [4]. In most instances, the dose of smoking is linearly related to the excess risk. Studies have also demonstrated higher cancer risks for smokers of nonfilter cigarettes compared with filter cigarettes and diminishing risk with increasing time since cessation of smoking [5–7].

Differences by gender and by primary site have been noted both in the magnitude of the risk estimates and in the gradients of the dose-response. Some studies have reported higher cancer risks for women than for men at each successive pack-year stratum [7,8]. Higher smoking-associated risk estimates for laryngeal malignancies compared with oral cavity cancers are also reported [8].

In our own experience at M. D. Anderson Cancer Center, risk estimates for cigarette smoking among male head and neck cancer patients increased linearly with each successive pack-year stratum from 1.8 to 4.0 to 7.5 in the heaviest smokers [8]. For women, the corresponding risks were 1.5, 9.0, and 12.0. In both instances, linear trend analysis was statistically significant [8]. We also noted subsite-specific differences in cigarette smoking risk estimates. The highest odds ratio estimate (OR = 15.1) was documented for laryngeal cancers, and the lowest risk was noted for oral cancers (OR = 2.1). These findings suggest a variable susceptibility, possibly sex and site dependent, to carcinogenic action.

Risk is also related to the type of tobacco used. Higher risks of laryngeal cancers were noted for users of dark tobacco than for users of light (flue-cured) tobacco [10]. It is reported that black tobacco contains higher concentrations of carcinogens, including N-nitroso compounds and aromatic amines.

Cigar and pipe smoking

Although smokers of cigars and pipes tend to inhale less than do cigarette smokers (as reflected in lower carboxyhemoglobin levels relative to cigarette smokers), they are at increased risk for the development of oral, oropharyngeal, hypopharyngeal, and laryngeal cancers [11]. The risk estimates approximate those of cigarette smokers for buccal cavity but not pharyngeal malignancies [12]. For laryngeal cancers, Wynder et al. [13] demonstrated a 12-fold increase in risk associated with cigar and pipe smoking compared with nonusers.

Snuff use

The Advisory Committee to the Surgeon General on the health consequences of smokeless tobacco concluded that 'the evidence is strong that the use of snuff can cause cancer in humans' and that the 'evidence for causality is strongest for cancer of the oral cavity' [14]. They also cited an almost 50-fold elevated risk for cheek and gum cancers in long-term snuff users. Snuff use has been implicated in the etiology of oral cavity cancers and, to a lesser extent, pharyngeal cancers [8,14]. One study documented a fourfold elevated risk of oral and pharyngeal cancer in white women who dipped snuff; this study also showed a strong dose-response relationship [15]. The major carcinogens identified in snuff are polonium-210 and volatile, nonvolatile, and tobacco-specific nitrosamines [16].

The Advisory Committee also noted 'that smokeless tobacco is responsible for the development of a portion of oral leukoplakias in both teenage and adult users' [13]. It should be noted that the production of smokeless tobacco has increased by an estimated 42% in the past two decades [17].

Alcohol use

Cohort and case-control studies have consistently demonstrated that alcohol consumption increases the risk of cancers of the oropharynx and larynx [18]. An interaction between tobacco smoking and alcohol in head and neck cancers has been demonstrated. This interaction appears to be multiplicative for laryngeal cancers [19], but more variable for oral and pharyngeal cancers. The separate effects of alcohol and tobacco use have been difficult to distinguish because the consumption of these products is so closely correlated. However, a recent population-based study documented an independent effect for alcohol and showed a dose-response relationship after controlling for exposure to tobacco [6]. The authors estimated that tobacco smoking and alcohol drinking combined account for approximately three quarters of all oral and pharyngeal cancers in the United States [6].

Marijuana smoking

There is much theoretical evidence that marijuana should be carcinogenic. Marijuana smoke is qualitatively similar to cigarette smoke but results in a greater tar burden to the respiratory tract [20]. Marijuana smoking may have a greater carcinogenic effect on the upper aerodigestive tract than on the lower airways, especially in light of the rapid, deep inhalation used in smoking the product [20]. However, there is little direct evidence of marijuana's role in cancer etiology because most abusers of marijuana are also exposed to tobacco and alcohol, and reliability of self-reported data are likely to be suspect.

Several authors have also described the occurrence of cancers in patients who have been nonsmokers and nonusers of alcohol. One study involved older women; another focused on adults less than 40 years [21,22]. Both noted that lesions were less likely (than in smokers) to involve the 'zone of risk,' that is, the horseshoe-shaped area of the oral mucosa [23].

Mouthwash use

A few reports in the literature have suggested that mouthwash use is associated with risk of oral cancer, although no relevant trends regarding frequency or duration of use were described [24,25]. These studies also raised concerns about the role of preclinical oral cancer symptoms that might have stimulated the practice of mouthwash use. However, a recent population-based case-control study documented significantly excess risk of oral cavity cancer among both men (OR = 1.4) and women (OR = 1.6) users of mouthwash high in alcohol content, even after adjusting for the effects of tobacco and alcohol consumption [26]. In this study, risk tended to increase with increasing duration and frequency of use, and was not attributed to recently initiated use (such as because of early symptomatic oral cancer) [26]. The authors stated that oral swishing with mouthwash containing 25% ethanol might provide an exposure to the mucosa similar to that of drinking 100-proof alcohol diluted with an equal amount of water. The interaction of the effects of using mouthwash and tobacco smoking requires further investigation.

Poor oral hygiene

Poor oral hygiene and dentition have been implicated for a long time in oral cavity cancer risk [26]. However, it has often not been possible to disentangle the effects of alcohol and tobacco use. In a study of snuff dipping and oral cancer [15], two- to threefold elevated risks were noted for persons who had lost 10 or more teeth after controlling for the wearing of dentures. However, once the effects of tobacco, alcohol, and socioeconomic status were controlled, no strong association could be detected. In the large population-based study of oral and pharyngeal cancers, no associations were noted for denture wearing, prior periodontal disease, cold sores, sores in the mouth, or bleeding gums [26].

Occupational risk factors

The evidence supporting an association between laryngeal cancer and asbestos exposure is fairly substantial, although few studies have effectively controlled for the confounding effect of tobacco exposure. These studies have been extensively reviewed and document odds ratios ranging from 1.4 to 15.0 [4,27]. Nickel exposure in smelting operations has also been implicated in the etiology of laryngeal cancer [28] but has not been associated with increased risk in other studies [29]. Workers occupationally exposed to sulfuric acid [30], workers involved in the manufacture of mustard gas [31], and machinists [29] are also said to be at increased risk of developing laryngeal cancer. Elevated oral cancer rates have been demonstrated in a variety of occupations, including plumbers and metal, textile, and steel workers [32]. A recent study implicated wood dust and exposure to organic compounds and coal products as increasing the risk for these cancers [33].

Diet

Considerable laboratory and epidemiologic evidence suggests that carotenoids act as dietary inhibitors of epithelial carcinogenesis. Vitamin A and synthetic retinoids have been shown to modulate the growth and differentiation of normal, premalignant, and malignant cells both in vivo and in culture. In early epidemiologic investigations of dietary vitamin A intake and cancer risk, the form of vitamin A was not distinguished. More recently, both case-control and prospective studies have found an inverse association between total vitamin A and carotene intake and lung cancer risk. Similar results have been reported for laryngeal cancer (carotene) [34], oral cancer (vitamin A) [35], and oral and pharyngeal cancers (fruit consumption) [36].

A recent report on oral and pharyngeal cancers in China showed that men in the highest tertile of intake of fruits and vegetables had about 30–50% of the risk of those in the lowest tertile, with a less pronounced effect for women [37]. In a study of oral and pharyngeal cancers conducted among women in North Carolina, there was a 50% reduction in risk associated with frequent consumption of fresh fruits and vegetables [38]. Fruits and vegetables contribute vitamin C, beta-carotene, and other carotenoids, all of which are antioxidants. Dark green and yellow vegetables are especially rich in carotene and lutein [39].

Few studies have evaluated possible interactions between cigarette smoking and these dietary factors. Stefani et al. demonstrated that tobacco use and low fruit intake exerted an effect that was greater than additive in laryngeal cancer risk [40]. A study in Texas suggested that carotene exerted its protective effect among smokers who had stopped smoking 2–10 years previously [34]. Zheng et al. present data from a case-control study in China reporting that the combined effects of smoking and diet were more than additive [41]. Intervention trials using these compounds have provided strong evidence for the potential of cancer chemoprevention.

Herpes simplex virus

Only limited evidence exists linking herpes simplex virus (HSV) to oral cancer. In one study, 42% of oral cancer patients (compared with none of the control subjects) exhibited HSV type 1 (HSV-1) protein [42]. Another study implicated two different late antigens of HSV-1, one recognized by IgA antibody and the other by IgM antibody [43]. There is also experimental evidence of an interaction between viral infection and tobacco carcinogenesis. Oral cancer was induced in 50% of hamster buccal pouches in the presence of both HSV infection and simulated snuff dipping, although neither HSV nor tobacco alone induced neoplastic changes [44].

Human papillomavirus

The possible role of human papillomavirus (HPV) infection in the etiology of oral squamous cell cancer is currently being explored by a number of research groups. Using the polymerase chain reaction (PCR) technique, HPV DNA has been detected in from 32% to 100% of oral squamous cell cancers [45–48]. The differences in prevalence are likely because of different experimental conditions. HPV types 6, 11, 16, and 18 were detected, with types 16 and 18 reported most frequently. The latter two types have been investigated most extensively because of their association with genital cancer. HPV types 6, 11, and 16 have also been detected in oral leukoplakia [49]. It has been estimated that the prevalence of HPV infection in the oral mucosa of normal adults is 40–45% [50].

Genetic susceptibility

While tobacco and alcohol exposures are major determinants of risk of upper aerodigestive tract cancers, host-specific factors also influence the risk for cancer development. Few ecogenetic studies have specifically targeted head and neck cancers. Because of the excess risk of lung cancers in these patients, it is appropriate to extrapolate the research focused on lung cancer to the upper aerodigestive tract. Based on the magnitude of the attributable risk of tobacco in these cancers, one could define susceptibility in the context of this specific exposure. The lifetime risk of developing lung cancer in men who smoke 20 or more cigarettes per day is only 15% [51]. Varying host susceptibility must therefore be inferred. An important factor in the estimate of carcinogen risk is consideration of these interindividual differences in susceptibility to carcinogenesis.

Metabolic factors in susceptibility

Animal studies clearly demonstrate that the rate of carcinogen metabolism is of central importance to carcinogenesis [52]. The concentration of mutagens depends on a delicate balance between the rate of activation and the rate of detoxification.

Many tobacco carcinogens, including polycyclic aromatic hydrocarbons (PAHs) and N-nitrosamines, require metabolic activation before exerting their carcinogenic effect. For example, the cytochrome P-450-dependent mono-oxygenase systems catalyze the initial oxidation of PAHs to electrophilic intermediates capable of binding to DNA and cellular proteins. Much of the interindividual variability in carcinogen metabolism may be explained by variable patterns of P450 isozymes in tissues of different individuals [53]. Studies of polymorphic variability are currently a focus of considerable interest. Most studies of metabolic markers have been of the case-control design and are confounded by the inducibility of some of these enzymes.

One particular P-450 enzyme, aryl hydrocarbon hydroxylase (AHH; associated with CYP 1A1 isozyme), has been extensively studied [54]. Patients with lung cancer were shown to have predominantly intermediate and high AHH inducibility phenotypes [54] in peripheral lymphocyte assays. The rationale advanced was that individuals with high inducibility could more readily activate the promutagens and procarcinogens in cigarette smoke. There were initial difficulties in reproducing these results, but they have since been corroborated [55]. More recently, a positive association between cigarette smoking and *CYP 1A1* gene expression was noted in normal human lung tissue, and altered gene regulation was documented in lung cancer patients [56].

Human debrisoquine activity is also known to be polymorphic. Autosomal recessive poor metabolizers constitute about 9% of the white population [57]. One study found an increased lung cancer risk in extensive metabolizers of debrisoquine [58], although no procarcinogens have been identified as substrates for debrisoquine-4-hydroxylase enzyme, and negative and ambiguous results have also been reported. The gene coding for CYP 2D6 has been cloned, and it is now possible with PCR-based assays to distinguish poor metabolizers from extensive or intermediate metabolizers [59].

There is also considerable interindividual variation in the activity of detoxifying isozymes of glutathione S-transferases (GST), which metabolize PAH constituents of tobacco smoke. These enzymes catalyze the detoxification of mutagenic electrophiles that are generated by the cytochrome P-450−mediated oxidation reactions. It is therefore highly likely that differences in GST expression would yield differences in susceptibility to carcinogenic exposure [52]. Data from a recent study suggest that high or intermediate enzyme activity has a moderately protective effect in persons heavily exposed to tobacco smoke [60]. This study included 15 patients with oral and pharyngeal cancers, but site-specific data were not presented.

DNA repair capability

Much of the evidence linking DNA repair deficiency and cancer risk is from the autosomal recessive DNA repair–deficient syndromes that in homozygotes are associated with high cancer rates. Despite the rarity of these diseases, their unique cytogenetic and biochemical characteristics have thrown much light on the issue of genetic predisposition to cancer.

Ataxia telangiectasia (AT) is a unique human model for studying genetic susceptibility to cancer because it is determined by a single gene that has been localized to 11q [61]. AT homozygotes are three times more sensitive to ionizing radiation than are normal individuals. Skin fibroblasts from heterozygotes show radiation dose-response curves that are intermediate between those of normal individuals and those of homozygotes. AT cells exhibit high frequencies of spontaneous chromosome breakage and collateral sensitivity to radiomimetic drugs such as bleomycin. Obligate AT heterozygotes are thought to be at eightfold increased risk of breast cancer [62].

Human tumor cells and cells from cancer-prone individuals (e.g., persons with AT, Fanconi's anemia) show a higher incidence of radiosensitivity during G_2 irradiation than do cells from normal individuals [63]. This radiosensitivity (manifested as chromatid breaks) may reflect greater radiation-induced damage. There is biochemical evidence for the correlation of DNA repair deficiency with induced chromatid aberration incidence [59]. Pero et al. [64] noted reduced in vitro, unscheduled DNA synthesis in cells from cancer patients and genetically predisposed individuals.

Xeroderma pigmentosum patients exhibit extreme ultraviolet sensitivity and are defective in excision repair of bulky adducts induced by ultraviolet radiation. In patients with Bloom's syndrome, DNA ligase I is deficient [65].

A working hypothesis developed by Hsu presupposes a spectrum of DNA repair capability within the general population [66]. To demonstrate the existence of differences in mutagen sensitivity, Hsu developed an assay in which quantification of chromosomal breakage induced by in vitro exposure to the radiomimetic drug bleomycin is used as an indirect measure of repair capability [67]. The principal test cells for the assay are primary cultures of peripheral lymphocytes that actively proliferate, yielding a good supply of mitotic cells for chromosomal study. The radiomimetic agent, bleomycin, was chosen as the test mutagen because it induces DNA breaks that express, within a short time period, as chromatid breaks. The protocol includes treating the cells of the culture with bleomycin (0.03 units/ml) for 5 hours and then harvesting the cells wth conventional cytogenetic methods. A minimum of 50 well-spread metaphases is examined, the breaks counted, and the data recorded as the average breaks per cell (b/c).

Bleomycin-induced sensitivity and environmental exposures have been assessed in 75 patients with previously untreated upper aerodigestive malignancies and 62 healthy control subjects [68]. Fifty-four patients, compared with only 13 of the controls, were sensitive to bleomycin-induced mutagenesis (i.e., had more than 0.8 average breaks per cell) [68]. On logistic regression analysis, mutagen sensitivity remained a strong and independent risk factor after adjustment for potential confounding from age, sex, and tobacco and alcohol consumption (OR = 4.3; 95% confidence limits = 2.0, 10.2; Table 1) [68].

We have recently confirmed these initial observations in a second case-control study involving 108 additional patients with newly diagnosed upper aerodigestive tract cancers (Table 1). Mutagen sensitivity (b/c >0.8) remained an independent risk factor on multivariate analysis, after controlling for the effects of alcohol and tobacco use [69]. The magnitude of the univariate and adjusted risk estimates for mutagen sensitivity were less in the second study, although still statistically significant. Both studies also

Table 1. Risk estimates for mutagen sensitivity, cigarette smoking, and alcohol use

	Odds ratio	
	Study 1, 1989[a,c] (n = 137)	Study 2, 1992[b,c] (n = 216)
Mutagen sensitivity		
Crude	3.9 (1.6, 9.1)	2.7 (1.1, 6.6)
Adjusted[d]	4.3 (2.0, 10.2)	2.2 (1.0, 5.1)
Cigarette smoking (cigarettes per day)		
1–14	0.7 (0.2, 2.2)	4.2 (1.4, 12.8)
15–24	2.8 (1.1, 6.9)	7.9 (3.2, 19.1)
25+	12.7 (13.8, 42.3)	11.0 (4.4, 27.4)
Alcohol use (drinks per day)		
1–2	1.9 (0.6, 5.7)	1.0 (0.7, 1.6)
3–6	5.0 (1.4, 17.9)	1.7 (0.7, 4.1)
>6	44.5 (2.5, 793.9)	14.0 (4.2, 47.0)

[a] From Spitz et al. [68], with permission.
[b] From Spitz et al. [69], with permission.
[c] Confidence limits in parentheses.
[d] Adjusted for sex, age, smoking, and alcohol use.

Table 2. Risk estimates for strata of cigarette smoking, alcohol use, and mutagen sensitivity (b/c >0.8)

	Odds ratios	
	Study 1, 1989[a,c] (n = 137)	Study 2, 1992[b,c] (n = 216)
Smoking/mutagen sensitivity		
No/no	1.0	1.0
No/yes	5.8 (1.3, 25.1)	3.2 (0.6, 18.7)
Yes/no	5.4 (1.5, 19.5)	8.1 (1.7, 37,7)
Yes/yes	19.8 (4.6, 84.8)	23.0 (5.0, 106.0)
Alcohol/mutagen sensitivity		
No/no	1.0	1.0
No/yes	3.6 (1.2, 11.1)	3.0 (1.4, 6.4)
Yes/no	5.4 (1.6, 18.3)	3.0 (1.2, 7.8)
Yes/yes	17.1 (4.1, 70.6)	5.6 (2.3, 14.2)

[a] From Spitz et al. [68], with permission.
[b] From Spitz et al. [69] with permission.
[c] 95% confidence limits in parentheses.

demonstrated dose-response relationships for cigarette smoking and alcohol use (Table 1).

To evaluate the independent effect of mutagen sensitivity and its interaction with cigarette smoking and alcohol consumption, risk estimates for various combinations of these factors were computed in stratified analyses (Table 2). These analyses were restricted to study participants for whom all relevant information was available. The referent category was study participants who were not mutagen sensitive and were nonusers of either cigarettes or alcohol. Mutagen sensitivity was a risk factor in the absence of both smoking and alcohol use (threefold to fivefold), and there were significantly elevated risks associated with smoking or alcohol use in mutagen-resistant persons. The combined effects of cigarette smoking and mutagen sensitivity seemed to be multiplicative. The data for alcohol and mutagen sensitivity were less consistent.

The second study also provided data suggestive of familial aggregation of cancer in first-degree relatives of mutagen-hypersensitive patients (b/c >1.0). Odds ratios were 2.8 (95% confidence limits = 1.1, 7.2) for one first-degree relative with cancer and 7.0 (95% confidence limits = 1.8, 27.1) for two or more first-degree relatives with cancer [70].

Populations of individuals with cancers other than head and neck cancer have also been evaluated for mutagen sensitivity [67]. The original hypothesis was that the assessment of such individuals would provide an explanation for site specificity of tumor development. Fifty of 71 patients (70%) with confirmed lung cancer and 58 of 83 patients (70%) with colon cancer expressed b/c counts above 0.8 [67].

82

The assay may also have predictive potential. Eighty-four previously untreated head and neck cancer patients were evaluated for sensitivity to bleomycin and then followed longitudinally for multiple primary malignancies (median follow-up of 20 months) (Table 3) [71]. Four of the 51 nonsensitive patients (8%) developed second primary malignancies, compared with 9 of 33 patients (27%) in the hypersensitive group (b/c >1.0). The relative risk of multiple primary cancers among the latter group was 4.4 (95% confidence limits = 1.2, 15.8). We have recently enlarged this study, accruing 278 patients followed from 1987 through 1993 [72]. The mean break/cell value for patients developing second malignancies was 1.17 (±0.54) compared with 0.98 (±0.44) for patients with only one primary (P = 0.004). The relative risk for developing second cancers was 2.67 (1.22, 5.79). This study also showed no differences in the distribution of mutagen sensitivity by smoking status, pack-years or tumor stage [71]. Cloos et al. have shown similar findings in their studies of head and neck cancer patients [73]. These findings have clinical and prognostic relevance, since second malignant tumors are the most important cause of mortality in early stage disease.

The finding of suggestive synergistic effects of alcohol use and mutagen sensitivity in our case-control study stimulated further in vitro studies of the effect of alcohol in this test assay system [74]. Cultured human cells were treated with a fixed concentration of bleomycin together with ethanol at concentrations varying from 0.1% to 4%. The frequency of chromosome breaks, compared with that in the bleomycin control, was unchanged at 0.1% and 0.5% ethanol but was markedly elevated beginning at 1% ethanol [74]. This series of experiments indicated that alcohol, although itself not a clastogen, could potentiate the genotoxic property of bleomycin with a dose-dependent effect.

We have also tested the potentiation property of ethanol on mutagens with different molecular mechanisms [74]. Four additional mutagens were chosen: the base analogue cytosine arabinoside, the ultraviolet-radiomimetic carcinogen 4-nitroquinoline-1-oxide, the alkylating agent triethylene-melamine, and a sample of cigarette smoke condensate. In all cases, ethanol enhanced their genotoxicity. Thus, it appears that the potentiation effect of

Table 3. Risk of multiple primary cancer in patients with head and neck cancer by mutagen hypersensitivity status

Mutagen hypersensitivity	No. of patients	Second malignancies (%)	Relative risk	(95% confidence limits)
>1.0 breaks per cell	33	9 (27.3)	4.4	1.2, 15.8
≤1.0 breaks per cell	51	4 (7.8)		

From Schantz et al. [74], with permission.

alcohol is a general phenomenon, not the formation of a particular molecular complex that increases the potency of a mutagen. This finding may explain the cocarcinogenic properties of alcohol in head and neck cancer etiology.

Summary

Tobacco use is such a major determinant of head and neck cancer risk that classical epidemiologic techniques were more than adequate to document and characterize the etiologic association. However, the new emphasis in epidemiologic research is multidisciplinary, centering on the role of interindividual differences in susceptibility to carcinogenic exposures and particularly on the interaction of genetic susceptibility and environmental forces, that is, ecogenetics. For upper aerodigestive tract cancers, measurements of carcinogen metabolic activation and DNA repair capability are especially relevant. These susceptibility markers will enable the identification of highrisk population subgroups who can be targeted for the most intensive primary and secondary preventive strategies.

Acknowledgments

This work was supported in part by NCI grant R03 CA50945.

References

1. Shields PG, Harris CC. Molecular epidemiology and the genetics of environmental cancer. JAMA 266:681–687, 1991.
2. American Cancer Society. Cancer Facts and Figures – 1994. Atlanta: American Cancer Society, p. 6, 1994.
3. Miller BA, Ries LAG, Hankey BF, Kosary CL, Edwards BK. Cancer statistics review: 1973–1989. Washington DC: National Cancer Institute NIH publication 92-2789, 1992.
4. Rothman KJ, Cann CI, Flanders D, et al. Epidemiology of laryngeal cancer. Epidemiol Rev 2:195–209, 1980.
5. Wynder EL, Covey LS, Mabuchi K, et al. Environmental factors in cancer of the larynx: A second look. Cancer 38:1591–1601, 1976.
6. Blot WJ, McLaughlin JK, Winn DM, et al. Smoking and drinking in relation to oral and pharyngeal cancer. Cancer Res 48:3282–3287, 1988.
7. Wynder EL, Stellman SD. Impact of long-term filter cigarette usage on lung and larynx cancer risk: a case-control study. J Natl Cancer Inst 62:471–477, 1979.
8. Spitz MR, Fueger JJ, Goepfert H, Hong WK, Newell GR. Squamous cell carcinoma of the upper aerodigestive tract: a case-comparison analysis. Cancer 61:203–208, 1988.
9. Maier H, Dietz A, Gewelke U, Heller WD, Weidauer H. Tobacco and alcohol and the risk of head and neck cancer. Clin Invest 70:320–327, 1992.
10. De Stefani E, Correa P, Oreggia F, et al. Risk factors for laryngeal cancer. Cancer 60:3087–3091, 1987.

11. Tobacco Smoking. IARC Monograph on the Evaluation of the Carcinogenic Risk of Chemicals to Humans, Vol. 380. Lyon: IARC, 1986.
12. Kahn HA. The Dorn study of smoking and mortality among US veterans: Report on eight and one-half years of observation. Natl Cancer Inst Mongr 19:1–125, 1966.
13. Wynder EL, Bross IJ, Day E. A study of environmental factors in cancer of the larynx. Cancer 9:86–110, 1956.
14. The Health Consequences of Using Smokeless Tobacco: A Report of the Advisory Committee to the Surgeon General. Washington DC: U.S. Department of Health and Human Services, National Cancer Institute NIH publication 86-2874, 1986.
15. Winn DM, Blot WJ, Shy CM, et al. Snuff dipping and oral cancer among women in the southern United States. N Engl J Med 304:745–749, 1981.
16. Hoffman D, Harley NH, Fisenne I, et al. Carcinogenic agents in snuff. J Natl Cancer Inst 76:435–437, 1986.
17. Cullen JW, Blot W, Henningfield J, et al. Health consequences of using smokeless tobacco. Summary of the advisory committee's report to the surgeon general. Public Health Rep 101:355–373, 1986.
18. Tuyns AJ. Alcohol. In: D Schottenfeld, JF Fraumeni, eds. Cancer Epidemiology and Prevention. Philadelphia: WB Saunders, 1982, pp 293–303.
19. Saracci R. The interactions of tobacco smoking and other agents in cancer etiology. Epidemiol Rev 9:175–193, 1987.
20. Caplan GA, Brigham BA. Marijuana smoking and carcinoma of the tongue. Is there an association? Cancer 66:1005–1006, 1990.
21. Moore C, Catlin D. Anatomic origins and locations of oral cancer. Am J Surg 114: 510–513, 1967.
22. Wey PD, Lotz MJ, Triedman LJ. Oral cancer in women nonusers of tobacco and alcohol. Cancer 60:1644–1650, 1987.
23. Schantz SP, Byers RM, Goepfert H, Shallenberger RC, Beddingfield N. The implication of tobacco use in the young adult with head and neck cancer. Cancer 62:1374–1380, 1988.
24. Wynder EL, Kabat GC, Rosenthal S, Levenstein M. Oral cancer and mouthwash use. J Natl Cancer Inst 70:255–260, 1983.
25. Blot WJ, Winn DM, Fraumeni JF. Oral cancer and mouthwash. J Natl Cancer Inst 70:255–260, 1983.
26. Winn DM, Blot WJ, McLaughlin JK, Austin DF, Greenberg RS, Preston-Martin S, et al. Mouthwash use and oral conditions in the risk of oral and pharyngeal cancer. Cancer Res 51:3044–3047, 1991.
27. Burch JD, Howe GR, Miller AB, et al. Tobacco, alcohol, asbestos, and nickel in the etiology of cancer of the larynx: A case-control study. J Natl Cancer Inst 67:1219–1224, 1981.
28. Shannon HS, Julian JA, Roberts RS. A mortality study of 11,500 nickel workers. J Natl Cancer Inst 73:1251–1258, 1984.
29. Zagraniski RT, Kelsey JL, Walter SD. Occupational risk factors for laryngeal carcinoma: Connecticut, 1975–1980. Am J Epidemiol 124:67–76, 1986.
30. Soskolne CL, Zeighami EA, Hanis NM, et al. Laryngeal cancer and occupational exposure to sulfuric acid. Am J Epidemiol 120:358–369, 1984.
31. Wada S, Nishimoto Y, Miyanishi M, et al. Mustard gas as a cause of respiratory neoplasia in man. Lancet 1:1161–1163, 1968.
32. Mahboudi E, Sayed GM. Oral cavity and pharynx. In: D Schottenfeld, JF Fraumeni Jr., eds. Cancer Epidemiology and Prevention. Philadelphia: WB Saunders, 1982, pp 583–595.
33. Maier H, Dietz A, Gewelke V, Heller WD. Occupational exposure to hazardous substances and risk of cancer in the area of the mouth cavity, oropharynx, hypopharynx and larynx. A case-control study. Laryngol Rhin Otol 70:93–98, 1991.
34. Mackerras D, Buffler PA, Randall DE, Nichaman MZ, Pickle LW, Mason TJ. Carotene intake and the risk of laryngeal cancer in coastal Texas. Am J Epidemiol 128:980–988, 1988.

35. Marshall J, Graham S, Mettlin C, Shedd D, Swanson M. Diet in the epidemiology of oral cancer. Nutr Cancer 3:145–149, 1982.
36. McLaughlin JK, Gridley G, Block G, et al. Dietary factors in oral and pharyngeal cancer. J Natl Cancer Inst 80:1237–1243, 1988.
37. Zheng W, Blot WJ, Xiao-Ou S, et al. Risk factors for oral and pharyngeal cancer in Shanghai with emphasis on diet. Cancer Epidemiol Biomarkers Prev 1:441–448, 1992.
38. Winn DM, Ziegler RG, Pickle LW, Gridley G, Blot WJ, Hoover R. Diet in the etiology of oral and pharyngeal cancer among women from the southern United States. Cancer Res 44:1216–1223, 1984.
39. Micozzi MS, Belcher GR, Taylor PR, Okhachik F. Carotenoid analysis of selected raw and cooked foods associated with a lower risk for cancer. J Natl Cancer Inst 82:282–285, 1990.
40. Stefani ED, Correa P, Oreggia F, et al. Risk factors for laryngeal cancer. Cancer 60:3087–3091, 1987.
41. Zheng W, Blot WJ, Xiao-Ou S, et al. Diet and other risk factors for laryngeal cancer in Shanghai, China. Am J Epidemiol 136:178–179, 1992.
42. Kassim KH, Daley TD. Herpes simplex virus type proteins in human oral squamous cell carcinoma. Oral Surg Oral Med Oral Pathol 65:445–448, 1988.
43. Shillitoe EJ, Greenspan D, Greenspan JS, Silverman S Jr. Antibody to early and late antigens of herpes simplex virus type 1 in patients with oral cancer. Cancer 54:266–273, 1986.
44. Park NH, Sapp JP, Herbosa EG. Oral cancer induced in hamsters with herpes simplex infection and simulated snuff dipping. Oral Surg Oral Med Oral Pathol 42:164–168, 1986.
45. Maitland NJ, Bromidge T, Cox MF, Crane IJ, Prime SS, Scully C. Detection of human papillomavirus genes in human oral tissue biospies and cultures by polymerase chain reaction. Br J Cancer 59:698–703, 1988.
46. Watts SL, Brewer EE, Fry TL. Human papillomaviruses DNA in squamous cell carcinomas of the head and neck. Oral Surg Oral Med Oral Pathol 71:701–707, 1991.
47. Yeudall WA, Campo MS. Human papillomavirus DNA in biopsies of oral tissues. J Gen Virol 72:173–176, 1991.
48. Woods KV, Shillitoe EJ, Spitz MR, Schantz SP, Adler-Storthz K. Analysis of human papilloma-virus DNA in oral squamous cell carcinomas. J Oral Pathol Med 22:101–108, 1993.
49. Kashima HK, Kutcher M, Kesis T, Levin LS, de Villiers EM, Shak K. Human papillomavirus in squamous cell carcinoma, leukoplakia lichen planus, and clinically normal epithelium in the oral cavity. Ann Otol Rhinol Laryngol 99:55–61, 1989.
50. Jenison SA, Xiu-ping Y, Valentine JM, et al. Evidence of prevalent genital type human papillomavirus infections in adults and children. J Infect Dis 162:60–69, 1990.
51. Law MR. Genetic predisposition to lung cancer. Br J Cancer 61:195–206, 1990.
52. Wolf CR. Metabolic factors in cancer susceptibility. Cancer Surv 9:437–474, 1990.
53. Vahakangas K, Pelkonen O. Host variations in carcinogen metabolism and DNA repair. In: HT Lynch, T Hirayama, eds. Genetic Epidemiology of Cancer. Boca Raton, FL: CRC Press, 1989, pp 35–54.
54. Kellermann G, Luyten-Kellermann M, Jett JR, Moses HL, Fontana RS. Aryl hydrocarbon hydroxylase in man and lung cancer. Hum Genet 1(Suppl):161–168, 1978.
55. Kouri RE, McKinney CE, Slomianry DT, et al. Positive correlation between aryl hydrocarbon hydroxylase activity and primary lung cancer as analyzed in cryopreserved lymphocytes. Cancer Res 42:5030–5037, 1982.
56. McLemore TL, Adelberg S, Liu MC, et al. Expression of *CYP 1A1* gene in patients with lung cancer: evidence for cigarette smoke-induced gene expression in normal lung tissue and for altered gene regulation in primary pulmonary carcinoma. J Natl Cancer Inst 82:1333–1339, 1990.
57. Peart GF, Boutagy J, Shenfield GM. Debrisoquine oxidation in an Australian population. Br J Clin Pharmacol 21:465–471, 1986.

58. Ayesh R, Idle JR, Ritchie J, et al. Metabolic oxidative phenotypes as markers for susceptibility to lung cancer. Nature 312:169–170, 1984.
59. Sugimura H, Caporaso NE, Shaw GL, et al. Human debrisoquine hydroxylase gene polymorphisms in cancer patients and controls. Carcinogenesis 11:1527–1530, 1990.
60. Heckbert SR, Weiss NS, Hornung SK, Eaton DL, Motulsky AG. Glutathione S-transferase and epoxide hydroxylase activity in human leukocytes in relation to risk of lung cancer and other smoking-related cancers. J Natl Cancer Inst 84:414–422, 1992.
61. Gatti RA. Localizing the genes for ataxia-telangiectasia: a human model for inherited cancer susceptibility. Adv Cancer Res 56:77–104, 1991.
62. Swift M, Reitrauer PJ, Morrell D, Chase CL. Breast and other cancers in families with ataxia-telangiectasia. N Engl J Med 316:1289–1294, 1987.
63. Gantt R, Parshad R, Price FM, Sanford KK. Biochemical evidence for deficient DNA repair leading to enhanced G2 chromatid radiosensitivity and susceptibility to cancer. Radiat Res 108:117–126, 1986.
64. Pero RW, Miller DG, Lipkin M, et al. Reduced capacity for DNA repair synthesis in patients with or genetically predisposed to colorectal cancer. J Natl Cancer Inst 70:867–875, 1982.
65. Chan JY, Becker FF, German J, Ray JH. Altered DNA ligase I activity in Bloom's syndrome cells. Nature 325:357–359, 1987.
66. Hsu TC. Genetic predisposition to cancer with special reference to mutagen sensitivity. In Vitro Cell Dev Biol 23:591–603, 1987.
67. Hsu TC, Johnston DA, Cherry LM, Ramkissoon D, Schantz SP, Jessup JM, et al. Sensitivity to genotoxic effects of bleomycin in humans: possible relationship to environmental carcinogenesis. Int J Cancer 43:403–409, 1989.
68. Spitz MR, Fueger JJ, Beddingfield NA, Annegers JF, Hsu TC, Newell GR, et al. Chromosome sensitivity to bleomycin-induced mutagenesis: an independent risk factor for upper aerodigestive tract cancers. Cancer Res 49:4626–4628, 1989.
69. Spitz MR, Fueger JJ, Halabi S, Schantz SP, Sample D, Hsu TC. Mutagen sensitivity in upper aerodigestive tract cancer: a case-control analysis. Cancer Epidemiol Biomarkers Prev 2:329–333, 1993.
70. Bondy ML, Spitz MR, Halabi S, Fueger JJ, Schantz SP, Sample D, Hsu TC. Association between family history of cancer and mutagen sensitivity in upper aerodigestive tract cancer patients. Cancer Epidemiol Biomarkers Prev 2:103–106, 1993.
71. Schantz SP, Spitz MR, Hsu TC. Mutagen sensitivity in patients with head and neck cancers: a biologic marker for risk of multiple primary malignancies. J Natl Cancer Inst 82:1773–1775, 1990.
72. Spitz MR, Hoque A, Trizna Z, Schantz SP, Amos CI, Bondy ML, Hong WK, Hsu TC. Mutagen sensitivity as a risk factor for second malignant tumors following upper aerodigestive tract malignancies. J Natl Cancer Inst, in press, 1994.
73. Cloos J, Braakhuis BJM, Steen I, et al. Increased mutagen sensitivity in head and neck squamous cell carcinoma patients, particularly those with multiple primary tumors. Cancer Lett 74:161–165, 1993.
74. Hsu TC, Furlong C, Spitz MR. Ethyl alcohol as a cocarcinogen with special reference to the aerodigestive tract: a cytogenetic study. Anticancer Res 325:357–359, 1991.

5. Biology and reversal of aerodigestive tract carcinogenesis

Scott M. Lippman, Gary L. Clayman, Martin H. Huber, Steven E. Benner, and Waun Ki Hong

Squamous cell carcinoma of the upper aerodigestive tract is a cosmetically, functionally, and economically devastating class of diseases yet to come under control with standard approaches to prevention, early detection, or therapy [1,2]. Three principle modalities are currently used to control this disease: tobacco/alcohol cessation programs, surgery and radiotherapy for early and local-regional advanced disease, and chemotherapy in advanced, recurrent, and metastatic disease.

The major aerodigestive tract cancers (head and neck, lung, and esophagus) are linked by a single causative agent — tobacco. The worldwide incidence of upper aerodigestive tract cancers has remained unchanged for two decades despite the availability of tobacco-cessation programs. Tobacco-use figures are staggering. Worldwide, there are approximately one billion smokers and 600 million chewers. Respective figures for the United States alone are 50 million smokers and 12 million chewers, and dissappointing recent Centers for Disease Control (CDC) figures indicate that, for the first time in many years, overall U.S. smoking rates are increasing [3]. This is a recent and worrisome trend, occurring in the face of increasingly intensive somking-cessation efforts. These figures indicate the exigent need for chemoprevention approaches as adjuncts to continued smoking-cessation research, to control this group of tobacco-related cancers.

During the past 20–30 years, only marginal improvement in overall survival has occurred for patients with early and locally advanced squamous cell carcinoma of the head and neck. This is true even though standard therapy of surgery and/or radiotherapy and newer neoadjuvant chemotherapy can effectively control primary tumors [1,2].

Despite successful primary therapy of advanced local and regional disease, 50–60% of head and neck cancer patients wil die from local recurrences, 20–30% will die from distant metastases, and 10–40% will die from second primary tumors. Although patients with early stage disease can be

Hong, Waun Ki and Weber, Randal S., (eds.), Head and Neck Cancer. © 1995 Kluwer Academic Publishers. ISBN 0-7923-3015-3. All rights reserved.

treated effectively with single modality local therapy (surgery or radio-therapy), these patients have an additional 4–7% annual risk of developing second primary tumors, the principle cancer-related cause of death in early-stage disease [4]. Long-term survivors, regardless of disease stage, are subject to the development of second primary tumors [5]. These troubling data reveal the need for effective chemopreventive approaches to increase survival for 'cured' head and neck cancer patients.

There is a great effort, therefore, directed to the development of effective new strategies to control these cancers. One new approach under study is cancer chemoprevention, the use of specific agents to stop carcinogenesis and to prevent the development of invasive cancer [6–13]. This field of clinical investigation emerged from laboratory and epidemiologic studies indicating the presence of thousands of potential inhibitors of carcinogenesis. The basic concepts of field carcinogenesis and multistep carcinogenesis underlie the expanding arena of chemoprevention.

Tumor biology

The basic concepts of multistep carcinogenesis and field carcinogenesis have opened the door for modern intervention research in the head and neck region. Epithelial carcinogenesis involves the progressive accumulation of genetic alterations, dysregulated epithelial proliferation and cell differention, the selected outgrowth of premalignant cells, invasion, and metastasis. The clinical premise of chemoprevention is that carcinogenesis, at least in early (premalignant) stages, is reversible, a concept supported by preclinical and epidemiologic data [14–31].

A central theme that links the upper aerodigestive tract and lung is the concept of field carcinogenesis — the multifocal development of pre-malignant (and malignant) lesions at various stages of carcinogenesis and that progress at various rates within the entire aerodigestive tract or 'field', exposed to diffuse and repeated primarily tobacco-related carcinogenic assault. Local therapy is inadequate in the face of these fieldwide developments.

Field carcinogenesis was initially described in the oral mucosa by Slaughter et al. [32]. Using standard histologic methods, Slaughter found widespread microscopic abnormalities in resected tissue specimens taken from epithelia surrounding the area of the primary carcinoma in patients with squamous cell carcinoma of the head and neck. The primary abnormalities described were epithelial hyperplasia (an increase in the number of rows in the epithelium), hyperkeratinization, and dyskaryosis (atypia). Several sections were also found to contain carcinoma in situ. Furthermore, when serial sections of the entire surgical specimen were studied, separate foci of carcinoma in situ or invasive carcinoma were frequent findings overall and found in all cases in which the primary tumor was less than 1 cm in diameter. Based on these observations, Slaughter coined the term *field cancerization* to describe the phenomenon of diffuse carcinogenic changes surrounding cancer. This finding implies a wide tissue area of risk that transcends the margins of the primary cancer. This phenomenon has also been referred to as *field carcinogenesis* and the *condemned mucosa syndrome*.

This field effect concept is certainly supported by prospective studies of head and neck cancer that have documented second primary tumor rates of 6–7% per year [5]. Furthermore, the site patterns of second primary tumor development indicate that over 80% occur within the tissue field of presumed risk from direct tobacco and alcohol exposure, the major aero-digestive tract carcinogens.

Forty years after Slaughter's initial report, this concept has been studied at the cellular and molecular level. Our group and others have used the same basic approach of assessing nonmalignant epithelia surrounding squamous cell carcinoma from resected tumor specimens using sensitive biologic probes to detect phenotypic (proliferation and differentiation) and genotypic abnormalities [33–39]. In addition, we and others are using these molecular and cellular probes to dissect the diverse nature of the clinical-histologic premalignant lesion.

Our studies of resected tumor specimens analyzed adjacent epithelia grouped by histologic stage of carcinogenesis: adjacent 'normal' tissue, hyperplasia, and dysplasia. The results of these phenotypic and genotypic marker studies were compared with each case's squamous carcinoma and with a true normal control (tissue from a volunteer without cancer).

We have studied two growth-related markers: proliferating-cell nuclear antigen and epidermal growth factor receptor. Proliferating-cell nuclear antigen is associated with DNA synthesis and cell cycle regulation, and therefore a potential marker of tissue dysregulation of proliferation. Proliferating-cell nuclear antigen, as determined by monoclonal antibody labeling, increased with histologic progression [36]. Furthermore, there was also evidence of proliferative dysregulation occurring from the basal to superficial epithelium. Epidermal growth factor receptor expression was studied as a marker of cell growth regulation. Again using monoclonal antibody techniques, dysregulation of epidermal growth factor receptor expression was increasingly observed with histologic progression to invasive squamous carcinoma.

In addition to the phenotypic changes described above, we have analyzed head and neck cancers and surrounding nonmalignant tissue for genotypic alterations that may be associated with field and multistep carcinogenesis. Using in situ hybridization techniques with centromeric probes to chromosomes 7 and 17, increasing polysomy was associated with the transition from histologically normal mucosa to invasive cancers [35]. Supporting the definition of a premalignant state and the concept of field carcinogenesis were genetic changes detected in regions of histologically normal epithelium in one third of cases studied. Chromosome polysomy was not found in mucosa of healthy nonsmoking volunteers.

We have also studied the tumor suppressor gene p53. Wild-type p53 has tumor suppressor function, while some mutations of the p53 gene have tumor promotor activity. We found marked variability of p53 expression in different areas of the cancer, which further indicates the marked heterogeneity of tumors. Furthermore, the frequency of p53 gene mutations increased with histologic progression. Detection of p53 mutations in hyperplasia and dysplasia adjacent to squamous cell carcinoma and in oral premalignant lesions [40] may indicate that p53 loss is an early molecular genetic event in head and neck carcinogenesis, and differs from colon and bladder carcinogenesis, in which p53 mutation occurs late [41,42].

The presence of p53 mutations in carcinogenic lesions has been previously documented in other tumors of the aerodigestive tract [43–45]. Sozzi et al. [38,39] identified p53 mutations in adjacent dysplastic lesions in three patients whose primary lung cancer had a p53 mutation using immunohistochemistry. Single-strand conformational polymorphism analysis in two cases revealed that the same exon was affected in both the primary tumor and the adjacent dysplastic tissue.

The presence of p53 alterations has also been demonstrated in preneoplastic lesions of the oral mucosa. Girod et al. [40] used an antibody to p53 protein to demonstrate p53 protein accumulation in premalignant lesions of the oral mucosa. The antibody was initially shown to stain positive in the presence of a p53 mutation; then, tissue sections of oral premalignant lesions and squamous cell carcinomas of the oral mucosa were evaluated.

P53 accumulation was not only present in invasive squamous cell cancers of the head and neck, but was also found in premalignant lesions. While 53% of all 104 sections containing squamous cell carcinomas were positive, 28.4% of the 64 sections with premalignant alterations without carcinoma also contained p53 protein [40]. In addition, investigators have also identified oncogenes in head and neck squamous carcinoma, including *int*-2, k-*ras*, c-*myc*, and *bcl*-1 [46–53].

The best available molecular data supporting the concept of field carcinogenesis comes from a recent report by Chung et al. [54], who evaluated p53 mutations in head and neck squamous cell carcinoma and their second primary tumors of either squamous cell carcinoma or other histologies. This study found the primary lesion and second primary tumors to have discordant mutations. In this study, tissue samples were collected from 31 patients who had surgery for squamous cell carcinomas of the head and neck and later developed second primary cancers of either the head and neck, esophagus, or lung. Second primary tumors were defined as occurring at least 3 years after the initial primary occurrence and geographic separation from the original site by at least 2 cm. Head and neck second primary tumors occurred in 17 patients, lung second primary tumors in 12 patients, and esophagus tumors in 2.

A total of 66 samples from the 31 patients were analyzed using single-strand conformation polymorphism analysis. Mutations of p53 were identified in 13 of the 31 (42%) initial primary tumors and 13 of 35 (37%) second primary tumors. Twenty-one of the patients had p53 mutation in either the initial primary tumors and/or their second primary tumors. Only 5 of these 21 patients had a p53 mutation in both the primary head and neck cancer and in their second primary tumor, and in each of these cases, regardless of histologic subtype, the p53 mutations were shown to be discordant.

This study provides supportive evidence at the molecular level for field carcinogenesis in head and neck squamous cell carcinoma. It is possible, however, that the apparent discordance reflects tumor heterogeneity, that is, differences in p53 mutation within a single tumor. Presumably cancer cells with a mutated p53 gene have a selective growth and metastatic advantage. Molecular characterization of p53 may become an important tool in the differential diagnosis of recurrence (local, regional, or distant) versus second primary tumors in lesions of squamous cell histology.

Clinical trials and promising agents

Multiple-site primary prevention trials

These large trials are attempting to demonstrate an association between chemoprevention and a reduction in cancer incidence. The trial design assumes that the beneficial effects of the agent in cancer prevention will result in an overall reduction in cancer incidence. In the United States, the Physicians' Health Study was designed to study the effects of beta-carotene and aspirin on the incidence of cancer and cardiovascular disease [55]. The study is a randomized, double-blind, placebo-controlled trial, begun in 1982, involving 22,071 male physicians. A more recently begun trial, the Women's Health Study, will determine the impact of beta-carotene, vitamin E, and aspirin on cancer and cardiovascular disease in 40,000 female nurses [56]. These broad multiple-site primary prevention trials are quite large and require long-term follow-up, which adds to expense and logistical difficulties. If the trials have positive results, however, they could have a significant public health impact.

Upper aerodigestive tract and lung

To date, the best-studied system for cancer chemoprevention in humans is the epithelial malignancies of the upper aerodigestive tract and lungs. In the United States, these malignancies account for 30% of cancer deaths [57]. The field cancerization hypothesis [32,58], which predicts diffuse epithelial injury as the result of inhaled carcinogens, has guided the development of these sutdies. Clinical evidence for field carcinogenesis is found in the occurrence of premalignant lesions and multiple primary tumors. Recent molecular studies of *p53* mutations, reviewed above, provide further evidence for field carcinogenesis in the upper aerodigestive tract.

Large randomized clinical trials in a general population testing chemoprevention agents specifically directed at reducing the incidence of head and neck cancer are logistically difficult to perform. First, because the incidence of head and neck cancer in the general U.S. population is very low, massive numbers of subjects would be required. Second, the primary endpoint, the development of cancer, will require 5–10 + years to occur and therefore require long-term follow-up and compliance. Last, since only a few subjects in a general population will develop a malignancy, a large number of subjects will be exposed to possible drug toxicity, with potential benefit to only a few. The logistical difficulty and cost of such a trial is therefore not reasonable or practical to assess primary chemoprevention strategies for head and neck cancer. Studies have thus been directed at individuals with premalignant or early stage lesions (treated) in the chemoprevention of invasive cancers (or reversal of premalignant lesions) and second primary malignancies, respectively.

Trials in premalignant lesions

Premalignant lesions serve as excellent models for chemoprevention studies. The occurrence of the lesions themselves identifies individuals at high risk for invasive cancer. Changes in the size or extent of the lesions may be used to assess the efficacy of the chemopreventive agent. In the oral cavity, leukoplakia has been used to study both clinical and histologic responses to therapy.

Oral leukoplakia, the most common premalignant lesion in the upper aerodigestive tract, has undergone extensive chemoprevention study. The lesion is essentially a diagnosis of exclusion, defined clinically as a white mucosal patch anywhere in the oral cavity or oropharynx that cannot be rubbed off and not otherwise classified into another specific disease entity [59–62]. In clinical trials, we use the term *oral premalignancy* to refer to the clinical spectrum of oral lesions from whitish (low-risk) to reddish (erythroplakia) or red-white (mixed; erythroleukoplakia) high-risk lesions, with further classification and stratification based upon histology (presence and degree of dysplasia).

Many characteristics of oral premalignancy make it an excellent human system for the study of chemoprevention. First, it is a well-described precursor of oral cancer. Second it is commonly found in patients with oral cancer. Leukoplakia has been found near oral cancer in as high as 100% (median, 30–40%) of cases in some series [61]. Furthermore, prospective series have documented the association of leukoplakia with a high risk of later development of oral cancer. The largest U.S. series (over 250 patients), conducted by Silverman et al. [60], found that the long-term overall transformation rate was 18%. Transformation rates in this and other series doubled in high-risk dysplastic lesions. The natural history of leukoplakia and other premalignant conditions has been further defined by randomized studies involving placebo arms and periodic biopsies and observation. Up to 30–40% of lesions may spontaneously regress, however, rarely completely. Contrastingly, over 50% of patients presenting with leukoplakia may experience histologic progression. Most importantly, marked histologic heterogeneity may present within lesions ranging from hyperkeratosis without dysplasia to areas of severe dysplasia and carcinoma in situ. Thus clinical trials must provide close observation and repeated histologic analysis to ensure patient safety from disease progression. The variable natural history, especially the substantial spontaneous regression rates, underscore the need for randomization in clinical chemoprevention trials of oral premalignancy.

The second major attribute of this system is that the oral cavity and oropharnx are easily and noninvasively monitored, which contrasts with the colon and lung, which require invasive procedures (e.g., colonoscopy and bronchoscopy) to detect and monitor the carcinogenic process. The accessibility of these lesions and the ease of performing repeat biopsies has led to the frequent incorporation of intermedate marker studies into these trials [34].

Third, and perhaps the most important attribute of this model system, is its implications for other aerodigestive tract epithelial cancers. Oral premalignancy chemoprevention studies already have contributed to the design of a retinoid trial discussed later that achieved significant suppression of second primary tumors in head and neck cancer patients.

Although high-risk dysplastic lesions account for only 10–20% of all oral premalignant lesions, this represents hundreds of thousands of individuals worldwide. A significant percentage of cases with advanced premalignant lesions are not amenable to local approaches because of the diffuse field carcinogenic process with multiple precancerous foci. Therefore, a systemic intervention within the premalignant process, or chemoprevention, is necessary for control of many high-risk lesions. No standard systemic approach now exists.

Retinoids

This class of over 3000 natural derivatives and synthetic analogues of vitamin A includes the best studied agents in preclinical and clinical chemoprevention testing [8,63–65]. Retinoids have potent effects on premalignant, and malignant cell growth and differentiation in many human systems that are thought to be the result of modulation of gene expression. By far, the major advance in the understanding of the molecular mechanism of action by which retinoids affect gene expression is the discovery of nuclear retinoid receptors [64–66]. The first nuclear receptor, identified and reported independently and simultaneously by two steroid receptor laboratories, was named *retinoic acid receptor* (RAR) *alpha*. Subsequently, two additional receptors in this class (beta and gamma) have been identified from human cells. The three RAR subtypes have sequence homology to the steroid receptor family, which is strongest in the DNA-binding domain. More recently, another nuclear retinoic acid class was identified and named *retinoid-X receptor* (RXR), with the X used only to distinguish this class from RARs, which have a vastly different DNA sequence. RXR-α, -β, and -γ subtypes have also been identified. To further complicate the nuclear retinoid receptor class, each receptor subtype (e.g., RAR-α) has multiple isoforms, the significance of which is not yet known.

These two fundamentally different receptor classes may represent distinct retinoid response pathways. Nuclear retinoid receptors act as ligand-activated DNA-binding proteins that modulate gene transcription by interacting with responsive elements in the promotor region of specific genes. Current data suggest that different receptor subtypes have distinct functions because of their different tissue distributions and retinoid binding affinity patterns. For example, RAR-α specifically binds to *trans*-retinoic acid with high affinity and the only known natural RXR ligand is 9-*cis*-retinoic acid. Intensive current efforts are presently directed to evaluate nuclear retinoid receptor-targeted retinoids alone and in combination (i.e., combining RAR- and RXR-specific retinoid analogs). It appears likely that these nuclear receptors are the primary mediators of retinoid's effects on carcinogenesis, although direct evidence to support this is limited.

Chemoprevention trials in oral premalignancy were initially reported in the late 1950s [67–69]. Early trials focused on systemic or topical vitamin A. Subsequent trials have explored the efficacy of other retinoids. To date, over 350 patients with leukoplakia have been treated with eight different retinoids in prospective studies [63,67–77]. Response rates have in each case exceeded 50% (median response rate >70%). The activity of retinoids in this setting are unquestioned and have been established in five randomized trials (Table 1). However, dose-related mucocutaneous toxicity is the major issue to contend with in this class of agents.

The first study of synthetic retinoids in oral leukoplakia was reported by Koch [71]. Seventy-five patients with leukoplakia (with or without epithelial dysplasia) were treated with all-*trans*-retinoic acid, 13-*cis* retinoic acid, or etretinate. The study design included an 8 week induction followed by a lower dose maintenance period. The induction response rates were 59%, 87%, and 91%, respectively. With 2–6 years of follow-up, over 40% of patients (43%, 45%, and 51%, respectively, for the three retinoid groups) remained in prolonged remission.

Among the five randomized trials reported involving four different retinoids — 13-*cis*-retinoic acid (two trials), natural vitamin A, and two retinamides — three of these are placebo-controlled induction trials and two are maintenance trials. All have observed statistically significant retinoid activity.

96

Table 1. Completed randomized chemoprevention trials: Head and neck cancer

Author (year)	Study setting	Design (N)	Agents	Result
Hong (1986)	Oral leukoplakia	Phase IIb (44)	Isotretinoin	Positive
Stich (1988)	Oral leukoplakia	Phase IIb (65)	Vitamin A	Positive
Han (1990)	Oral leukoplakia	Phase IIb (61)	Retinamide	Positive
Lippman (1993)	Oral leukoplakia	Phase IIb (70) (maintenance)	Isotretinoin	Positive
Chiesa (1993)	Oral leukoplakia	Phase IIb (80) (maintenance)	Fenretinide	Positive
Hong (1990)	Prior SCC	Phase III (103)	Isotretinoin	Positive (SPT)

SPT = second primary tumor; SCC = squamous cell carcinoma.

Induction trials

Hong et al. [73] determined the effects of 13-*cis*-retinoic acid on oral leuko-plakia in a randomized trial in 44 patients. Patients were required to have histologically confirmed oral leukoplakia and were excluded if they were consuming megadoses of vitamin A. Patients were randomized to receive either 13-*cis*-retinoic acid, 1–2 mg/kg/day, or placebo for 3 months followed by 6 months of follow-up off treatment. Cheilitis, facial erythema, and dryness and/or peeling of the skin were noted in 19 of 24 patients (79%), conjunctivitis in 13 of 24 (54%), and hypertriglyceridemia in 17 of 24 (71%) receiving retinoic acid, but the toxicity was generally tolerable as only 2 of the 24 patients randomized to receive 13-*cis*-retinoic acid were unable to complete the study. Two patients were inevaluable in the placebo arm, though none secondary to toxicity.

Major responses, complete or partial remissions, were noted in 16 of the 24 patients randomized to receive 13-*cis*-retinoic acid, whereas only 2 of the 20 patients on placebo had similar responses. This difference was highly significant, p = 0.0002. Thirteen of the 24 patients on 13-*cis*-retinoic acid had reversal of their dysplasia on biopsy, which was noted in only 2 of the 20 patients on placebo. Several of the patients relapsed in the follow-up portion of the trial, typically within 2–3 months. This study, therefore, clearly demonstrated the efficacy of 13-*cis*-retinoic acid in treating oral leukoplakia, but also raised several other questions. While quite effective, relapses off drug were frequent, which indicates a possible need for maintenance therapy, which was addressed in a subsequent study. Second, while 1–2 mg/kg/day is tolerable for a short period of time, it was unlikely to be as well tolerated for longer time periods; therefore, further exploration to identify the optimal dose was needed. Finally, while the premalignant lesion, oral leukoplakia was reversed, larger patient populations and longer follow-up will be required to determine if the reversal of the premalignant lesion is associated with a decreased risk of developing cancer.

The second randomized trial used N-4-(hydroxycarbophenyl) retinamide as a cancer prevention agent for the treatment of oral leukoplakia [74]. Patients were randomized to receive either the retinamide 40 mg orally per day and 40 mg topically per day or placebo. Major responses were noted in 27 of the 31 patients on treatment (87.1%), including patients with complete remissions. Only 5 of the 30 patients on placebo (16.7%) had major responses and none were complete remissions. Toxicity was noted to be minimal and consisted of minor elevations of serum transaminases in two patients. No data on skin toxicity are available. These data are of import as this compound is very similar to another synthetic retinoid, 4-hydroxphenyl retinamide, which is currently being evaluated in several clinical trials.

Stich et al. [75] evaluated the effects of vitamin A in 65 tobacco users or betel nut chewers with oral leukoplakia in India. This sample population has a high exposure to carcinogens, as they maintain a quid containing tobacco and betel leaf against their oral mucosa. Thirty participants were randomly assigned to receive 100,000 IU of vitamin A twice weekly, and 35 individuals were randomly assigned to placebo. Little change in their oral habits was noted during the course of the study, and compliance was excellent in the patients who completed the trial, as medication was administered under nursing supervision. However, only 21 of the 30 patients randomized to receive vitamin A were evaluable, and the authors do not account for this discrepancy. Among these 21 patients in the vitamin A group, 12 subjects (57.1%) had complete remissions, 9 (42.9%) had no change, and no patients developed new leukoplakia lesions. Among the 33 evaluable subjects in the placebo group, only one patient (3.0%) had a complete remission, lesions of 25 subjects (75.8%) did not change, and 7 (21.2%) progressed. The results of this study again confirm the efficacy of retinoids in inducing remissions of oral leukoplakia lesions.

Maintenance trials

We recently reported the effects of low dose 13-*cis*-retinoic acid versus β-carotene as maintenance therapy after high-dose 13-*cis*-retinoic acid [76]. Seventy patients with biopsy proven oral leukoplakia received 13-*cis*-retinoic acid 1.5 mg/kg/day for 3 months. Sixty-six of these patients were evaluable at the end of induction therapy, and 59 of these who had either remission or stable disease were randomized to receive either β-carotene, 30 mg/day, or 13-*cis*-retinoic acid, 0.5 mg/kg/day. Only 2 of the 24 who completed 9 months of 13-*cis*-retinoic acid progressed, whereas 16 of the 29 on β-carotene progressed (p < 0.001).

In a second study, Chiesa et al. [77] randomized 115 patients following resection of oral leukoplakia to receive either N-(4-hydroxyphenyl)-

retinamide (fenretinide; 4HPR) 200 mg/day or placebo for 1 year. The initial report of this study identified 12 local relapses or new lesions in the 41 patients in the control, whereas only three patients relapsed among the 39 patients receiving fenretinide. Toxicity was minimal and consisted primarily of dermatitis and mild hyperbilirubinemia.

The randomized trials by our group and the Milan group are comparable in that both studies defined the efficacy of synthetic retinoids in preventing relapses following primary therapy of oral leukoplakia. The studies differ in design in that the first trial follows patients after induction with higher dose retinoid therapy, whereas the second study follows surgical remissions. However, the final results are similar and statistically significant. First, the β-carotene in our trial and the placebo arm in the Italian trial had high relapse (or progression) rates at 1 year, 55% and 29%, respectively. Second, the treatment arms in both trials had very similar low progression rates, 8% and 7.7%, respectively.

Nonrandomized trials

β-carotene

The rationale for studying this agent includes its strong epidemiologic data in squamous cell carcinoma of the lung, antioxidant structure and pro-vitamin A activity in vivo, lack of clinical toxicity, low cost, and wide availability. Perhaps its greatest attribute for chemoprevention is its lack of acute clinical toxicity. It only produces a dose-dependent yellowing of the skin. However, a potentially adverse micronutrient interaction has been reported with profound suppression of plasma vitamin E levels after pharmacological β-carotene dosing in animals and humans [78].

Several nonrandomized trials have tested β-carotene in oral leukoplakia [79–81]. These trials included diverse groups of patients (smokers, snuff, betel nut), response criteria and evaluation, doses, and schedules. Response rates have varied widely, with no apparent relationship to dose.

Stich et al. [79] first reported the effects of β-carotene on oral leukoplakia in a three-arm trial in tobacco/betel nut chewers. A total of 130 individuals were divided into three groups and received either β-carotene 180 mg per week, vitamin A 100,000 IU per week and β-carotene 180 mg per week, or placebo. Only one patient (3.0%) of the 33 evaluable patients in the placebo group had a complete remission at the end of 6 months of therapy, and seven patients (21.2%) progressed. In the β-carotene only group 27 patients were evaluable, and 4 patients (14.8%) were in complete remission and 4 patients (14.8%) developed new leukoplakia. Finally, in the 51 evaluable patients receiving both agents, 14 (27.5%) were in complete remission and only 4 (7.8%) developed new lesions. The combination of both agents was significantly better than placebo with regards to complete remission rates (p = 0.004). The difference between β-carotene alone and placebo was not statistically significant.

α-tocopherol

This vitamin is another nontoxic lipid-phase antioxidant under intensive study in chemoprevention. The only oral leukoplakia study, reported recently, suggested drug activity. Forty-three participants with either symptomatic lesions or epithelial dysplasia were treated with α-tocopherol 400 IU twice daily for 24 weeks on a Community Clinical Oncology Program (CCOP) study [82,83]. This trial, the first multicenter oral leukoplakia chemoprevention trial, reported substantial logistic problems, raising important feasibility issues for multicenter studies of this premalignant lesion. Unfortunately, 12 subjects were not evaluable for clinical response. Clinical complete responses were observed in 10 subjects (23%) and partial responses in 10 subjects (23%), giving an overall major response rate of 46%.

The study effectively monitored plasma drug levels and reported a two- to threefold increase in plasma levels with the 800 IU per day dose. Toxicity was minimal. Only one subject reported grade 2 headache, and the remaining 14 complaints of toxicity were evaluated as grade 1.

As with β-carotene and all promising new agents, randomized trials (placebo-controlled) will be required to establish the activity of α-tocopherol in oral chemoprevention. Preclinical and clinical data support the study of α-tocopherol plus β-carotene. In addition, this agent may play an important role in combination with 13cRA based on its apparent independent activity and its reported ability to ameliorate mucocutaneous and lipid retinoid toxicities.

Our current oral leukoplakia study is an evolutionary stage following two previous randomized studies. These predecessor trials established the efficacy of a high dose of 13-cis-retinoic acid in reversing oral premalignant lesions and the efficacy of low-dose 13-cis-retinoic acid in maintaining response. Our current goal is to establish either less or completely nontoxic chemoprevention for long-term use in the oral region. This study disposed entirely of the toxic, high-dose 13-cis-retinoic acid phase present in our earlier studies. Our current long-term randomized trial is comparing low-dose 13-cis-retinoic acid and the combination of the two natural, nontoxic agents, vitamin A (retinyl palmitate) and β-carotene.

The study has three main objectives. First, we will evaluate the chemopreventive efficacy of the vitamin A–β-carotene combination. Second, we will evaluate the efficacy and toxicity of long term low dose 13-cis-retinoic acid. Third, this study will contribute data and tissue samples to the evaluations of a series of potential biomarkers of intermediate endpoints of carcinogenesis.

Selection of the β-carotene plus vitamin A regimen for this trial is based on favorable activity and toxicity data from both preclinical and clinical studies. Preclinical studies of the regimen have occurred in two epithelial systems. Combined β-carotene and retinol are active and synergistic in inhibiting certain types of carcinogen-induced lung cancer. Similar positive results have been reported in the ultraviolet-B mouse-skin model [84].

Data are available from two clinical chemoprevention trials employing this combination. In a large-scale trial of subjects at high risk for lung cancer, investigators from Seattle have established that this regimen is safe and nontoxic for at least 5 years [85]. Only one clinical trial has reported efficacy results. The trial by Stich and coworkers [79], discussed earlier, achieved a 28% complete remission rate with this combination in Asian betel nut chewers. This activity rate was twofold higher than that of their β-carotene group and ninefold higher than that of placebo. However, Stich's trial was not strictly randomized and the results were unconfirmed histologically.

Unresolved issues

Three unresolved issues face investigators of chemoprevention regimens for oral premalignancy. The major clinical issue is that of the delicate balance between toxicity and efficacy. Our approach to this problem over the past 10 years has been to evolve trials with larger study populations, decreasing drug doses of 13-*cis*-retinoic acid and longer term intervention. Our first randomized trial included 44 subjects treated for 3 months with high-dose 13-*cis*-retinoic acid. Our second randomized trial included 70 subjects treated for 12 months with a lower dose of 13-*cis*-retinoic acid or β-carotene. Our current randomized trial will include 120 subjects treated for 3 years with even lower dose of 13-*cis*-retinoic acid or the promising nontoxic combination of vitamin A plus β-carotene. This long-term trial will provide assessments of early marker changes against late marker and clinical evaluations, possibly even against invasive cancer. This study's low-dose retinoid and nontoxic natural agent regimens will provide consistent doses throughout study.

Another major unresolved issue is the impact of diet and tobacco on the natural history of this disorder. Current studies in this setting should include rigorous monitoring of dietary assessment and plasma micronutrient levels as a means for studying this issue. Intensive smoking cessation counseling and biochemical monitoring (e.g., cotinine levels) should also be formally integrated into these trials.

The last major unresolved issue concerns the biology of preneoplasia. A better understanding of this biology is required to develop fundamentally new and better approaches for its control. Clinical trials in this premalignancy setting must include systematic studies of genomic, proliferation, and differentiation markers to provide data on the biology of multistep carcinogenesis and chemoprevention.

Several lung chemoprevention trials used progressive changes in the bronchial epithelium, such as metaplasia or dysplasia, as a study endpoint [86–
90] (Table 2). Gouveia et al. [88] reported an uncontrolled trial of etretinate
(25 mg per day) for 6 months. They found this agent to be highly effective
in reversing squamous metaplasia read from biopsy specimens in heavy
smokers. They reported a reduction in metaplasia index in 29 of 40 participants; the mean metaplasia index decreased from 34.75% before treatment
to 26.96% following the retinoid therapy.

A recent chemoprevention trial, using isotretinoin, also employed histologic studies of bronchoscopic biopsies to examine the intermediate endpoint
of squamous metaplasia [89]. This study also included randomization to
isotretinoin or placebo groups in order to confirm the activity reported in
the earlier uncontrolled trial. The authors reported a substantial reduction
in the extent of squamous metaplasia in 35 isotretinoin-treated patients
(54.3%) and 34 placebo-treated patients (58.8%), indicating that isotretinoin
at the given dose and schedule had no impact on reversal of squamous
metaplasia, re-emphasizing the critical importance of controlled trials in
studies using intermediate endpoints or in studies that hope to verify preliminary findings of positive drug activity.

Arnold et al. reached a similar conclusion in a recently reported randomized trial of etretinate for the reversal of metaplasia read from sputum
samples [90]. Of the 138 participants in this study who completed 6 months
treatment with etretinate (25 mg per day) or placebo, 32.4% of the 71
etretinate-treated patients and 29.8% of the 67 placebo-treated patients had
improvement in sputum atypia.

These trials have established that retinoids have no effect on metaplasia,
but the significant response of metaplasia to smoking cessation and its
significant spontaneous variability indicate that metaplasia may be one

Table 2. Completed randomized chemoprevention trials: Lung cancer

Author (year)	Study setting	Design (N)	Agents	Result
Heimburger (1988)	Metaplasia (sputum)	Phase IIb (73)	Vitamin B12, folic acid	Positive (atypia)
Arnold (1992)	Metaplasia (sputum)	Phase IIb (150)	Etretinate	Negative
Van Poppel (1992)	Micronuclei (sputum)	Phase IIb (114)	β-carotene	Positive
Lees (1993)	Metaplasia (biopsy)	Phase IIb (87)	Isotretinoin	Negative
Pastorino (1993)	Prior NSCLC	Phase III (307)	Retinyl palmitate	Positive (SPT)

NSCLC = Non-small cell lung cancer; SPT = second primary tumor.

of the earliest stages in the carcinogenic process. Retinoids have shown activity in later stages of the carcinogenic process, and it is therefore possible that they are active in later stages of lung premalignancy. The activity of retinoids in the chemoprevention of lung cancer remains to be established in future trials using intermediate biomarkers that more directly reflect stages of carcinogenesis.

Intermediate endpoints

Aerodigestive tract epithelial carcinogenesis is an extremely complex multistep process. Rather late, clinical and histologic markers (e.g., dysplastic oral leukoplakia) of this process are not capable of detecting the subtle cellular, molecular, and biochemical changes occurring in the earliest preneoplastic phases. New markers of subtle intermediate stages, or endpoints, of the multistep process are being developed in preclinical and clinical studies. Called *intermediate endpoint biomarkers*, these markers may provide far earlier and more specific indicators of cancer risk and drug efficacy in prevention trials than current standard clinical and histologic evaluations [34].

The data regarding oral leukoplakia, which represents the intermediate clinical marker with the strongest association with the development of head and neck cancer, has been reviewed above. However, other biomarker intermediate endpoints are being evaluated as indicators of the development of malignancy. Ideally, a specific molecular alteration associated with the development of cancer would be known and reversal of that marker would be associated with reversal of cancer risk, but as previously discussed, the steps in the development of squamous cell carcinoma of the head and neck remain unknown. The most commonly studied intermediate endpoint, to date, in head and neck cancer, aside from oral leukoplakia, is the presence of micronuclei.

Biomarkers in chemoprevention studies

Micronuclei are the best studied potential intermediate endpoint biomarker in subjects at high risk for oral cancer [84]. This genotoxic marker is strongly associated with chromosomal breakage and is formed from chromosome fragments created by clastogenic events (including carcinogenic damage to DNA) in proliferating cells [84,91]. Therefore, the marker reflects ongoing genetic damage. Elevated micronuclei frequencies have been shown to correlate with cancer risk at many sites, including the aerodigestive tract (head and neck, lung, esophagus), cervix, and bladder [83,84,91]. Furthermore, within high risk tissue regions, the micronuclei frequencies are generally higher at lesion sites and sites with the most intense carcinogen exposure, such as where betel quids are held within the mouth. Furthermore, subjects with more intense carcinogen exposure also have higher micronuclei frequencies by an order of magnitude than subjects with less intense exposures (e.g., cigarette smokers). This site-specific and dose-response relationship between carcinogen (clastogen) exposure and micronuclei frequency is an important characteristic of a potential intermediate endpoint marker. The increased micronuclei frequency in normal-appearing oral sites in high risk subjects (betel nut, tobacco exposure) also supports the concept of field carcinogenesis.

Many investigators have used micronuclei data as a short-term in vivo marker as an adjunct to standard clinical and histologic assessments to help screen for active anticarcinogenic agents in animal and human systems. Micronuclei data have been important to the early study of vitamin A and β-carotene as potential chemopreventive agents. Important logistical features that support the study of micronuclei (as part of a marker panel) within the context of a chemoprevention trial include the ability to obtain samples from oral mucosal scrapings (noninvasive) and to measure micronuclei frequency quantitatively.

Stich et al. [92] demonstrated that the frequency of micronuclei in cells obtained from oral mucosa scrapings of betel nut chewers decreased threefold with the administration of retinol and β-carotene. A second trial by Stich et al. [93] evaluated the effects of β-carotene intervention on micronuclei in Inuits who used smokeless tobacco. This population has a diet that leads to normal retinol levels, reflecting the tight homeostasis of serum retinol levels, but results in low levels of β-carotene; therefore, this population allows one to test the hypothesis that restoration of normal β-carotene levels would lead to a decrease in the number of cells containing micronuclei. Twenty-four of the initial 27 subjects who began the trial were evaluable, and in these 24 subjects the mean frequency of cells with micronuclei decreased from 1.87% to 0.74% following 10 weeks of treatment. Finally, in the multi-arm trial of placebo versus β-carotene alone versus β-carotene and retinol by Stich et al. [79] discussed above, the frequency of micronuclei decreased dramatically in both treatment arms and did not decrease significantly in the placebo arm. Also, the decrease in micronuclei was noted in both the leukoplakia lesion and in the surrounding normal mucosa.

Studies of micronuclei and other markers are useful in that they allow the rapid identification of biologic activity for a chemoprevention strategy. However, as discussed in the section on oral leukoplakia, until intermediate endpoints are validated in larger trials with the development of cancer as a primary endpoint, it is critical that these studies not be used as surrogates for prospective randomized trials evaluating the prevention of tumor development.

The most critical long-term issue facing investigators in the new field of intermediate endpoint biomarker research is the establishment of biomarkers that are valid measures of carcinogenesis and chemoprevention. This issue of validation is extremely complicated and difficult, as illustrated by the micronuclei data. Vitamin A, β-carotene, vitamin E, and 13-*cis*-retinoic acid have been reported to produce clinical, and in some studies, histologic, responses. These same agents have achieved reductions in micronuclei frequency. However, there is no association, at least in the short term, between lesion response and suppression of micronuclei. All are early or intermediate markers, and even premalignant lesions are variable. These lesions can progress but not result in invasive cancer, or can regress in advance of cancer.

The correlations between micronuclei and lesion results in several chemo-prevention trials involving different agents is not significant. Over time, discrepancies between micronuclei frequencies and lesion response may disappear. Epithelial carcinogenesis is a multistep process associated with the accumulation of specific genetic alterations and driven by DNA damage, which may be indicated by micronuclei frequency. It seems likely, therefore, that long-term suppression of micronuclei frequency may be associated with a reduction in cancer incidence, the only valid endpoint. In other words, an earliest micronuclei change may be established as correlating with a dysplastic lesion response or invasive cancer occurring years later, at which time the micronuclei changes may have entered an unrelated phase. We anticipate that long-term relationships between biomarkers of various stages of carcinogenesis and its modulation by agents will form the bases of valid panels of intermediate endpoint biomarkers. To date, no markers currently under study have been established as valid intermediate endpoint biomarkers [34,94].

Ideal markers will be those that express early patterns of modulation that correlate directly with later stages of invasive cancer. The immediate task is therefore to continue to pursue positive data from the most promising biomarker candidates for future long-term validation studies.

Second primary tumor prevention

As mentioned above, patients with head and neck cancer are at very high risk of developing a second primary tumor of the upper aerodigestive tract [95]. Retrospective studies of patients with head and neck cancer have identified an increased incidence of second primary tumors [96–101]. The concept of a second malignancy in patients cured of one malignancy is not new, as it was initially described by Bilroth in 1883.

Several recent studies have identified an increased incidence of second primary tumors in patients with a history of head and neck cancer. Christensen et al. [98] identified 21 patients from a series of 415 patients with primary laryngeal cancer who developed second primary tumors of the lung. The overall risk of developing lung cancer was 2.66 in the group with glottic tumors and 6.73 in patients with supraglottic tumors. In a series of 235 patients with laryngeal cancer who received radiation therapy as part of their management, McDonald et al. [101] identified 50 patients who developed 61 second primary tumors, which represented an overall relative risk of developing a second primary tumor of 9.9 compared to a control population. Lung cancer and second head and neck tumors were the most frequent. Cooper et al. [100] evaluated 928 patients treated with radiation therapy for head and neck cancer at all sites and identified 110 second primary tumors, of which 64% developed in the upper aerodigestive tract for an overall risk of developing a second primary tumor of 23% at 8 years. Licciardillo et al. [96] identified an annual incidence of second primary tumors of 4% in some subgroups of patients with head and neck cancer, and an annual incidence as high as 6% in patients with primary cancers of the floor of the mouth. As high as these figures are, retrospective trials are likely to underestimate the true incidence of second primary tumors. For example, in a group of patients followed prospectively following definitive local therapy of stage III or IV head and neck cancers, Vikram et al. [102] identified a 5.3% annual incidence of second primary tumors of the lung, which represented 82% of all second primary tumors in this population.

According to these accumulated data, the overall per-year second primary tumor rate in head and neck cancer patients is constant; surviving patients cannot expect their risk of developing second primary tumors to improve over time. Therefore, the cumulative incidence of second primary tumors is greatest in early stage head and neck cancer patients, who survive the longest after primary treatment. As diagnostic techniques, supportive care measures and treatment of primary lesions continue to improve, however, second primary tumor rates and survival impacts will increase in patients with all types of upper aerodigestive tract and lung epithelial cancers. Current local and systemic approaches do not eliminate or ameliorate the field, or multifocal, cancerization process.

Based mostly on positive oral leukoplakia data, Hong et al. [103] designed an adjuvant chemoprevention study in head and neck cancer patients to determine the efficacy of 13-*cis*-retinoic acid. After definitive local therapy of head and neck cancer with radiotherapy and/or surgery, 103 patients were randomized to receive either 13-*cis*-retinoic acid or placebo for 12 months. Of the first 44 patients randomized, 13 (30%) required dose reductions from $100\,mg/m^2$ to $50\,mg/m^2$ due to toxicity. Therefore, the protocol was modified to a starting dose of $50\,mg/m^2$ for the remaining 59 patients. The major endpoints were primary disease recurrence, the development of a second primary tumor (defined as being of a different histologic type, at a site more than 2 cm from the previous disease, or occurring more than 3 years after the initial diagnosis), and survival. At a median follow-up of 32 months, only 2 of the 51 patients receiving 13-*cis*-retinoic acid developed second primary tumors, whereas 12 of the 49 patients receiving placebo developed second primary tumors (p = 0.005).

In a recent update of this trial (median follow-up of 55 months), 16 patients in the placebo arm had developed second primary tumors, compared with only 7 patients in the retinoid group who developed second primary tumors (31% vs. 14%, p = 0.04) [104]. In a subset analysis of only second primaries within the high-risk field (head and neck, lung and esophagus), a persistent chemopreventive effect was observed on the recent follow-up. This provocative apparent long-lasting retinoid activity (on targeted second primaries) is unprecedented for other clinical or preclinical retinoid carcinogenesis studies. Current studies of larger scale and longer follow-up will further examine this phenomenom.

The applicability of these head and neck findings to other tobacco-related cancers is suggested by a recent report by Pastorino et al. [105] of high dose vitamin A adjuvant therapy in stage-I non-small cell lung cancer. The lung findings are remarkably similar to those of the head and neck cancer study. Both Pastorino et al. and Hong et al. observed a reduction in second primary tumor rates in the retinoid arm. The annual second primary tumor rate was 3.1% in the retinoid arm of both studies. The control arm annual second primary tumor rates were 4.8% for Pastorino's lung study (median follow-up 46 months), and 6.8% for Hong's head and neck study (median follow-up 55 months).

Retinoid treatment, therefore, achieved a 35% reduction in the annual second primary tumor rate in the lung and a 54% reduction in the annual rate of second primary tumor development in the head and neck. It should be noted that the control arm rates of both studies would be higher if the total number of second primary tumors were included, since multiple second primary tumors developed in three patients in the lung study (all in the control group) and in five patients in the head and neck study (four in the placebo group). In both studies, over 70% of second primary tumors occurred in the tobacco-exposed field, and the time to the development of tobacco-related second primary tumors significantly favored the retinoid arms. Primary disease recurrence (local, regional, or distant) was not significantly different between the arms. Neither study was associated with a survival improvement, however, which in part reflects effective surgical salvage of second primary tumors in these prospectively followed patients.

The results of the studies by Pastorino et al. and Hong et al. should serve as an indicator that the problem of second primary tumors in patients with head and neck and lung cancer may currently be under-rated. Both Pastorino et al. and Hong et al. used rigorous criteria to define second primary tumor; in both cases, these criteria were applied to prospectively followed patients, either blindly or by an independent review group. Although the data are limited, it seems significant that both studies have reported control arm second primary tumor rates for head and neck and lung cancer that are roughly twofold higher than retrospective or tumor registry data.

Although smoking indisputably is a major risk factor for the development of primary cancers of the upper aerodigestive tract and lung, the influence of smoking cessation on the rate of second primary tumor development is controversial [106]. Reports by Moore [107,108] and Silverman [109,110] and most other studies do suggest that smoking cessation reduces the incidence of second primary tumors [111–113]. These reports, however, have experienced difficulties in collecting accurate smoking-related data and have lacked biochemical confirmation of smoking behavior (i.e., serum cotinine levels) and therefore do not render a clear quantitative assessment of smoking's impact on second primary tumor development. Some investigators have gone so far as to question the unconfirmed association between smoking and second primary tumor risk [114].

In the Hong and Pastorino studies, smoking had only a minor effect on second primary tumor rate. Smoking cessation may have a greater beneficial effect at earlier stages of the multistep carcinogenic process, or stages that precede advanced premalignant or malignant primary lesions. Other environmental and genetic factors may have influences on second primary tumor development equal to or greater than that of smoking.

All these smoking data indicate that an effective chemopreventive is needed for the prevention of second primary tumors in head and neck cancer patients as an adjunct to the important primary preventive measure of smoking cessation. Although the data are limited, analysis of clinical studies of bronchial metaplasia suggest that the chemopreventive activity of retinoids is enhanced by smoking cessation.

Retinoid toxicity data and the need for long-term therapy suggest the need for continued investigation of new chemopreventive approaches. Promising preclinical results with vitamin E and β-carotene and positive pilot clinical data resulting from vitamin A- and β-carotene treatments of oral leukoplakia suggest these relatively nontoxic natural agents as candidates for future studies in the prevention of second primary tumors in early stage head and neck cancer patients. Also, future adjuvant trials should investigate the efficacy of newer, less-toxic synthetic retinoids. Currently, several large, randomized trials are underway worldwide to determine the efficacy of retinoids in preventing head and neck and lung associated second primary tumors.

The lifetime risk of second primary tumors following early stage head-and-neck or lung cancer is 20–40%. This high rate allows second primary tumor chemoprevention trials to have smaller sample sizes than primary prevention trials. A trial to study the efficacy of low-dose isotretinoin (30 mg/day) to prevent second primary tumors following early stage (I and II) head and neck cancer is being carried out through the Radiation Therapy Oncology Group. In this randomized, double-blind, placebo-controlled trial, 1000 participants will receive 3 years of treatment and an additional 4 years of follow-up. A reduction in the incidence of second primary tumors is the study endpoint. A U.S. intergroup study is using the same design in patients who have had a successful resection of a stage I non-small cell lung cancer.

A European multicenter study, the Euroscan trial, is also studying the efficacy of chemoprevention following head and neck or lung cancer. The Euroscan study consists of two parallel trials, one for each organ site, and is using a 2 × 2 factorial design to study the efficacy of retinyl palmitate and the antioxidant N-acetyl-cysteine.

Primary chemoprevention trials in lung cancer have studied individuals at increased risk for the development of lung cancer as the result of smoking or asbestos exposure. A large randomized trial of Finnish male smokers will study the efficacy of α-tocopherol and β-carotene in reducing lung cancer incidence. The study will require long-term follow-up of over 20,000 participants. A trial of β-carotene and vitamin A, termed the *CARET trial*, is being performed through United States centers.

Conclusions

Squamous cell carcinoma of the head and neck continues to be a major worldwide health problem that has not changed its disease control in over 30 years despite prevention and screening efforts and multimodality therapeutic approaches. Even though patients may be cured by surgery and/or radiotherapy, the threat of second primary malignancies remains burdensome, justifying further chemoprevention studies. Chemoprevention is therefore a promising new strategy to manage these disease processes, and head and neck cancer is an excellent model.

Several randomized trials now indicate that several retinoids can induce and maintain remission in oral premalignant lesions; therefore, suggesting great promise for this approach in head and neck chemoprevention. Before retinoids may be accepted as a standard therapy for oral leukoplakia, however, trials will need to be completed to evaluate the relative roles of retinoids and surgery in controlling this process. Additionally, while retinoids may be capable of maintaining remission, the prevention of recurrence of leukoplakia will need to be correlated with a decreased risk of developing cancers. Completion of large randomized trials evaluating the efficacy of these agents will allow us to provide an answer to the role of these agents in clinical practice. Oral premalignancy appears to be a good model system for the upper aerodigestive tract. In oral carcinogenesis, significant activity with high doses of 13-*cis*-retinoic acid has translated to a reduction of second primary tumors in head and neck cancer patients.

The future successes in chemoprevention will require studies defining intermediate endpoints and the biologic processes involved in multistep carcinogenesis and field cancerization. These studies may then be used to assist in patient treatment selection, biologic predictive capabilities, and the development of novel chemoprevention strategies, such as gene therapy.

The enthusiasm for chemoprevention generated by the early positive retinoid results in reducing head-and-neck and lung-associated second primary tumors should be focused toward enrolling more patients on the currently ongoing large-scale phase-III studies. In the United States, three major NCI studies of low-dose 13-*cis*-retinoic acid: Two in early stage head and neck cancer (MDACC/RTOG 91-15, ECOG C0590) and one in stage I non-small cell lung cancer (intergroup NCI 91-0001) are ongoing. The impact of smoking is critical, albeit difficult, to assess in these studies. The current large scale U.S. trials are stratified by smoking status, and one study includes biochemical validation of smoking cessation, which will add important new data on this issue. In Europe, a large scale multicenter trial to include 2000 early stage head and neck and lung cancer patients is ongoing. The enthusiasm in this area has led to the widespread and easy access for patients worldwide to enter clinical trials. The results of these large-scale phase-III retinoid upper aerodigestive tract and lung trials will have important implications for standard clinical practice.

References

1. Vokes EE, Weichselbaum RR, Lippman SM, Hong WK. Head and neck cancer. N Engl J Med 328:184–194, 1993.
2. Wolf G, Lippman SM, Laramore G, Hong WK. Head and neck cancer. In: JF Holland, E Frei, RC Bast Jr, et al. eds. Cancer Medicine, 3rd ed. Philadelphia: Lea & Febiger, 1211–1275, 1993.
3. Centers for Disease Control. Cigarette smoking among adults — United States, 1991. MMWR 42:230–233, 1993.
4. Lippman SM, Hong WK. Second malignant tumors in head and neck squamous-cell carcinoma: The overshadowing threat for patients with early-stage disease. Int J Radiat Oncol Biol Phys 17:691–694, 1989.
5. Lippman SM, Hong WK. Not yet standard: Retinoids versus second primary tumors. J Clin Oncol 1204–1207, 1993.
6. Sporn MB, Dunlop NM, Newton DL, Smith JB. Prevention of chemical carcinogenesis by vitamin A and its synthetic analogs (retinoids). Fed Proc 35:1332–1338, 1976.
7. Boone CW, Kelloff GJ, Malone WE. Identification of candidate cancer chemopreventive agents and their evaluation in animal models and human clinical trials: A review. Cancer Res 50:2–9, 1990.
8. Lippman SM, Benner SE, Hong WK. Cancer chemoprevention. J Clin Oncol 12:851–873, 1994.
9. Toth BB, Martin J, Lippman SM, Hong WK. Chemoprevention as a form of cancer control. J Am Dent Assoc 124:243–246, 1993.
10. Lippman SM, Spitz MR. Intervention in the premalignant process. Cancer Bull 43:473–474, 1992.
11. Benner SE, Lippman SM, Hong WK. Retinoid chemoprevention of second primary tumors. Semin Hematol 31 (Suppl 5):26–30, 1994.
12. Hong WK, Doos WG. Chemoprevention of head and neck cancer. Otolaryngol Clin North Am 18:543–549, 1985.
13. Boone CW, Kelloff GJ, Steele VE. Natural history of intraepithelial neoplasia in humans with implications for cancer chemoprevention strategy. Cancer Res 52:1651–1659, 1991.
14. Hong WK, Lippman SM, Wolf GT. Recent advances in head and neck cancer – larynx preservation and cancer chemoprevention: The Seventeenth Annual Richard and Hinda Rosenthal Foundation Award Lecture. Cancer Res 53:1–8, 1993.
15. Hirayama T. Diet and cancer. Nutr Cancer 1:67–81, 1979.
16. Shekelle RB, Lepper M, Liu S, Maliza C, Raynor WJ Jr, Rossof AH. Dietary vitamin A

and risk of cancer in the Western Electric study. Lancet 2:1185–1190, 1981.

17. Kvale G, Bjelke E, Gart JJ. Dietary habits and lung cancer risk. Int J Cancer 31:397–405, 1983.
18. Wang L, Hammond EC. Lung cancer, fruit, green salad, and vitamin pills. Chin Med J (Engl) 98:206–210, 1985.
19. Krombout D. Essental micronutrients in relation to carcinogenesis. Am J Clin Nutr 45:1361–1367, 1987.
20. Paganini-Hill A, Chao A, Ross RK, Henderson BE. Vitamin A, β-carotene, and the risk of cancer: A prospective study. J Natl Cancer Inst 79:443–448, 1987.
21. Menkes MS, Constock GW, Vuilleumier JP, et al. Serum β-carotene, vitamins A and E, selenium and the risk of lung cancer. N Engl J Med 315:1250–1254, 1986.
22. Willett WC, Polk BF, Underwood BA, et al. Relation of serum vitamins A and E and carotenoids to the risk of cancer. N Engl J Med 310:430–434, 1989.
23. Peto R, Doll R, Buckley JD, et al. Can dietary β-carotene materially reduce human cancer rates? Nature 290:201–208, 1981.
24. Farber E. The multistep nature of cancer development. Cancer Res 44:4217–4223, 1984.
25. Slaga TJ, Jimenez Conti IB. An animal model for oral cancer. J Natl Canc Inst Monogr 13:55–61, 1992.
26. Santis H, Shklar G, Chauncey HH. Histochemistry of experimentally induced leukoplakia and carcinoma of the hamster buccal pouch. Oral Surg Oral Med Oral Pathol 17:84–95, 1964.
27. Shklar G, Schwartz J, Grau D, et al. Inhibition of hamster buccal pouch carcinogenesis by 13-cis-retinoic acid. Oral Surg 50:45–52, 1980.
28. Lee JS, Kim SY, Hong WK, et al. Detection of chromosomal polysomy in oral leuko- plakia, a premalignant lesion. J Natl Cancer Inst 85:1951–1954, 1993.
29. Shklar G. Oral mucosal carcinogenesis in hamster: Inhibition by vitamin E. J Natl Cancer Inst 68:791–797, 1982.
30. Moon RC, Rao KVN, Detrisac CJ, Kelloff GJ. Animal models for chemoprevention of respiratory cancer. J Natl Cancer Inst 13:45–49, 1992.
31. Sporn MB. Carcinogenesis and cancer: Different perspectives on the same disease. Cancer Res 51:6215–6218, 1991.
32. Slaughter DP, Southwick HW, Smejkal W. Field cancerization in oral stratified squamous epithelium: Clinical implications of multicentric origin. Cancer 6:963–968, 1953.
33. Lee JS, Lippman SM, Hong WK, et al. Determination of biomarkers for intermediate end points in chemoprevention. Cancer Res 52(Suppl):S2707–S2710, 1992.
34. Lippman SM, Lee JS, Lotan R, Hittelman W, Wargovich MJ, Hong WK. Biomarkers as intermediate endpoints in chemoprevention trials. J Natl Cancer Inst 82:555–560, 1990.
35. Voravud N, Shin DM, Ro JY, et al. Increased polysomies of chromosomes 7 and 17 during head and neck multistage tumorigenesis. Cancer Res 53:2874–2883, 1993.
36. Shin DM, Voravud N, Ro JY, et al. Sequential increase of proliferating cell nuclear antigen expression in head and neck tumorigenesis: A potential biomarker. J Natl Cancer Inst 85:971–978, 1993.
37. Nees M, Homann N, Discher H, Andl T, Enders C, Herold C, Schuhmann A, Bosch FX. Expression of mutated p53 tumor-distant epithelia of head and neck cancer patients: Molecular basis for the development of multiple tumors. Cancer 53:4189–4196, 1993.
38. Sozzi G, Miozzo M, Tagliabue E, et al. Cytogenetic abnormalities and overexpression of receptors for growth factors in normal bronchial epithelium and tumor samples of lung cancer patients. Cancer Res 51:400–404, 1991.
39. Sozzi G, Miozzi M, Donglhi R, et al. Deletions of 17p and *p53* mutations in preneoplastic lesions of the lung. Cancer Res 52:6079–6082, 1992.
40. Girod SC, Fischer U, Rollins BJ. p53 as a prognostic factor in neoplastic and preneoplastic lesions of the oral mucosa. Proc Am Assoc Cancer Res 34:103, 1993.
41. Hollstein M, Sidransky D, Vogelstein B, et al. p53 mutations in human cancers. Science 253:49–53, 1991.

42. Vogelstein B, Fearon ER, Hamilton SR. Genetic alterations during colorectal tumor development. N Engl J Med 319:525–532, 1988.
43. Takahashi T, Nau MM, Chiba I, et al. p53: A frequent target for genetic abnormalities in lung cancer. Science 246:491–494, 1989.
44. Iggo R, Gatter K, Bartek J, et al. Increased expression of mutant forms of p53 oncogene in primary lung cancer. Lancet 335:675–679, 1990.
45. Vahakangas KH, Samet JM, Metcalf RA, et al. Mutations of p53 and ras genes in rado-associated lung cancer from uranium miners. Lancet 339:576–580, 1992.
46. Branchman DG, Graves D, Vokes E, et al. Occurrence of p53 gene deletions and human papilloma virus infection in human head and neck cancer. Cancer Res 52:4832–4836, 1992.
47. Gusterson BA, Anbazhagan R, Warren W, et al. Expression of p53 in premalignant and malignant squamous epithelium. Oncogene 6:1785–1789, 1991.
48. Zhou DJ, Casey G, Cline MJ. Amplification of human int-2 in breast cancers and squamous carcinomas. Oncogene 2:279–282, 1988.
49. Somers KD, Cartwright SL, Schechter GL. Amplification of the int-2 gene in human head and neck squamous cell carcinomas. Oncogene 5:915–920, 1990.
50. Merritt WD, Weissler MC, Turk BF, Gilmer TM. Oncogene amplification in squamous cell carcinoma of the head and neck. Arch Otolaryngol Head Neck Surg 116:1394–1398, 1990.
51. Berenson JR, Yang J, Mickel RA. Frequent amplification of the bcl-1 locus in head and neck squamous cell carcinomas. Oncogene 4:1111–1116, 1989.
52. Cowan JM, Beckett MA, Ahmed-Swan S, Weichselbaum RR. Cytogenetic evidence of the multistep origin of head and neck squamous cell carcinomas. J Natl Cancer Inst 84:793–797, 1992.
53. Somers KD, Merrick MA, Lopez ME, et al. Frequent p53 mutations in head and neck cancer. Cancer Res 52:5997–6000, 1992.
54. Chung KY, Mukhopadhyay T, Kim J, et al. Discordant p53 gene mutations in primary head and neck cancers and corresponding second primary cancers of the upper aerodigestive tract. Cancer Res 53:1676–1683, 1993.
55. Hennekens CH. Issues in the design and conduct of clinical trials. J Natl Cancer Inst 73:1473–1476, 1984.
56. Buring JE, Hennekens CH. The Women's Health Study: Summary of the study design. J Myocard Ischemia 4:27–29, 1992.
57. Boring CC, Squires RS, Tong T. Cancer statistics, 1993. Ca Cancer J Clin 43:7–26, 1993.
58. Strong MS, Incze J, Vaughan CW. Field cancerization in the aerodigestive tract — Its etiology, manifestation, and significance. J Otolaryngol 13:1–6, 1984.
59. Kramer IR, Luca RB, Pindorg JJ, et al. Definition of leukoplakia and related lesions: An aid to studies on oral precancer. Oral Surg Oral Med Oral Pathol 46:518–539.
60. Silverman S, Gorsky M, Lozada F. Oral leukoplakia and malignant transformation a follow-up study of 257 patients. Cancer 53:563–568, 1984.
61. Burquot JE, Weiland LH, Kurland LT. Leukoplakia and carcinoma in situ synchronously associated with invasive oral/oropharyngeal carcinoma in Rochester, Minn., 1935–1984. Oral Surg Oral Med Oral Pathol 65:199–207, 1988.
62. Banoczy J, Cisba A. Comparative study of the clinical picture and histopathologic structure of oral leukoplakia. Cancer 29:1230–1234, 1972.
63. Lippman SM, Kessler JF, Meyskens FL. Retinoids as preventive and therapeutic anticancer agents. Cancer Treat Rep 71:391–405, 493–515, 1987.
64. Smith MA, Parkinson DR, Cheson BD, Friedman MA. Retinoids in cancer therapy. J Clin Oncol 10:839–864, 1992.
65. Sporn MB, Roberts AB, Goodman DS, eds. The Retinoids: Biology, Chemistry and Medicine, 2nd ed. New York: Raven Press, 1994.
66. Evans R. The steroid and thyroid hormone receptor super family. Science 240:889–895, 1988.

112

67. Silverman S, Renstrup G, Pindborg JJ. Studies in oral leukoplakia. Acta Odontol Scand 21:271–292, 1963.
68. Silverman S, Eisenberg E, Renstrup G. A study of the effects of high doses of vitamin A on oral leukoplakia (hyperkeratosis), including toxicity, liver function and skeletal metabolism. J Oral Ther Pharmacol 2:9–23, 1965.
69. Wolf K. Zur vitamin A behandlung der leukoplakien. Arch Klin Exp Derm 206:495–498, 1957.
70. Raque CJ, Biondo RV, Keeran MG, et al. Snuff dippers kekratosis (snuff-induced leukoplakia). South Med J 68:565–568, 1975.
71. Koch HF. Effet of retinoids on precancerous lesions of oral mucosa. In: CE Orfanos, O Braun-Falco, EM Farbert, et al. (eds). Retinoids: Advances in Basic Reasearch and Therapy. Berlin: Springer-Verlag, 1981, pp 307–312.
72. Shah JP, Strong Ew, DeCosse JJ, et al. Effect of retinoids on oral leukoplakia. Am J Surg 146:466–470, 1983.
73. Hong WK, Endicott J, Itri LM, et al. 13-cis-retinoic acid in the treatment of oral leukoplakia. N Engl J Med 315:1501–1505, 1986.
74. Han J, Lu Y, Sun Z, et al. Evaluation of N-4-(hydroxycarbophenyl) retinamide as a cancer prevention agent and as a cancer chemotherapeutic agent. In Vivo 4:153–160, 1990.
75. Stich HF, Hornby AP, Mathew B, et al. Response of oral leukoplakia to the administration of vitamin A. Cancer Lett 40:93–101, 1988.
76. Lippman SM, Batsakis JG, Toth BB, et al. Comparison of low-dose isotretinoin with beta carotene to prevent oral carcinogenesis. N Engl J Med 328:15–20, 1993.
77. Chiesa F, Tradati N, Morazza M, et al. Prevention of local relapses and new localisations of oral leukoplakias with the synthetic retinoid ferentinide (4-HPR). Preliminary results. Oral Oncol Eur J Cancer 28B:97–102, 1992.
78. Xu JM, Plezia PM, Alberts DS, et al. Reduction in plasma or skin alpha-tocopherol concentration with long-term oral administration of beta carotene in humans and mice. J Natl Cancer Inst 84:1559–1565, 1992.
79. Stich HF, Rosin MP, Hornby AP, et al. Remission of oral leukoplakia and micronuclei in tobacco/betel quid chewers treated with beta carotene and with beta carotene plus vitamin A. Int J Cancer 42:195–199, 1988.
80. Garewal HS, Meyskens FL, Killen D, et al. Responses of oral leukoplakia to β-carotene. J Clin Oncol 8:1715–1720, 1990.
81. Toma S, Albanese E, DeLorenzi M, et al. β-carotene in the treatment of oral leukoplakia. Proc Am Soc Clin Oncol 9:179, 1990.
82. Benner SE, Winn RJ, Lippman SM, et al. Regression of oral leukoplakia with alpha-tocopherol: A Community Clinical Oncology Progrem (CCOP) chemoprevention study. J Natl Cancer Inst 85:44–47, 1993.
83. Benner SE, Wargovich MJ, Lippman SM, et al. Reduction in oral mucosa micronuclei frequency following alpha-tocopherol treatment of oral leukoplakia. Cancer Epidemiol Biomarkers Prevent 3:73–76, 1994.
84. Lippman SM, Hong WK. Differentiation therapy for head and neck cancer. In: G Snow, JR Clark, eds. Multimodality Therapy for Head and Neck Cancer. Verlag Press, 1992, pp 160–181.
85. Omenn GS, Goodman GE, Thornquist MD, et al. The carotene and retinol efficacy trial (CARET) to prevent lung cancer in high-risk populations: Pilot study with asbestos-exposed workers Cancer Epidemiol Biomarkers Prevent 2:2381–387, 1993.
86. Heimburger DC, Alexander B, Birch R, et al. Improvement in bronchial squamous metaplasia in smokers treated with folate and vitamin B_{12}. Report of a preliminary randomized, double-blind intervention trial. JAMA 259:1525–1530, 1988.
87. van Poppel G, Kok FJ, Hermus RJJ. Beta-carotene supplementation in smokers reduces the frequency of micronuclei in sputum. Br J Cancer 66:1164–1168, 1992.
88. Gouveia J, Mathe G, Hercend T, et al. Degree of bronchial metaplasia in heavy smokers

113

and its regression after treatment with a retinoid. Lancet 1:710–712, 1983.

89. Lee JS, Lippman SM, Benner SE, et al. Randomized placebo-controlled trial of iso-tretinoin in chemoprevention of bronchial squamous metaplasia. J Clin Oncol 12:937–945, 1994.

90. Arnold AM, Browman GP, Levine MN, et al. The effect of the synthetic retinoid etretinate on sputum cytology: Results from a randomised trial. Br J Cancer 65:737–743, 1992.

91. Rosin MP, Dunn BP, Stich HF. Use of intermediate end points in quanitating the response of precancerous lesions to chemopreventive agents. Cana J Physiol Pharmacol 65:483–487, 1987.

92. Stich HF, Rosin MP, Vallejera MO. Reduction with vitamin A and beta-cartene administration of proportion of micronucleated buccal mucosal cells in Asian betel nut and tobacco chewers. Lancet 1:1204–1206, 1984.

93. Stich HF, Hornby AP, Dunn BP. A pilot β-carotene invervention trial with Inuits using smokeless tobacco. Int J Cancer 36:321–327, 1985.

94. Schatzkin A, Freedman LS, Schiffman MH, et al. Validation of intermediate end points in cancer research. J Natl Cancer Inst 82:1746–1753, 1990.

95. Warren S, Gates O. Multiple primary malignant tumors: A survey of the literature and statistical study. Am J Cancer 51:1358–1403, 1932.

96. Licciardillo JT, Spitz MR, Hong WK. Multiple primary cancer in patients with cancer of the head and neck: Second cancer of the head and neck, esophagus and lung. Int J Radiat Oncol Biol Phys 17:467–476, 1989.

97. Ihde DC, Tucker MA. Secondary primary malignancies in small-cell lung cancer: A major consequence of modest success. J Clin Oncol 10:1511–1513, 1992.

98. Christensen P, Joergensen K, Munk J, Oesterlind A. Hyperfrequency of pulmonary cancer in a population of 415 patients treated for laryngeal cancer. Laryngoscope 97:612–614, 1987.

99. Tepperman BS, Fitzpatrick PJ. Second respiratory and upper digestive tract cancers after oral cancer. Lancet 2:547–549, 1981.

100. Cooper JS, Pajak TF, Rubin P, et al. Second malignancies in patients who have head and neck cancer: Incidence, effect on survival and implications for chemoprevention based on the RTOG experience. Int J Radiat Oncol Biol Phys 17:449–465, 1989.

101. McDonald S, Haie C, Rubin P, Nelson D, Divers LD. Second malignant tumors of laryngeal carcinoma: Diagnosis, treatment, and prevention. Int J Radiat Oncol Biol Phys 17:457–65, 1989.

102. Vikram B. Changing patterns of failure in advanced head and neck cancer. Arch Otolaryngol 110:564–565, 1984.

103. Hong WK, Lippman SM, Itri LM, et al. Prevention of second primary tumors with isotretinoin in squamous-cell carcinoma of the head and neck. N Engl J Med 323:795–801, 1990.

104. Benner SE, Pajak TF, Lippman, et al. Prevention of second primary tumors with isotre-tinoin in squamous cell carcinoma of the head and neck: Long-term follow-up. J Natl Cancer Inst 86:140–141, 1994.

105. Pastorino U, Infante M, Mioli M, et al. Adjuvant treatment of stage I lung cancer with high-dose vitamin A. J Clin Oncol 11:1216–1222, 1993.

106. Lippman SM, Hong WK. Retinoid chemoprevention of upper aerodigestive tract car-cinogenesis. In: VT DeVita, S Hellman, SA Rosenberg, eds. Important Advances in Oncology. Philadelphia: JB Lippincott, 1992, pp 93–109.

107. Moore C. Smoking and cancer of the mouth, pharynx, and larynx. JAMA 191:107–110, 1965.

108. Moore C. Cigarette smoking in cancer of the mouth, pharynx, and larynx — A continuing study. JAMA 218:553–558, 1971.

109. Silverman S, Griffith M. Smoking characteristics of patients with oral carcinoma and the risk for second oral primary carcinoma. J Am Dental Assoc 85:637–640, 1972.

110. Silverman S, Gorsky M, Greenspan D. Tobacco usage in patients with head and neck carcinomas: A follow-up study on habit changes and second primary oral/oropharyngeal cancers. J Am Dental Assoc 106:33–35, 1983.
111. Wynder EL, Dodo H, Bloch DA, Gantt RC, Moore OS. Epidemiologic investigation of multiple cancer in the upper alimentary and respiratory tracts. Cancer 24:730–739, 1969.
112. Hellquist H, Lundgren J, Olofosson J. Hyperplasia, keratosis, dysplasia, and carcinoma in situ of the vocal cords. Clin Otolaryngol 7:11–27, 1982.
113. Gillis TM, Incze J, Strong MS, Vaughan CW, Simpson Gy. Natural history and management of keratosis, atypia, carcinoma in situ and microinvasive cancer of the larynx. Am J Surg 146:512–519, 1983.
114. Castigliano SC. Influence of continous smoking on the incidence of second primary cancers involving mouth, pharynx and larynx. J Am Dent Assoc 77:580–585, 1968.

6. Mechanisms of invasion by head and neck cancers

Douglas D. Boyd and Garth L. Nicolson

Local and regional spread of squamous cell carcinoma (SCC) of the upper aerodigestive tract represents a major challenge to the oncologist, since it carries a high risk of regional recurrence and a high mortality rate. The invasiveness of these tumors frequently requires surgical resections that impair important physiological functions, including speech and swallowing. The therapy of SCC may be approaching a plateau, as the efficacy and toxicity of the agents used for treatment, particularly chemotherapy, seems to be optimal given present knowledge; therefore, understanding the mechanisms that underlie the invasiveness of SCC is required to develop novel treatments that attenuate the local spread of these tumors. Such anti-invasive agents would not be used alone, but rather in conjunction with existing therapies to improve the overall therapy of head and neck SCC.

While the process of tumor invasion by SCC is poorly understood, breachment of the basement membrane, to which the squamous cells are attached, and destruction of the surrounding extracellular matrix represent the first steps in local invasion (Figure 1) [1,2]. Basement membrane structures are made up of a diverse set of molecules, including laminin, fibronectin, collagens, entactin, and proteoglycans such as heparan sulfate proteoglycan [1]. The acquisition of an invasive phenotype by the SCC tumor cells is thought to depend, in part, on their ability to hydrolyze these components, thereby removing an obstacle to their tissue infiltration [1,2].

Degradative enzymes in tumor cell invasion

Because of the diversity of the extracellular matrix components, it is thought that the coordinated expression of multiple proteases by the invading tumor cells is required for the effective degradation of the extracellular matrix. Several hydrolases have been implicated in extracellular matrix destruction, including the plasminogen activator (PA), urokinase (UK), metallopro-

Hong, Waun Ki and Weber, Randal S., (eds.), Head and Neck Cancer. © 1995 Kluwer Academic Publishers.
ISBN 0-7923-3015-3. All rights reserved.

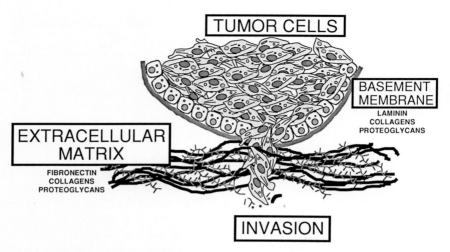

Figure 1. Tumor cell invasion of basement membranes and tissue extracellular matrix. Tumor invasion requires the synthesis of degradative enzymes and cellular motility.

teinases (MMP) such as type I and IV collagenases, endoglycosidases (of which heparanase is the most important), and cathepsins (Figure 2) [1,3–5].

An important property of metastatic cells is their ability to solubilize extracellular matrix and to penetrate this structure [4–6]. Higher levels of matrix-degradative enzymes are more often found in malignant tumors than in surrounding normal tissues or benign lesions [reviewed in 1–3,5,6]. Some of these enzymes may be involved in activating, inhibiting, or regulating the activities of other enzymes released by normal or tumor cells (Figure 2). Invasion does not appear to be mediated by individual degradative enzymes; it is thought to involve multiple degradative activities operating in an enzymatic cascade in which certain enzymes are required to activate other enzymes that are secreted in inactive proenzyme forms [7].

Since highly metastatic cells synthesize various classes of degradative enzymes and release them at higher concentrations or activities than their poorly metastatic or nonmetastatic counterparts, it is important to determine which enzymes are actually required for malignant cell invasion. In many studies, the exact subclass of individual degradative enzymes was not determined; however, the overall levels of activity for at least some enzyme classes were higher in the more highly metastatic cells and tissues. For example, higher levels of plasminogen activators have been found in more metastatic cells and metastatic tissues [8,9]. Furthermore, the highest concentrations of degradative enzymes are usually found in tumor-invasive regions [10]. The importance of tumor degradative enzymes against basement-membrane molecules for extracellular matrix penetration has been demonstrated with natural substrates, such as subendothelial matrix,

118

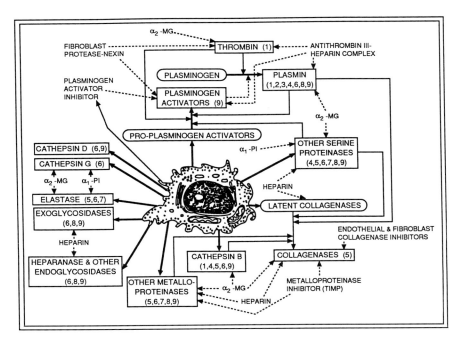

Figure 2. Tumor-associated degradative enzymes and plasma proteinases and inhibitors. The bold solid lines indicate release of degradative enzymes or activation of proenzymes. The numbers indicate the possible roles of degradative enzymes in (1) platelet aggregation, (2) fibrinolysis, (3) lamininolysis, (4) fibronectinolysis, (5) collagenolysis, (6) proteoglycanolysis, (7) elastinolysis, (8) host cell lysis, and (9) other activities. The broken lines indicate possible inhibitory mechanisms. α_1-PI = α_1-proteinase inhibitor; α_2-MG = α_2-macroglobulin; TIMP = tissue inhibitor of metalloproteinase. (Modified from Nakajima et al. [5], with permission.)

amnion membrane, lens capsule, and Matrigel-coated filters [reviewed in 11]. However, even though degradative enzymes are important in these processes, not all degradative enzymes are expressed by malignant cells in amounts proportional to their metastatic potentials. Most researchers monitor only a few degradative enzymes and do not analyze appropriate matrix-degrading enzymes (or their inhibitors). This has resulted in an incomplete picture of the degradative capacities of certain tumors and, in some cases, incorrect conclusions that there is an inconsistent relationship between the amounts of degradative enzymes and invasive properties.

There are several possible reasons for concluding the relationship is inconsistent [12]. These include tumor heterogeneity, host-cell contamination, rate-limiting steps in the metastatic process, and the presence of endogenous inhibitors against degradative enzymes. Fragments of tissues are often used for examining enzymatic activities; in such tissues it is often difficult to distinguish between degradative enzymes released by tumor cells and enzymes released by tumor-associated normal cells, since tumor-infiltrating host cells, such as lymphocytes, macrophages, mast cells, and fibroblasts, can synthesize and release high concentrations of degradative enzymes, especially in the tumor area [14,15]. For example, fibroblasts in the tumor area can be stimulated by tumor cells, tumor-activated macrophages, or lymphocytes to secrete high levels of collagenases [14]. In a few cases the tumor-released molecules responsible for stimulating host-cell degradative enzymes have been isolated. Baici et al. [16] isolated two rabbit V2 carcinoma cytokines that were activated by proteolysis and stimulated cathepsin B release by malignant tumor cells.

Role of degradative enzyme inhibitors in tumor invasion

Inhibitors of degradative enzymes have been used to block invasion and metastasis formation. They have also proved useful in demonstrating a functional role for degradative enzymes in metastasis formation. Using antibodies to UK-type plasminogen activator, Ossowski and Reich [17] were able to inhibit organ colonization by hepatoma cells in a chick embryo model of tumor cell colonization. Furthermore, addition of degradative enzymes can enhance invasion and metastasis. For example, addition of UK-type plasminogen activator can under certain circumstances enhance spontaneous lung metastasis in experimental tumor systems, and administration of the plasminogen activator inhibitor tranexamic acid inhibits metastasis formation of animal tumor cells [18]. A variety of protease inhibitors have also been used to inhibit metastasis [19], as well as tumor cell invasion of intact [20] or reconstituted basement membranes (Matrigel) [21]. Other degradative enzymes, such as the endoglycosidase heparanase that cleaves the heparan sulfate side chains of the basement membrane heparan sulfate proteoglycans, are also important in tumor invasion. Using chemical derivatives of heparin that block heparanase activity, we were able to inhibit murine melanoma lung colonization, indicating the important role of endoglycosidases in malignant cell invasion [5,22].

Normal host cells, and even tumorigenic or metastatic cells, can produce inhibitors of degradative enzymes. The most widely reported of these are the tissue inhibitors of metalloproteinases (TIMPs) [reviewed in 23,24]. These natural inhibitors block collagenases by combining with the activated or inactivated proenzyme forms of the enzymes to regulate enzymatic activity. Although TIMPs are very active in inhibiting collagenases, they are not active against serine-, cysteine-, and aspartic-type proteinases. They are not unique to tumor cells and can be produced by a variety of normal cells [23,24]. Malignant cells that produce TIMPs apparently do so in inverse proportion to their metastatic potentials [25]. In a more direct demonstration of its possible role in regulating tumor cell invasion, purified TIMP has been used to block invasion [26]. In other experiments, transfection of a

TIMP antisense gene construct into nontumorigenic, noninvasive cells resulted in cell transformation. In addition, the transformed cells acquired invasive, tumorigenic, and metastatic properties [27].

Tumor urokinase and basement membrane degradation

An important degradative enzyme in head and neck SCC invasion is UK. The UK-type plasminogen activator, encoded by a 6.4-kb gene, is secreted by tumor and some normal cells as a single-chain glycosylated proenzyme (SC-UK) of 55 kD [28,29]. It can promote tumor cell invasion by catalyzing the conversion of the inactive zymogen, plasminogen, which is abundant in extracellular fluids, into the active serine-type protease plasmin [30,31]. Plasmin degrades extracellular matrix components, such as laminin, a major component of basement membranes [32]. In addition, UK can activate type IV procollagenase into its fully active form, which in turn catalyzes the hydrolysis of type IV collagen, a major structural component of basement membranes [33]. There have also been reports that plasmin can cleave type IV collagen [34]. Thus UK may play a pivotal role in activating basement membrane degradative enzymes.

Two lines of evidence implicate UK in tumor cell invasion. First, UK is elevated in several malignacies, most dramatically at the leading edge of invading cancers [35–37]. Secondly, as mentioned above, UK antibodies can, in some instances, inhibit the metastasis of tumor cells to secondary sites [17,38].

Since UK is an important enzyme in tumor cell invasion, regulation of UK activity is important in invasive tumors. There are two principal ways in which UK activity is regulated. First, the expression of the plasminogen activator can be elevated, leading to an increased rate of plasminogen activation and a concomitant increase in extracellular matrix hydrolysis [39,40]. Alternatively, a variety of physiological inhibitors for UKs, including PAI-1, PAI-2, and protease nexin, bind to the catalytic moiety of UK, thus neutralizing the enzyme [41,42]. Decreased expression of one or more of these inhibitors (relative to that of the plasminogen activator) would, in effect, lead to an increase in the overall proteolytic potential of tumor cells.

In vitro invasion of the oral cavity by SCC requires
UK plasminogen activator

Studies by our group using cultured SCC have indicated that these cells are avid secretors of UK and highly invasive in vitro. This is very much reminiscent of the behavior of head and neck SCC in vivo [42]. Indeed, UK overexpression is associated with the tumor cells located at the leading edge of the cancer in vivo. More important, we have found that the in vitro invasive capacities of cultured SCC cell lines can be substantially compromised by antibodies directed at the catalytic moiety of the UK molecule [43]. Niedbala and Sartorelli [44] had previously reported a reduced degradation of subendothelial extracellular matrix in SCC cells cultured in the presence of anti-UK antibodies, suggesting that the reduced invasion by SCC was a consequence of attenuated extracellular matrix degradation.

Levels of UK and its inhibitior, PAI-1, in SCC partly reflect overexpression of UK

We have speculated that in SCC cells an imbalance in the expression of UK and UK inhibitors could culminate in the enhanced proteolysis required for the invasive phenotype of SCC cells. To demonstrate this we compared the amounts of UK and its inhibitor, PAI-1, in the medium conditioned by two invasive SCC cell lines. On a molar basis there was an excess of UK over UK inhibitors in the culture supernatant. Overexpression of UK by SCC could explain this disparity. Indeed, we found that highly invasive SCC cell lines have increased levels of UK mRNA encoding the plasminogen activator. Thus the increased concentrations of UK were a consequence of transcriptional activation rather than amplification of the UK gene or an increase in mRNA stability [43]. Other possible mechanisms of regulation of UK expression are discussed in the last section of this chapter.

Collagenases in tumor invasion and metastasis

While plasminogen activation by UK is thought to play a central role in basement membrane hydrolysis, there is ample evidence implicating a family of enzymes collectively designated the MMPs in SCC invasion [1,45,46]. The major function of these enzymes is the degradation of plasmin-resistant collagens that are integral components of basement membranes and interstitial extracellular matrix [1,47]. Several lines of evidence have implicated the MMP family of hydrolases in tumor invasion and metastasis.
1. The release of several MMPs, including the type IV collagenases, correlates well with the invasive and metastatic phenotypes of several tumor types and cell lines [48–51].
2. Inhibition of the expression or activity of these enzymes leads to reduced invasive and metastatic capacity [52,53].
3. The expression of an antisense cDNA to the type IV collagenase inhibitor TIMP promoted the invasive and metastatic behavior of 3T3 cells [54,55].

The activity of the MMPs is mainly directed toward digestion of collagens that form an integral part of the structures of basement membranes and interstitial extracellular matrix. In this regard, two collagenases, MMP-9 and MMP-2, digest type IV and type V collagens in basement membranes, whereas stromelysin (MMP3) predominantly cleaves several collagens [47].

One of the MMPs, stromelysin, is also capable of degrading the glycoprotein matrix component laminin and is found in cultures of oral SCC cells [55].

Role of matrix metalloproteinases in oral cavity SCC invasion

An important class of basement membrane-degradative enzymes released by SCC cells is represented by the MMPs. Kusukawa et al. [55], using western blotting and zymography, demonstrated the secretion of MMP-2, MMP-3, and MMP-9 by cultured SCC cell lines. In a separate study, Muller et al. [56] found higher levels of the mRNA for two MMP stromelysin genes, type I collagenase and PUMP-1, in resected SCC than in normal adjacent tissue. These data are consistent with the findings of Kusukawa et al. [55], who examined the production of MMP-2 and MMP-3 in head and neck SCC cells. Using in situ hybridization, Pollete et al. [57] found high levels of mRNA for stromelysin 2 in head and neck SCC cells and also in stromal cells in contact with the malignant cells. In examining two invasive SCC cell lines (UM-SCC-1 and MDA-TU-138) for the presence of MMPs, we found an activity in the conditioned medium that was indistinguishable from MMP-9 in its molecular mass and other properties. The role of this MMP in tumor invasion was confirmed in experiments in which the MMP inhibitor TIMP-2 significantly reduced the in vitro invasion of the cultured SCC cells through a reconstituted basement membrane matrix.

Our observation of MMP-9 secretion by UM-SCC-1 and MDA-TU-138 oral cavity SCC cells was somewhat at variance with the reports of Kusukawa et al. [55] and Muller et al. [56] that implicated MMP-2 and MMP-3 in SCC invasion. One possible explanation for this could be the heterogeneous nature of the disease, in which different cell clones express one or more collagenases. Indeed, our recent studies have indicated that MMP-2 is the predominant collagenase elaborated by another SCC cell line (UM-SCC-6). Alternatively, the expression of one or more of the MMP collagenases could reflect tumor cell-stromal cell interactions in vivo that lead to induction of MMPs. Indeed, the findings of Polette et al. [57] would agree with this contention, insofar as mRNA for stromelysin 2 was found predominantly in the stromal cells proximal to the tumor cell population.

Regulation of UK and MMP-9 type IV collagenase in SCC

The mechanisms that determine the overexpression of UK and collagenases in SCC cells are unclear at present. Our preliminary findings indicate that overexpression of both UK and MMP-9 by SCC cells reflect, at least in part, activation of protein kinase C (PKC)-dependent signal transduction pathway(s). For example, incubation of the SCC cells with calphostin C, a selective inhibitor of PKC, led to substantial reduction in the mRNA and amounts of secreted UK and MMP-9. It is unlikely that this inhibition represented a toxic effect of the agent, because we could induce the expression of both proteases by treatment of the SCC cells with the phorbol ester PMA, a specific PKC agonist.

The observations above may provide some insight into potential mechanisms by which UK and collagenase gene activation could occur. It is well accepted that PKC is activated by several growth factors, including EGF, TGF-α, FGF, TNF-α, interferons, and TGF-β [58–61], and these mitogens can also induce the expression of UK [62–65] and several of the collagenases in a variety of cell types [66–69]. Since cancer cells are often characterized by their ability to elaborate and respond to their own growth factors (autocrine stimulation), it is very possible that the expression of UK and MMP-9 in SCC cells is driven by peptide substances expressed by the tumor cells themselves. This contention is supported by the observation of overexpression of the EGF receptor and the *int*-2 oncogene, which encodes an FGF-like molecule, [70] by SCC cells. This receptor receives its signal from EGF or TGF-α [71]. Alternatively, stimulating growth factors could originate in the stromal compartment and stimulate protease expression in the tumor cells through a paracrine stimulation pathway.

Tumor cell motility, chemotaxis, and haptotaxis

The invasive behavior of malignant cells is due to a number of properties, including cell adhesion, motility, destruction of host tissues, and growth [72,73]. Malignant cells that have the correct combination of these properties should be able to selectively invade particular host tissues. Although loose connective tissues and bone are readily invaded by most malignant tumors, cartilage, aorta, cornea, lens, and other tissues are relatively resistant to invasion [74]. The resistance of certain tissues to tumor invasion is thought to be due to tissue structural properties as well as to tissue molecules that can inhibit tumor cell invasion. As discussed in a previous section, malignant tumors can use normal host molecules during invasion of resistant tissue structures by stimulating surrounding mast cells, fibroblasts, and other host cells to secrete degradative enzymes, but normal host cells and tissues also possess inhibitors of degradative enzymes.

Malignant cell invasion requires degradative enzymes but is also determined by selective and directed chemotaxis mediated by tissue-specific chemotatic and haptotactic factros. The directed cell movement stimulated by soluble chemotactic or insoluble haptotactic factors, which can be small proteolytic fragments derived from collagen, complement molecules, and extracellular matrix constituents [75], is especially important in malignant cell invasion. For example, metastatic fibrosarcoma cells respond and move toward a gradient of the complement C5a peptide, whereas nonmetastatic cells are unresponsive to C5a [76]. Intact molecules or fragments of extracellular-matrix molecules, such as fibronectin, laminin, and collagen, are important sources of tumor chemotatic or haptotactic factors, and these molecules can stimulate the directed movements of malignant cells into various tissues.

The directed motility of tumor cells can also be driven by immobilized factors (haptotaxis). For example, immobilized fibronectin in extracellular matrix stimulated the directed movement of melanoma cells, suggesting that this molecule can function as a haptotactic signal in basement membranes and tissue extracellular matrix [77]. Laminin and its fragments can also stimulate haptotaxis [78], and an antibody against the laminin receptor blocked laminin-mediated attachment and haptotaxis of human melanoma cells on laminin-coated but not fibronectin-coated surfaces [79].

Different chemotactic factors have been isolated from various organs and tissues, and these may be involved in paracrine-stimulated malignant cell invasion (bone, brain, liver, and lung). For example, brain-colonizing melanoma cells responded to brain-derived chemotactic factors, lung-colonizing fibrosarcoma cells to lung-derived factors, and liver-colonizing monocytic tumor cells to liver-derived chemotactic molecules. Furthermore, human breast adenocarcinoma cells responded to extracts from bone and brain (which are possible targets for metastatic colonization in this tumor system), but were not chemotactically stimulated by lung or liver chemotatic molecules [80]. Bresalier et al. [81] showed that highly metastatic liver-selected tumor lines were significantly more responsive to isolated liver chemotactic factors than lung or brain factors in chemotaxis assays, and Cerra and Nathanson [82] found that after extracting lung and liver extra-cellular matrix and testing the extracts on lung-colonizing tumor cell lines, only lung matrix yielded molecules that induced lung-colonizing tumor cell motility. Thus, tissue chemotactic factors may be involved in stimulating malignant-cell differential tissue invasion.

Tumor cells can also synthesize their own autocrine motility factors to stimulate cell movement. Autocrine motility factors of $\sim$53 kD have been isolated from metastatic melanoma [83] and mammary carcinoma cells [84]. This autocrine factor stimulates random cell movements but is not a chemo-attractant for normal neutrophils. Highly metastatic mammary adenocarci-noma cells synthesize large amounts of the autocrine motility factor, which then stimulates chemokinetic movements of poorly metastatic clones that do not synthesize the autocrine factor [84]. The autocrine motility factor receptor has recently been identified as a $\sim$74-kD cell-surface molecule expressed by melanoma and other tumor cells [85].

Although paracrine and autocrine motility factors are important in malig-nant cell invasion, little information is available on head and neck SCC cell motility. Using SCC and adenocarcinoma lines established from non-small cell lung cancers, Erdel et al. [86] examined cell interactions and cell moti-lity. They found that the cell lines possessed differences in self-adhesive properties, adhesion to extracellular matrix components, and expression of cell-surface adhesion components, such as integrins. An important property was the ability to respond to haptotatic factors, particularly basement membrane components, such as fibronectin and laminin. Salge et al. [87] investigated the motility of three SCC and three large-cell carcinoma cell lines. They found heterogeneous cell motilities among the cell lines, and the tumor promotor phorbol-12-myristate-13-acetate generally increased the expression of differentiation markers on the cell lines of low differentiation grade and inhibited cell adhesion and motility. In contrast, cell lines of high differentiation grade did not respond to the tumor promoter, and their cell adhesion and motility properties were unchanged.

Conclusions

It is clear that the expression of proteases, in particular, UK and the MMP collagenases, by SCC cells and their ability to move into surrounding tissues are critical determinants of their invasive capacities. Further studies will be necessary to determine whether other hydrolases (heparanses, cathepsins) are also required for this phenotype. In preliminary studies we have found that the expression of heparanase is enhanced in SCC compared with surrounding tissues. Equally important is the need for studies that address the mechanism by which these degradative enzymes are overexpressed in SCC of the head and neck. In addition, there is an almost complete lack of information on the motility responses of oral cavity SCC. The abilities of SCC cells to respond to paracrine and autocrine motility factors and to move into surrounding tissues are critical properties of tumor invasion. Identifying the motility molecules and their receptors on SCC cells should be an important step in understanding SCC cell invasive behavior. The acquisition of such knowledge on SCC degradative enzymes and motility responses could ultimately lead to the development of novel treatments that block the invasiveness of these tumors and increase the quality of life and survival of patients with head and neck SCC.

References

1. Tryggvason K, Höyhtyä M, Salo T. Proteolytic degradation of extracellular matrix in tumor invasion. Biochim Biophys Acta 907:191–217, 1987.
2. Nicolson GL, Cancer metastasis: Organ colonization and the cell surface properties of malignant cells. Biochim Biophys Acta 695:113–176, 1982.
3. Danø K, Andreasen PA, Grøndahl-Hansen J, Kristensen P, Nielsen LS. Plasminogen activators, tissue degradation, and cancer. Adv Cancer Res 44:139–266, 1985.
4. Nakajima M, Irimura T, Nicolson GL, Basement membrane degradative enzymes and tumor metastasis. Cancer Bull 39:142–149, 1987.
5. Nakajima M, Irimura T, Nicolson GL, Heparanases and tumor metastasis. J Cell Biochem 36:157–167, 1988.
6. Liotta LA, Rao CN, Wewer UM, Biochemical interactions of tumor cells with the basement membrane. Annu Rev Biochem 55:1037–1057, 1986.

7. Mignatti P, Robbins E, Rifkin DB. Tumor invasion through the human amniotic membrane: Requirement for a proteinase cascade. Cell 47:487–498, 1986.
8. Markus G, Takita H, Camiolo SM, Corasanti JG, Evers JL, Hobika GH. Content and characterization of plasminogen activators in human lung tumors and normal lung tissue. Cancer Res 40:841–848, 1980.
9. Carlsen SA, Ramshaw IA, Warrington RC. Involvement of plasminogen activator production with tumor metastasis in a rat model. Cancer Res 44:3012–3016, 1984.
10. Clavel C, Chavanel G, Birembaut P. Detection of the plasmin system in human mammary pathology using immunofluorescence. Cancer Res 46:5743–5747, 1986.
11. Starkey JR. Cell-matrix interactions during tumor invasion. Cancer Metastasis Rev 9: 113–123, 1990.
12. Duffy MJ. Do proteases play a role in cancer invasion and metastasis? Eur J Cancer Clin Oncol 23:583–589, 1987.
13. Biswas C. Tumor cell stimulation of collagenase production by fibroblasts. Biochem Biophys Res Commun 109:1026–1032, 1982.
14. Dabbous MK, North SM, Haney L, Nicolson GL. Macrophage and lymphocyte potentiation of syngeneic tumor cell and host fibroblast collagenolytic activity in rats. Cancer Res 48:6832–6836, 1988.
15. Dabbous MK, Wooley DE, Haney L, Carter LM, Nicolson GL. Host-mediated effectors of tumor invasion: Role of mast cells in matrix degradation. Clin Exp Metastasis 4:141–152, 1986.
16. Baici A, Knöpfel M, Keist R. Tumor-host interaction in rabbit V2 carcinoma: Stimulation of cathepsin B in host fibroblasts by a tumor-drived cytokine. Invasion Metastasis 8: 143–158, 1988.
17. Ossowski L, Reich E. Antibodies to plasminogen activator inhibit human tumor metastasis. Cell 35:611–619, 1983.
18. Tanaka N, Ogawa H, Tanaka K, Kinjo M, Kohga S. Effects of tranexamic acid and urokinase on hematogenous metastases of Lewis lung carcinoma in mice. Invasion Metastasis 1:149–157, 1981.
19. Pauli BU, Schwartz DE, Thonar EJM, Kuettner KE. Tumor invasion and host extracellular matrix. Cancer Metastasis Rev 2:129–152, 1983.
20. Persky B, Ostrowski LE, Pagast P, Ahsan A, Schultz RM. Inhibition of proteolytic enzymes in the in vitro amnion model for basement membrane invasion. Cancer Res 46:4129–4134, 1986.
21. Yagel S, Warner AH, Nellans HN, Lala PK, Waghorne C, Denhardt DT. Suppression by cathepsin L inhibitors of the invasion of amnion membranes by murine cancer cells. Cancer Res 49:3553–3557, 1989.
22. Irimura T, Nakajima M, Nicolson GL. Chemically modified heparins as inhibitors of heparan sulfate specific endo-β-glucoronidase (heparanse) or metastatic melanoma cells. Biochemistry 25:5322–5328, 1986.
23. Khokha R, Denhardt D. Matrix metalloproteinases and tissue inhibitor of metalloproteinases: Review of their role in tumorigenesis and tissue invasion. Invasion Metastasis 9:391–405, 1989.
24. Liotta LA, Steeg PS, Stetler-Stevenson WG. Cancer metastasis and angiogenesis: An imbalance of positive and negative regulation. Cell 64:327–336, 1991.
25. Hicks NJ, Ward RV, Reynolds JJ. Fibrosarcoma model derived from mouse embryo cells: Growth properties and secretion of collagenase and metalloproteinase inhibitor (TIMP) by tumour lines. Int J Cancer 33:835–844, 1984.
26. Schultz RM, Silberman S, Persky B, Bajkowski AS, Carmichael DF. Inhibition by human recombinant tissue inhibitor of metalloproteinases of human amnion invasion and lung colonization by murine B16-F10 melanoma cells. Cancer Res 48:5539–5545, 1988.
27. Khokha R, Waterhouse P, Yagel S, Denhardt D. Antisense RNA-induced reduction in murine TIMP levels confers oncogenicity on Swiss 3T3 cells. Science 243:947–950, 1989.
28. Verde P, Boast S, Franze A, Robbiati F, Blasi F. An upstream enhancer and a negative

element in the 5' flanking region of the human urokinase plasminogen activator gene. Nucleic Acids Res 16:10699–10715, 1988.

29. Nielsen L, Hansen J, Skriver L, Wilson E, Kaltoft K, Zenthen J, Danø K. Purification of zymogen to plasminogen activator from human glioblastoma cells by affinity chromatography with monoclonal antibody. Biochemistry 21:6410–6415, 1982.

30. Collen D, Verstraete M. Molecular biology of human plasminogen. II. Metabolism in physiological and some pathological conditions in man. Thrombosis Diathesis Haemorrhagica 34:403, 1975.

31. Robbins KC, Summaria L, Hsieh B, Shah R. The peptide chains of human plasmin. J Biol Chem 242:2333–2342, 1967.

32. Liotta L, Goldfarb R, Brundage R, Siegel G, Terranova V, Garbisa, S. Effect of plasminogen activator (urokinase), plasmin, and thrombin on glycoprotein and collagenous components of basement membrane. Cancer Res 41:4629–4636, 1981.

33. Matrisian L, Bowden T. Stromelysin/transin and tumor progression. Semin Cancer Biol 1:107–115, 1990.

34. Mackay AR, Corbitt RH, Hartzler JL, Thorgeirsson UP. Basement membrane type IV collagen degradation: Evidence for the involvement of a proteolytic cascade independent of metalloproteinases. Cancer Res 50:5997–6001, 1990.

35. Markus G, Takita H, Camiola S, Corasanti J, Evers J, Hobika G. Content and characterization of plasminogen activators in human lung tumors and normal lung tissue. Cancer Res 40:841–848, 1980.

36. Markus G, Camiolo SM, Kohga S, Madeja JM, Mittelman A. Plasminogen activator secretion of human tumors in short-term organ culture, including a comparison of primary and metastatic colon tumors. Cancer Res 43:5517–5525, 1983.

37. Skriver L, Larsson LI, Kielberg V, Nielsen LS, Andreasen PB, Kristensen P, Danø K. Immunocytochemical localization of urokinase-type plasminogen activator in Lewis lung carcinoma. J Cell Biol 99:752–757, 1984.

38. Hearing V, Law L, Corti A, Appella E, Blasi F. Modulation of metastatic potential by cell surface urokinase of murine melanoma cells. Cancer Res 48:1270–1278, 1988.

39. Sappino A, Busso N, Belin D, Vassalli J. Increase of urokinase-type plasminogen activator gene expression in human lung and breast carcinomas. Cancer Res 47:4043–4046, 1987.

40. Lund L, Ronne E, Roldan A, Behrendt N, Romer J, Blasi F, Danø K. Urokinase receptor mRNA level and gene transcription are strongly and rapidly increased by phorbol myristate acetate in human monocyte-like U937 cells. J Biol Chem 266:5177–5181, 1991.

41. Hekman CM, Loskutoff DJ. Endothelial cells produce a latent inhibitor of plasminogen activators that can be activated by denaturants. J Biol Chem 260:11581–11587, 1985.

42. Maddox WA, Urist MM. Histopathological prognostic factors of certain primary oral cavity cancers. Oncology 4:39–42, 1990.

43. Clayman G, Wang SW, Nicolson GL, El-Naggar A, Mazar A, Henkin J, Balsi F, Goepfert H, Boyd DD. Regulation of urokinase-type plasminogen activator expression in squamous cell carcinoma of the oral cavity. Int J Cancer 54:73–80, 1993.

44. Niedbala M, Sartorelli AC. Plasminogen activator-mediated degradation of subendothelial extracellular matrix by human squamous carcinoma cell lines. Cancer Commun 2:189–199, 1990.

45. Wilhelm SM, Collier IE, Marmer BL, Eisen AZ, Grant G, Goldberg G. SV40-transformed human lung fibroblasts secrete a 92-kDa type IV collagenase which is identical to that secreted by normal human macrophages. J Biol Chem 264:17213–17221, 1989.

46. Bejarano PA, Noekken ME, Suzuki K, Hudson BG, Nagase H. Degradation of basement membranes by human matrix metalloproteinase 3 (stromelysin). Biochem J 256:413–419, 1988.

47. Matrisian LM. Metalloproteinases and their inhibitors in matrix remodeling. Trends Genet 6:121–125, 1990.

48. Bernhard EJ, Muschel RJ, Hughes EN. M_r 92,000 gelatinase release correlates with the metastatic phenotype in transformed rat embryo cells. Cancer Res 50:3872–3877, 1990.

49. Ura H, Bonfil RD, Reich R, Pfeifer A, Harris CC. Expression of type IV collagenase and procollagen genes and its correlation with the tumorigenic, invasive, and metastatic abilities of oncogene-tranformed human bronchial epithelial cells. Cancer Res 49:4615–4621, 1989.

50. Garbisa S, Pozzatti R, Mushcel RJ, Saffiotti U, Ballin M, Goldfarb R, Khoury G, Liotta L. Secretion of type IV collagenase protease and metastatic phenotype: Induction by transfection with c-Ha-*ras* but not c-Ha-*ras* plus Ad2-Ela. Cancer Res 47:1523–1528, 1987.

51. Nakajima M, Welch DR, Belloni PN, Nicolson GL. Degradation of basement membrane type IV collagen and lung subendothelial matrix by rat mammary adenocarcinoma cell clones of differing metastatic potentials. Cancer Res 47:4869–4876, 1987.

52. DeClerck Y, Perez N, Shimada H, Boone T, Langley K, Taylor S. Inhibition of invasion and metastasis in cells transfected with an inhibitor of metalloproteinases. Cancer Res 52:701–708, 1992.

53. Schultz RM, Silberman S, Persky B, Bajkoski AS, Carmichael DF. Inhibition by human recombinant tissue inhibitor of metalloproteinases of human amnion invasion and lung colonization by murine B16–F10 melanoma cells. Cancer Res 48:5539–5545, 1988.

54. Khokha R, Waterhouse P, Yagel S, Lala P, Overall C, Norton G, Denhardt D. Antisense RNA-induced reduction in murine TIMP levels confers oncogenicity on Swiss 3T3 cells. Science 243:947–950, 1989.

55. Kusukawa J, Sasaguri Y, Shima I, Kameyama T, Morimatsu M. Production of matrix metalloproteinase 2 (gelatinase/type IV collagenase) and 3 (stromelysin) by cultured oral squamous cell carcinoma. J Oral Pathol Med 21:221–224, 1992.

56. Muller D, Breathnach R, Engelmann A, Millon R, Bronner G, Flesch H, Dumont P, Eber M, Abecassis J. Expression of collagenase-related metalloproteinase genes in human lung or head and neck tumours. Int J Cancer 48:550–556, 1991.

57. Polette M, Clavel C, Muller D, Abecassis J, Binninger I, Birembaut P. Detection of mRNA encoding collagenase I and stromelysin 2 in carcinomas of the head and neck by in situ hybridization. Invasion Metastasis 11:76–83, 1991.

58. Kudlow JE, Bjorge JD. TGF-α in normal physiology. Semin Cancer Biol 1:293–302, 1990.

59. Presta M, Tiberio L, Rusnati M, Dell'era P, Ragnotti G. Basic fibroblast growth factor requires a long-lasting activation of protein kinase C to induce cell proliferation in transformed fetal bovine aortic endothelial cells. Cell Regul 2:719–726, 1991.

60. Tiefenbrun N, Kimichi A. The involvement of protein kinase C in mediating growth suppressive signals of interferons in hematopoietic cells. Oncogene 6:1001–1007, 1991.

61. Schutze S, Machleidt T, Kronke M. Mechanisms of tumor necrosis factor action. Semin Oncol 19:16–24, 1992.

62. Murphy P, Hart D. Modulation of plasminogen activator and plasminogen activator inhibitor expression in the human U373 glioblastoma/astrocytoma cell line by inflammatory mediators. Exp Cell Res 198:93–100, 1992.

63. Presta M, Maier A, Rusnati M, Moscatelli D, Ragnotti G. Modulation of plasminogen activator activity in human endometrial adenocarcinoma cells by basic fibroblast growth factor and transforming growth factor β. Cancer Res 48:6384–6389, 1988.

64. Collart M, Belin D, Vassalli J, Kossodo S, Vassalli P. Gamma interferon enhances macrophage transcription of the tumor necrosis factor/cachetin, interleukin 1, and urokinase genes, which are controlled by short-lived repressors. J Exp Med 164:2113–2118, 1986.

65. Tienari J, Alanko T, Lehtonen E, Saksela O. The expression and localization of urokinase-type plasminogen activator and its type-1 inhibitor are regulated by retinoic acid and fibroblast growth factor in human teratocarcinoma cells. Cell Regul 2:285–297, 1991.

66. Okada Y, Tsuchiya H, Shimizu H, Tomita K, Nakanishi I, Sato H, Seike M, Yamashita K, Hayakawa T. Induction and stimulation of 92-kDa gelatinase/type IV collagenase production in osteosarcoma and fibrsarcoma cell lines by tumor necrosis factor α. Biochem Biophys Res Commun 171:610–617, 1990.

67. Salo T, Lyons JG, Rahemtulla F, Birkedal-Hansen H, Larjava H. Transforming growth factor-β up-regulates type IV collagenase expression in cultured human keratinocytes. J Biol Chem 266:11436–11441, 1991.

129

68. Unemori EN, Hibbs MS, Amento EP. Constitutive expression of a 92-kD gelatinase (type IV collagenase) by rheumatoid synovial fibroblasts and its induction in normal human fibroblasts by inflammatory cytokines. J Clin Invest 88:1656–1662, 1991.
69. Turksen K, Choi Y, Fuchs E. Transforming growth factor alpha induces collagen degradation and cell migration in differentiating human epidermal raft cultures. Cell Regul 2: 613–625, 1991.
70. Somers K, Cartwright SL, Schechter GL. Amplification of the *int-2* gene in human head and neck squamous cell carcinomas. Oncogene 5:915–920, 1990.
71. Santini J, Formento J, Francouai M, Milano G, Schneider M, Dassonville O, Demard F. Characterization, quantification, and potential clinical value of the epidermal growth factor receptor in head and neck squamous cell carcinomas. Head Neck 13:132–139, 1991.
72. Hart IR. Mechanisms of tumor cell invasion. Cancer Biol Rev 2:29–58, 1981.
73. Mareel MMK. Invasion in vitro: Methods of analysis. Cancer Metastasis Rev 2:201–218, 1983.
74. Nicolson GL, Poste G. Tumor cell diversity and host responses in cancer metastasis. I. Properties of metastatic cells. Curr Prob Cancer 7:1–83, 1982.
75. Varani J. Chemotaxis of metastatic cells. Cancer Metastasis Rev 1:17–28, 1982.
76. Orr FW, Varani J, Delikatny J, Jain N, Ward PA. Comparison of the chemotactic responsiveness of two fibrosarcoma subpopulations of differing malignancy. Am J Pathol 102:160–167, 1981.
77. Lacovara J, Cramer EB, Quigley JP. Fibronectin enhancement of directed migration of B16 melanoma cells. Cancer Res 44:1657–1663, 1984.
78. Graff J, Iwamoto Y, Sasaki M, Martin GM, Kleinman HK, Robey FA, Yamada Y. Identification of an amino acid sequence in laminin mediating cell attachment, chemotaxis, and receptor binding. Cell 48:989–996, 1987.
79. Wever UM, Taraboletti G, Sobel ME, Albrechtsen R, Liotta LA. Role of laminin in tumor cell migration. Cancer Res 47:5691–5698, 1987.
80. Hujanen ES, Terranova VP. Migration of tumor cells to organ-derived chemoattractants. Cancer Res 45:3517–3521, 1985.
81. Bresalier RS, Hujanen ES, Raper SE, Roll FJ, Itzkowitz SH, Martin GR, Kim YS. An animal model for colon cancer metastasis: Establishment and characterization of murine cell lines with enhanced liver-metastasizing ability. Cancer Res 47:1398–1406, 1987.
82. Cerra RF, Nathanson SD. Organ-specific chemotactic factors present in lung extracellular matrix. Surg Res 46:422–426, 1989.
83. Liotta LA, Mandler R, Murano G, Katz DA, Gordon RK, Chang PK, Schiffman E. Autocrine motility factors. Proc Natl Acad Sci USA 83:3302–3306, 1986.
84. Atnip KD, Carter LM, Nicolson GL, Dabbous MK. Chemotactic response of rat mammary adenocarcinoma cell clones to tumor-derived cytokines. Biochem Biophys Res Commun 146:996–1002, 1987.
85. Nabi IR, Watanabi H, Raz A. Identification of B16-F1 melanoma autocrine motility-like factor receptor. Cancer Res 50:409–414, 1990.
86. Erdel M, Spiess E, Trefz G, Boxberger HJ, Ebert W. Cell interactions and motility in human lung tumor cell lines HS-24 and SB-3 under the influence of extracellular matrix components and proteinase inhibitors. Anticancer Res 12:349–359, 1992.
87. Salge U, Kilian P, Newmann K, Elsasser HP, Havemann K, Heidtmann HH. Differentiation capacity of human non-small cell lung cancer cell lines after exposure to phorbol ester. Int J Cancer 45:1143–1150, 1990.

130

7. Cellular and molecular mechanisms of radioresistance

Ralph R. Weichselbaum, Michael A. Beckett, Everett E. Vokes,
David G. Brachman, Daniel Haraf, Dennis Hallahan, and Donald Kufe

Outstanding work on the cellular and molecular aspects of radioresistance has been published in the past 10 years [1,2]. The work presented herein does not attempt to be comprehensive but is a review of the work of our laboratory as it pertains to aspects of radioresistance with potential applicability to chemotherapy/cytokine radiotherapy interactions.

Cellular response of human tumor cells to radiation injury

Cellular radioresistance

Our group has analyzed radiation survival data from 23 early-passage epithelial tumor cell lines established from head and neck carcinoma patients (Table 1) and 13 early-passage mesenchymal cell lines established from patients with soft-tissue sarcomas (Table 2) prior to radiotherapy. Both patient groups were treated with curative intent radiotherapy and were subsequently followed [3,4]. Tumor cells cultured from head and neck cancer patients exhibited a wide range of radiosensitivities (D_0 = 107–333; mean D_0 = 185.5 ± 12.4). Overall, tumor cells derived from patients with soft-tissue sarcomas were more radiosensitive (D_0 = 126.1 ± 6.6) with a narrower range of radiobiologic parameters (D_0 = 94–182) than tumor cell lines derived from patients with head and neck carcinoma. More cell lines from patients with longer follow-up are necessary before conclusions can be drawn concerning in vitro radiobiologic parameters in relation to predicting patient outcome. However, the presence of radioresistant cells cultured from human tumors suggests that inherent tumor cell radioresistance may contribute to radiotherapy failure in some patients. The fact that tumor cells derived from head and neck cancer patients after they failed radiotherapy are more radioresistant than preradiotherapy-derived head and neck cancer cell lines and normal fibroblasts further supports this notion [5]. We hypo-

Hong, Waun Ki and Weber, Randal S., (eds.), Head and Neck Cancer. © *1995 Kluwer Academic Publishers.
ISBN 0-7923-3015-3. All rights reserved.*

Table 1. Radiobiological parameters for head and neck cell lines initiated prior to radiation therapy

Cell line	Site	D_0	ñ	Alpha
JSQ-11	Buccal cavity	173	2.5	0.19
HN-SCC-296A	Pyriform sinus	175	1.9	0.29
HN-SCC-170A	Subglottic	192	1.8	0.21
SQ-39	Retromolar trigone	213	1.0	0.47
HN-SCC-151	Anterior tongue	217	1.4	0.27
HN-SCC-135	Hard palate	227	1.6	0.24
HN-SCC-294	Oral tongue	227	1.6	0.27
HN-SCC-131	Anterior tongue	244	1.3	0.30
HN-SCC-58	Base of tongue	256	1.2	0.49
HN-SCC-161	Base of tongue	256	1.0	0.39
HN-SCC-166	Soft and hard palate	263	1.3	0.25
HN-SCC-143	Oropharynx	333	1.3	0.41
SCC-61	Anterior tongue	107	1.8	0.57
SCC-73	Retromolar trigone	108	1.2	0.91
HN-SCC-104	Pyriform sinus	119	2.5	0.23
SCC-66	Floor of mouth	129	2.1	0.34
HN-SCC-3	Soft palate	133	2.1	0.39
SCC-9	Anterior tongue	134	1.4	0.59
HN-SCC-288B	Larynx	139	2.0	0.96
HN-SCC-153	Larynx	143	2.7	0.24
SQ-38	Retromolar trigone	146	1.8	0.33
SCC-71	Soft palate	160	1.5	0.45
SQ-29	Retrolomar trigone	173	1.6	0.31
Mean ± SEM		185.5 ± 12.4	1.68 ± 0.1	0.40 ± 0.04

thesize that mutations conferring radioresistance occur during radiotherapy or that certain tumor cells are already resistant at the beginning of therapy. In either case, fractionated treatment would select for radio-resistant tumor cells. Because of the difficulties in experimentally producing radioresistant mutant human cell lines in vitro, we believe the former hypothesis to be unlikely.

Sublethal and potentially lethal damage repair

When a population of cells is exposed to radiation, some cells may not experience lethal damage and therefore are unaffected in the context of clonogenicity, whereas other cells may accumulate enough damage to cause death. If additional damage accumulates in a surviving cell before the initial sublethal lesion is repaired, the two may interact and cause cell death. Sublethal damage is defined operationally as the enhancement in survival when a radiation dose is divided over a period of time. The survival enhancement between radiation exposures is usually equal to the extrapolation number, ñ, of the survival curve [6–8]. Sublethal damage repair may be

Table 2. Radiobiological parameters for sarcoma cell lines initiated prior to radiation therapy

Cell line	Histology	Site	D_0	$\bar{n}$	Alpha
STSAR-26	Liposarcoma	Left triceps	94	2.6	0.67
STSAR-100	MFH	Left thigh	100	1.0	1.06
STSAR-84	Synovial sarcoma	Left palm	105	1.0	1.06
STSAR-91	Undifferent. sarcoma	Right pelvic region	112	2.0	0.21
STSAR-49	MFH	Left bicep	116	0.8	1.12
STSAR-13	Liposarcoma	Lateral aspect of right leg	117	1.2	0.63
STSAR-48	Malignant schwannoma	Left pelvic region	121	2.5	0.46
STSAR-8	MFH	Rt. deltoid pectoral groove	128	1.7	0.61
STSAR-255	Liposarcoma	Right arm	129	1.4	0.52
STSAR-217	Fibrosarcoma	Left thigh	140	1.0	0.77
HN-SCC-147	Osteosarcoma	Left mandible	146	1.1	0.72
STSAR-210	MFH	Lt. lateral thigh	149	1.0	0.66
HN-SCC-19	Neurosarcoma	Rt neck through neural foramina	182	2.1	0.19
Mean ± SEM			126.1 ± 6.6	1.49 ± 0.17	0.66 ± 0.08

important in radiotherapy because a shoulder region is recapitulated during a multifractionated treatment regimen, thereby greatly magnifying a small enhancement in survival following a single daily treatment. Most human fibroblasts and tumor lines studied in vitro have relatively small $\bar{n}$ [6,9–11]. Radiobiologists have characterized the low-dose region of the curve as the alpha parameter, which describes the initial slope of the radiation survival curve [12]. Whatever the description, a 30-fold to 40-fold magnification of the survival fraction following a single dose of radiotherapy may be important to clinical outcome.

Radiation-induced damage that is potentially lethal under a given set of environmental conditions may not be lethal if postradiation conditions are manipulated. For example, a delay in subculture after radiation in order to keep cells from initiating DNA synthesis (or dividing, depending upon experimental conditions) until the potentially lethal damage is repaired can enhance cell survival. This enhancement of survival following manipulations of postradiation conditions is referred to as *potentially lethal damage repair* (PLDR) [13–17]. This effect occurs principally in the G_1 phase of the cell cycle. Many human tumors have a relatively large component of noncycling G_1 (or G_0) cells, such that PLDR may be important clinically following fractionated radiotherapy.

Manipulation of radiosensitivity and repair by chemotherapeutic agents: Possible potential applications in head and neck cancer treatment

Because even a small change in the survival fraction after 2 Gy raised to the 30th or 40th power may have a profound effect on the ultimate survival fraction, one strategy for combining chemotherapeutic agents with radiation therapy is to alter radiation survival and/or repair parameters. Drugs that have been proposed to alter sublethal and potentially lethal damage repair include doxorubicin, Ara-A, cisplatin, and actinomycin-D. Reviews describing the strategy for combining chemotherapeutic agents and radiation in the context of altering radiation survival parameters have been published [18,19]. A large body of evidence suggests that cells vary in their radiosensitivity during various phases of the cell cycle. Although this variation depends on an individual cell line, cells are usually most radiosensitive during mitosis. Quiet et al. [20] recently confirmed this by showing that in radioresistant and radiosensitive human head and neck cancer cell lines, S phase cells were most radioresistant. Thus, the potential for elimination of radioresistant S phase cells in vivo may dominate the clinical response and may be useful in designing new chemotherapeutic agents and treatment regimens. The elimination of relatively radioresistant S phase cells is likely to be one basis for the success of the Vokes-Weichselbaum regimen, which combines the S-phase specific agents 5-fluorouracil and 6-hydroxyurea concomitantly with radiotherapy [21–25]. Cell kinetics and the relative sensitivity/resistance of cells in the cycle are important in designing alternative fractionated radiotherapy regimens.

Molecular aspects of radioresistance and DNA repair

Genes that repair gamma radiation-induced double-strand DNA breaks (the major lethal lesion produced by ionizing radiation) in mammalian cells have not been identified [26]. The product of one recently identified mammalian gamma repair gene, XRCC-1, participates in the repair of radiation-induced single-strand DNA lesions but does not correlate with cellular radiosensitivity [27,28]. Ionizing radiation inhibits cell cycle progression at the G_1/S and G_2/M transition points in the cell cycle. Such delays are referred to as *checkpoints* and are likely to represent active processes. For example, the RAD 9 gene product of *Saccharomyces cerevisiae* is responsible for the arrest of cells after DNA damage in the G_2 phase. Cells with a RAD 9 mutation that do not undergo G_2 arrest are x-ray sensitive, suggesting that cell-cycle–specific arrest is an important function in surviving radiation exposure [29]. It is likely that combinations of activation of cell-cycle arrest (checkpoint) and DNA repair genes function to allow survival following x-ray exposure.

The importance of identifying DNA repair genes for radiotherapy-induced damage is analogous to the discovery of genes that alter cell survival following exposure to chemotherapeutic agents. For example, amplification of genes that repair DNA damage and growth arrest may be responsible for tumor radioresistance or at least participate in the recovery from radiation damage. Inhibition of DNA repair gene function by chemotherapeutic agents might increase local tumor control by irradiation if the effects of these drugs could be concentrated in tumors. The cloning of DNA gamma repair genes and the subsequent screening for abnormalities of DNA and RNA from tumors may lead to a rapid, accurate prediction of tumor radiosensitivity. Genes having products that are involved with detoxification of radiation-induced free radicals may also be important in clinical radioresistance. These genes include superoxide dismutase, glutathione S-transferase, and glutathione S-peroxidase [30 for review].

The radical buffering system may be a potential molecular target to reverse radioresistance.

Oncogenes and cellular response to radiation

Fitzgerald et al. [31] reported that cells were made radioresistant by transfection with the oncogene N-*ras*, although the radioresistance was dependent on dose rate. Sklar [32] showed that the intrinsic radiation resistance of NIH/3T3 cells was increased by transfection with *ras* oncogenes activated by missense mutations, although the increase was a specific consequence of the *ras* mutations rather than transformation, since revertant cells that contained functional *ras* genes but were not transformed retained a radioresistant phenotype. Kasid et al. [33] noted that DNA from a radioresistant human laryngeal carcinoma cell line transfected into NIH/3T3 cells produced a c-*raf* transcript in the transformants. Kasid et al. [34] also transfected a radiation-resistant human laryngeal carcinoma line with a c-*raf*-1 cDNA fragment in the sense orientation and the c-*raf*-1 cDNA in reverse orientation so that antisense c-*raf*-1 RNA partially inhibited *raf* gene expression. Antisense c-*raf*-1 RNA partially suppressed both radioresistance and tumorigenicity of the laryngeal carcinoma line.

Pirollo et al. [35] noted that transfection of NIH/3T3 cells with Li-Fraumeni DNA containing the activated *raf* oncogene conferred radioresistance on fibroblasts as well as the transformed phenotype, and that both radioresistance and transformation were due to the presence of the activated c-*raf*-1 oncogene. These investigators also measured the effect of the oncogenes v-*mos*, v-*fes*, and v-*abl* on radioresistance. Transfection with the v-*mos* oncogene conferred radioresistance to NIH/3T3 cells, but transfection with v-*fes* and v-*abl* did not. The oncogenes v-*mos* and v-*raf* are serine-threonine protein kinases, whereas v-*fes* and v-*abl* are tryosine kinases. Pirollo et al. [35] proposed that activated oncogenes having gene products related to serine and threonine phosphorylation affect radioresistance. They also suggested that *ras* confers radioresistance because it transduces signals through direct regulation of protein kinase C (PKC), a serine-threonine kinase, in addition to its role as a G-protein and its effect on hydrolysis of phosphoinositides. Thus, alterations in the 'stress response' signal transduction pathway may alter a phenotypic response of cells to radiation. Protein kinases and molecular signalling pathways may be potential targets for inactivation by chemotherapeutic agents.

Signal transduction and the cellular radiation response

Alterations in intracellular signalling proteins (e.g., Raf and Ras) can alter cell survival following irradiation, suggesting that kinase-dependent signalling may be involved in the cellular response to radiation. Protein kinase C, which transduces signals from cell-surface receptors to the nucleus, is important in the cellular response to external stimuli such as growth factors, serum, and phorbol esters [36,37]. A recent study has suggested the participation of PKC and radiation-mediated gene induction [38]. Radiation directly activated PKC within 15–45 seconds. Depletion of PKC following prolonged exposure to the phorbol ester TPA results in attenuation of x-ray induction of genes encoding the transcription factors c-*jun* and *Egr*-1 [39]. Recently, Hallahan et al. [38] noted that PKC mediates the transcriptional induction of the tumor necrosis factor-α (TNF) gene by x-rays. Free radical intermediates generated in the cell membrane and/or DNA strand breaks following x-ray exposure are leading candidates as initial signals to propagate signalling; however, the exact mechanisms are unclear. Nontoxic doses of the purine analogue sangivamycin, which inhibits PKC by competing with adenosine triphosphate for enzyme binding, and the diacylglycerol competitor staurosporine both produced radiosensitization [40]. Therefore, kinase inhibitors may represent a new class of radiation sensitizers. With a better understanding of signal transduction following irradiation, additional targets may be identified for potential radiosensitization.

Cytokine induction and cellular response to radiation

Witte et al. [41] reported that platelet-derived growth factor (PDGF) and PDGF-like growth factors were released from the endothelium after irradiation. These authors suggested that PDGF-like factors secreted from the intima of blood vessels may serve as paracrine factors for the proliferation of smooth muscle cells observed in small arterioles after radiation in vivo. Similarly, fibroblast growth factor secreted after irradiation may participate in the abnormal proliferation of endothelial cells that has been reported to obliterate the lumina of small caliber arterioles and various organs. Thus, secretion of these growth factors may account for some of the long-term effects of radiation secondary to small vessel obliteration. Fibroblast growth factor has been reported to enhance the repair of radiation damage and is likely induced following activation of PKC [42].

Our group reported that irradiation induced a cytotoxic protein when culture medium decanted after irradiation of tissue cultures from some human sarcoma cells was cytotoxic to these as well as other tumor cell lines [43]. ELISA analysis indicated the level of tumor necrosis factor (TNF)-α in irradiated cultures was elevated over that in nonirradiated cultures. Monoclonal antibodies to TNF reversed the radiation-induced cytotoxicity. Increased levels of TNF-α were detected in TNF-α-producing cell lines after ionizing radiation. Nuclear run-on studies showed that radiation controlled TNF expression at the level of transcription [44]. The cytotoxicity of the medium from irradiated cells to other cell lines suggested a paracrine effect of TNF. We hypothesize that intracellular secretion of TNF after irradiation may also produce autocrine effects on the irradiated cells. Radiation survival experiments with TNF-producing and -nonproducing cell lines were carried out in the presence of varying concentrations of TNF-α. In some cell lines, sublethal concentrations of TNF enhanced killing by radiation, suggesting a radiosensitizing effect for TNF and a synergistic effect between TNF and x-rays [45]. In other cell lines, additive killing or independent effects occurred. The interactive effects of TNF and radiation are apparently cell specific. For example, Neta et al. [46] reported that TNF alone or in combination with interleukin 1 protects hematopoietic cells from the killing effects of radiation.

The concept of combining cytokines and radiation is currently being tested in a variety of centers. Tumor necrosis factor can be administered concomitantly during a course of radiotherapy, with the goal of protecting the hematopoietic microenvironment and/or sensitizing tumor cells. A phase I trial attempting to identify the maximally tolerated dose of TNF with radiotherapy is currently in progress at our institution.

Acknowledgments

This research was supported in part by NIH grants CA-41068 and CA-42596, The Center for Radiation Therapy, and a gift from the Passis Family.

References

1. Peters LJ, Brock WA, Johnson T, Meyn RE, Tofilon PJ, Milas L. Potential methods for predicting tumor radiocurability. Int J Radiat Oncol Biol Phys 12:459–467, 1986.
2. Brock WA, Baker FL, Wike JL, Sivon SL, Peters LJ. Cellular radiosensitivity of primary head and neck squamous cell carcinomas and local tumor control. Int J Radiat Oncol Biol Phys 18:1283–1286, 1990.

137

3. Weichselbaum RR, Dahlberg W, Beckett MA, Karrison T, Miller D, Clark J, Ervin TJ. Radiation-resistant and repair-proficient human tumor cells may be associated with radiotherapy failure in head and neck cancer patients. Proc Natl Acad Sci USA 83:2684–2688, 1986.

4. Weichselbaum RR, Beckett MA, Vijayakumar S, Simon MA, Awan AA, Nachman J, Panje WR, Goldman ME, Tybor AG, Moran WJ, Vokes EE, Ahmed-Swan S, Farhangi, E. Radiobiological characterization of head and neck sarcoma cells derived from patients prior to radiotherapy. Int J Radiat Oncol Biol Phys 19:313–319, 1990.

5. Weichselbaum RR, Beckett MA, Schwartz JL, Dritschilo A. Radioresistant tumor cells are present in head and neck carcinomas that recur after radiotherapy. Int J Radiat Oncol Biol Phys 15:575–579, 1988.

6. Weichselbaum RR, Nove J, Little JB. Radiation response of human tumor cells in vitro. In: RH Withers, R Meyn, eds. Radiation Biology and Cancer Research. New York: Raven Press, 1980, pp 345–351.

7. Elkind MM, Sutton H. X-ray damage and recovery in mammalian cells in culture. Nature 184:1293–1295, 1969.

8. Elkind MM. Fractionated dose radiotherapy and its relationship to survival curve shapes. Cancer Treat Rev 3:2–15, 1976.

9. Nilsson S, Carlsson J, Larsson B. Survival of irradiated glia and glioma cells studied with a new cloning technique. Int J Radiat Biol 37:267–279, 1980.

10. Weichselbaum RR, Dahlberg W, Little JB. Inherently radioresistant cells exist in some human tumors. Proc Natl Acad Sci USA 87:4732–4735, 1985.

11. Weichselbaum RR, Nove J, Little JB. X-ray sensitivity of 53 human diploid fibroblast cell strains from patients with characterized genetic disorders. Cancer Res 40:920–925, 1980.

12. Withers HR. Biological basis of radiation therapy. In: CA Peres, LW Brady, eds. Principles and Practice of Radiation Oncology. Philadelphia: JB Lippincott, 1987, pp 67–98.

13. Phillips RA, Tolmach LJ. Repair of potentially lethal damage in x-irradiated HeLa cells. Radiat Res 29:413–432, 1966.

14. Weichselbaum RR, Nove J, Little JB. Deficient recovery from potentially lethal radiation damage in ataxia telangiectasia and xeroderma pigmentosum. Nature 27:261–262, 1978.

15. Weichselbaum RR, Schmit A, Little JB. Cellular repair factors influencing radiocurability of human malignant tumors. Br J Cancer 45:10–16, 1982.

16. Weichselbaum RR, Little JB. The differential response of human tumors to fractionated radiation may be due to a post-irradiation repair process. Br J Cancer 46:532–537, 1982.

17. Weichselbaum RR, Beckett MA. The maximum recovery potential of human tumor cells may predict clinical outcome in radiotherapy. Int J Radiat Oncol Biol Phys 13:709–713, 1987.

18. Fu KK, Phillips TL. Biologic rationale of combined radiotherapy and chemotherapy. Hemotol/Oncol Clin North Am 5:737–751, 1991.

19. Vokes EE, Weichselbaum RR. Concomitant chemoradiotherapy: Rationale and clinical experience in patients with solid tumors. J Clin Oncol 8:911–934, 1990.

20. Quiet C, Weichselbaum RR, Gradina D. Variation in radiation sensitivity during the cell cycle to two human squamous cell carcinomas. Int J Radiat Oncol Biol Phys 20:733–738, 1991.

21. Vokes EE, Panje WR, Schilsky RL, Mick R, Awan AM, Moran WJ, Goldman MD, Tybor AG, Weichselbaum RR. Hydroxyurea, fluorouracil, and concomitant radiotherapy in poor-prognosis head and neck cancer: A phase I–II study. J Clin Oncol 7:761–768, 1989.

22. Haraf DJ, Vokes EE, Panje WR, Weichselbaum RR. Survival and analysis of failure following hydroxyurea, 5-fluorouracil and concomitant radiation therapy in poor prognosis head and neck cancer. Am J Clin Oncol 14:419–426, 1991.

23. Weppelmann B, Wheeler RA, Peters GE, Kim RY, Spencer SA, Meredith RF, Salter MM. Treatment of recurrent head and neck cancer with 5-fluorouracil, hydroxyurea and reirradiation. Int J Radiat Oncol Biol Phys 22:1051–1056, 1992.

24. Guillot T, Wibault P, Cvitkovit E, Luboinski E, Tellez B, Eschwege F, Schwaab G,

138

Armand JP. Treatment of 'favorable' recurrent (REC) head and neck squamous cell cancer (H+NSCC) with 5 days on/9 days simultaneous chemoradiotherapy (CH/RT) Vokes-Weichselbaum (VW) protocol (abstract #684). Proc Am Soc Clin Oncol 9:177, 1990.

25. Vokes EE, Beckett M, Karrison T, Weichselbaum RR. The interaction of 5-fluorouracil, hydroxyurea and radiation in two human head and neck cancer cell lines. Oncology 49:454–460, 1992.

26. Bohr VA, Evans MK, Fornace AJ. DNA repair and its pathogenetic implications. Lab Invest 61:143–161, 1989.

27. Thompson LH, Brookman KW, Jones NJ, Allen SA, Carrano AV. Molecular cloning of the human *XRCC-1* gene, which corrects defective DNA strand break repair and sister chromatid exchange. Mol Cell Biol 10:6160–6171, 1990.

28. Dunphy EJ, Beckett MA, Thompson LH, Weichselbaum RR. Expression of the polymorphic human DNA repair gene *XRCC-1* does not correlate with radiosensitivity in human head and neck tumor cell lines. Radiat Res 130:166–170, 1992.

29. Weinert TA, Hartwell LH. The *RAD9* gene controls the cell cycle response to DNA damage in *Saccharomyces cerevisiae*. Science 241:317–322, 1988.

30. Mitchell JB, Cook JA, DeGraff W, Glatstein E, Russo A. Glutathione modulation in cancer treatment: Will it work? Int J Radiat Oncol Biol Phys 16:1289–1295, 1989.

31. Fitzgerald TJ, Daugherty C, Kase K, Rothstein LA, McKenna M, Greenberger JS. Activated human n-*ras* oncogene enhances x-irradiation repair of mammalian cells in vitro less efficiently at low dose rates. Am J Clin Oncol 8:517–522, 1985.

32. Sklar MD. The *ras*-oncogenes increase the intrinsic resistance of NIH/3T3 cells to ionizing radiation. Science 239:645–657, 1989.

33. Kasid U, Pfeifer A, Weichselbaum RR, Dritschilo A, Mark GE. The *raf*-oncogene is associated with the radiation-resistant human laryngeal cancer. Science 237:1039–1041, 1987.

34. Kasid U, Pfeifer A, Brennan T, Beckett MA, Weichselbaum RR, Dritschilo A, Mark GE. Effect of anti-sense c-*raf*-1 on tumorigenicity and radiation sensitivity of a human squamous cell carcinoma. Science 243:1354–1356, 1989.

35. Pirollo KF, Garner R, Yuan SY, Li L, Blather WA, Chang EH. *Raf* involvement in the simultaneous genetic transfer of the radioresistant and transforming phenotypes. Int J Radiat Biol 55:783–796, 1989.

36. Horiguchi J, Spriggs D, Imamura K, Stone R, Leubbers R, Kufe D. Role of arachidonic acid metabolism in transcriptional induction of tumor necrosis factor gene expression by phorbol ester. Mol Cell Biol 9:252–258, 1989.

37. Rozengurt E, Rodriguez-Pena A, Coombs M, Sinnett-Smith J. Diacylglycerol stimulates DNA synthesis and cell division in mouse 3T3 cells: Role of Ca^+ 2-sensitive phospholipid-dependent protein kinase. Proc Natl Acad Sci USA 81:5748–5752, 1984.

38. Hallahan D, Virudachalam S, Sherman ML, Huberman E, Kufe DW, Weichselbaum RR. Tumor necrosis factor gene expression is mediated by protein kinase C following activation by ionizing radiation. Cancer Res 51:4565–4569, 1991.

39. Hallahan DE, Sukhatme VP, Sherman ML, Virudachalam S, Kufe D, Weichselbaum RR. Protein kinase C mediates x-ray inducibility of nuclear signal transducers, egr-1 and c-jun. Proc Natl Acad Sci USA 88:2152–2160, 1991.

40. Hallahan DE, Virudachalam S, Schwartz JL, Panje N, Mustafi R, Weichselbaum RR. Inhibition of protein kinases sensitizes human tumor cells to ionizing radiation. Radiat Res 129:345–350, 1992.

41. Witte L, Fuks Z, Haimovitz-Friedman A, Vlodavsky I, Goodman DS, Eldor A. Effects of radiation on the release of growth factors from cultured bovine, porcine, and human endothelial cells. Cancer Res 49:5066–5072, 1989.

42. Haimovitz-Friedman A, Vlodavsky I, Chaudhuri A, Witte L, Fuks Z. Autocrine effects of fibroblast growth factor in repair of radiation damage in endothelial cells. Cancer Res 51:2552–2558, 1991.

43. Hallahan DE, Spriggs DR, Beckett MA, Kufe DW, Weichselbaum RR. Increased tumor

139

necrosis factor-alpha mRNA after cellular exposure to ionizing radiation. Proc Natl Acad Sci USA 86:10104–10107, 1989.

44. Sherman ML, Datta R, Hallahan DE, Weichselbaum RR, Kufe DW. Regulation of tumor necrosis factor gene expression by ionizing radiation in human myeloid leukemia cells and peripheral blood monocytes. J Clin Invest 87:1794–1797, 1991.

45. Hallahan DE, Beckett MA, Kufe D, Weichselbaum RR. Interaction between recombinant human tumor necrosis factor and radiation in 13 human tumor cell lines. Int J Radiat Oncol Biol Phys 19:69–74, 1990.

46. Neta R, Oppenheim JJ, Schreiber RD, Chizzonite R, Ledney GD, Mac Vittie T. Role of cytokines (interleukin 1, tumor necrosis factor, and transforming growth factor beta) in natural and lipopolysaccharide-enhanced radioresistance. J Exp Med 173:1177–1182, 1991.

8. Early detection and screening for head and neck cancer

Jack L. Gluckman and Robert P. Zitsch

The concept of screening for cancer in order to facilitate early diagnosis has become quite popular in recent years. The stimulus for this interest is the increasing realization that the prognosis for cancers of the upper aerodigestive tract has improved very little over the past two decades, reflecting the late diagnosis of many of these tumors. Because the decline in smoking and drinking habits is only likely to have a direct impact on the incidence of this disease in 15–20 years, the need for early diagnosis is perceived as being essential to improve survival rates [1]. Our ability to formulate a satisfactory screening program is essential to achieve this end but, as will be evident from this chapter, this is no easy task.

The concept of screening for cancer is founded on several general principles. First, the cancer being screened must be accepted as being potentially life threatening if allowed to progress undetected. This is unquestioned in cancers of the upper aerodigestive tract but may be less clear in some other cancers, for example, well-differentiated thyroid cancer and prostatic cancer in the elderly.

Second, the asymptomatic cancer must, in some way, be detectable for the screening to be effective. In the mucosa of the head and neck, pre-malignant lesions usually present as leukoplakia or erythroplakia, while early frank invasive cancers may manifest as a small asymptomatic mucosal mass or ulcer. These are certainly capable of being detected by screening programs before they become symptomatic (detectable preclinical phase). By the time they have reached this size, however, the lesion may be quite advanced, and therefore it would be preferable if they could be diagnosed even earlier, perhaps at the molecular level (nondetectable preclinical phase). This is graphically demonstrated in Figure 1. Screening techniques for upper aerodigestive tract cancers are at present designed for detection of the clinically obvious tumors, with rudimentary efforts being made to detect abnormalities at the molecular level.

Third, effective cancer screening can only be performed if there is an

Hong, Waun Ki and Weber, Randal S., (eds.), Head and Neck Cancer. © *1995 Kluwer Academic Publishers. ISBN 0-7923-3015-3. All rights reserved.*

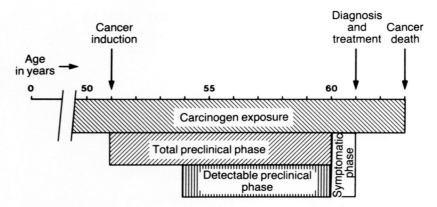

Figure 1. Diagram demonstrating asymptomatic and symptomatic phases of cancer development.

appropriate screening test. These tests should have a high degree of validity (as measured by sensitivity and specificity), be reliable, and be reproducible [1]. The screening test must also not be prohibitively complex or expensive and should have minimal morbidity.

The objective of a cancer screening program should be clearly understood. The ultimate objective is not to merely identify the cancer but to identify the tumor at a stage that treatment can affect the mortality rate of the detected cancer. This then has to be weighed against the cost and convenience of the screening process. Using the rates of cancer detection as justification for screening programs is *not* sufficient or acceptable. A lack of awareness and understanding of this basic issue has led to significant controversy regarding the effectiveness of screening for cancers of the upper aerodigestive tract.

The only absolutely valid gauge of success of a screening program would be to compare mortality rates of a screened population with expected mortality in the same population had they not undergone screening [2], that is, to evaluate two population groups concurrently or to compare the mortality of the 'at risk' population prior to the introduction of screening. These types of studies provide only oblique comparisons, which would suggest the probable effectiveness of the screening program, as a number of confounding variables may influence the outcome, for example, improved survival in the screened population may not be due to the screening procedure itself, but rather to an improved therapeutic regimen.

Other major problems encountered in evaluating a screening program are lead time bias and length bias. Both of these biases are common in groups of patients in whom asymptomatic disease is discovered by screening. Lead time is the period of time by which the diagnosis of the second cancer is temporally advanced (Figure 2). Any effective screening program will result in significant lead time because the cancer is being diagnosed earlier. This

142

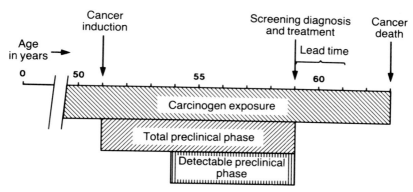

Figure 2. Diagram demonstrating the lead time of 2 years created by screening.

may effect survival data, as lead time bias will give an illusionary improved length of survival due to earlier diagnosis, but without actual postponement of death [1]. Lead time bias can be eliminated, however, if long-term survival is the criterion used for screening assessment.

Length bias also represents a significant problem in screening cancer patients [3]. This is due to the difference in cancer growth rates. Slowly growing, less aggressive cancers have a significantly longer detectable pre-clinical phase than rapidly growing aggressive cancers. This slow growth rate usually equates with a better prognosis. In any screening program, the slow growing lesions (with a favorable prognosis) would more likely be detected by screening, skewing comparison with those rapidly growing, aggressive tumors that are diagnosed late by symptoms alone [1].

Value of screening for cancer of the mucosa of the upper aerodigestive tract

The use of screening programs to identify cancers in the mucosa of the upper aerodigestive tract as a method of improving survival is a relatively new concept, even though 'at-risk goups' and 'field cancerization' with multicentric cancers have been recognized for many years [4–6], rendering the potential for screening an attractive concept. Of particular interest has been the knowledge that the mucosa has a propensity for multiple cancers to develop, significantly adversely affecting long-term survival.

These multiple cancers are classified temporally into
1. Simultaneous tumors: These are diagnosed at the time of the diagnosis of the index cancer.
2. Synchronous tumors: These are tumors that are not detected at the time of diagnosis of the initial cancer but are diagnosed within 6 months. These presumably were present initially but were just not clinically apparent.

3. Metachronous tumors: These are diagnosed after 6 months and may develop many years later.

The hypothesis for the development of these multicentric mucosal cancers in a 'field of growth' became clearer as tobacco emerged as the prime etiologic agent [7–10]. Once this etiologic relationship was established, it became obvious that tobacco users were at risk for the development of multicentric cancers and would need careful monitoring of the mucosa of the upper aerodigestive tract as well as other organ system.

Recommendations for close surveillance of patients with head and neck cancers did not await the identification of the responsible carcinogens, however. As early as 1943, radiographic evaluation of the total digestive tract was recommended for all patients in whom aerodigestive tract cancer had been diagnosed in order to detect later developing cancers [11]. Frequent lifelong follow-up examinations were also recommended as a means of detecting second cancers [12]. Likewise, a program of routine semiannual chest x-rays in patients with head and neck cancer, to detect metachronous lung cancers, was advocated [13]. The clear rationale behind these primitive screening programs was an attempt to improve survival rates by early detection.

Until 'field cancerization' and its association with multiple primary cancers was accepted [14,15], limited screening was the rule. This consisted at the initial evaluation of a thorough history and physical examination, including an attempt to visualize as much of the upper aerodigestive tract as possible, as well as chest x-ray. Close follow-up at regular intervals after treatment of the index primary lesion, looking not only for recurrence, but also for new cancers, became standard among oncologists treating head and neck cancer. Today, this approach, albeit rudimentary, continues to be the basic attempt at screening with the addition of fiberoptic endoscopy for inaccessible areas if indicated. Direct laryngoscopy, esophagoscopy, and bronchoscopy under general anesthesia have been added to the evaluation at the initial examination in most centers, but the value of these remains inconclusive as a worthwhile screening program. Endorsements have been based on the prevalence rates [16–20], with concomitant improved mortality rates usually being presumed but not proven [19–21]. The following aspects need to be considered when evaluating screening programs for cancer of the upper aerodigestive tract.

Patient selection for screening

Any screening program that has as its objective to reduce cancer mortality by earlier diagnosis of the disease must be performed on a group of patients with a sufficiently high disease incidence to justify the program. A screening program for cancer of the mucosa of the upper aerodigestive tract in the general population in the United States would certainly not be cost effective,

144

even if it was able to achieve a cancer-specific mortality reduction, because of the very low incidence of these cancers among the general population.

On the other hand, screening populations whose risk for these cancers is extremely high may be worthwhile. Populations in Iran, China, and Africa, where the risk of esophageal cancer is 20 times higher than in other population of the world, are such examples, as are the Chinese and Aleuts, who have a very high incidence of nasopharyngeal cancer. Unfortunately, as some of these countries are regarded as third world, the cost and logistics of instituting screening programs is often prohibitive.

Honing the at-risk group down to those exposed to known carcinogens, for example, tobacco and alcohol, is unfortunately still insufficient to justify screening from a cost-effectiveness standpoint. It has been suggested that workers exposed in industry to asbestos, coal soot, petroleum products, chromium, and iron oxide all have an increased incidence of upper aerodigestive tract cancer [22], but screening these workers has resulted in little return.

Some known medical disorders predispose to the development of esophageal cancer, and these high risk groups may be worth screening, for example, tylosis, a rare autosomal-dominant disorder, with affected family members having a 95% risk of developing esophageal cancer by age 65 [23], achalasia [24], chronic esophageal strictures following lye ingestion [25], Plummer-Vinson syndrome [26], celiac disease [27], and Barrett's esophagus due to chronic reflux [28]. Likewise, patients with overt lichen planus, submucosal fibrosis, and established leukoplakia should be subject to screening and certainly close follow-up of the established lesion.

In reality the only group in which a screening program can truly be justified are patients who have already developed an overt carcinoma of the upper aerodigestive tract mucosa. These patients have an extremely high incidence of second cancers (20–30%) [29–32]. In this group of patients, certain subgroups exist with an even higher risk of developing a second cancer, that is, those who continue to abuse tobacco and alcohol after treatment of the index cancer, and possibly those with the index cancer at certain sites. Moore determined that the incidence of a second upper aerodigestive tract cancer was only 6% in those patients who gave up the use of tobacco as compared to 40% in those who continued tobacco use [33]. Conversely, those patients with squamous cell carcinoma of the upper aerodigestive tract with no significant history of ethanol and tobacco use have been reported to have a comparatively reduced risk of second malignancies [34].

Those with primary cancers in the soft palate [35], and particularly the larynx [36–38], have a high incidence of second cancers, with the most common site of these malignancies being in the lung, oropharynx, and esophagus. On the other hand, sinonasal and nasopharyngeal cancers rarely occur as the second primary cancer [38,39], and an argument can be made not to include this area in any screening protocol.

While on the surface it would seem logical to screen all patients with one cancer for subsequently developing cancers, this issue is far from clear. For example, how should they be screened and how often? Should patients with advanced index cancers, with little chance for cure, also be included in this group, where determining the existence of a second cancer will have little bearing on the patient's survival?

Another population that could be considered for screening are those patients who have undergone prior radiation therapy to the head and neck area, looking for radiation-induced malignancies. The first recognition of head and neck malignancy secondary to radiation was in radium watch-dial painters, who were noted to have a high incidence of bone tumors, some of which occurred in the paranasal sinuses and mastoid [40]. The risk of developing head and neck malignancy from external beam irradiation, however, was not really appreciated until 40 years ago, when a greater than expected incidence of thyroid cancer was observed in patients who had been irradiated as children [41]. This observation was subsequently confirmed by further studies, and was noted particularly after low dose radiation treatment for benign conditions of the head and neck [42–44].

Although the development of thyroid cancers has attracted the most attention, tumors of the salivary glands, parathyroid, central nervous system, and mucosa of the upper aerodigestive tract have all been attributed to childhood irradiation [45–50].

While low dose irradiation has the greatest potential for inducing malignant transformation [51], the high dose therapeutic radiation used in the treatment of head and neck cancer has also been implicated as a possible cause of cutaneous, mucosal, salivary gland, bone, and soft tissue malignancies [52–56].

There is, however, contradictory evidence refuting the concept of radiation-induced aerodigestive tract carcinoma. Several retrospective investigations of head and neck cancer patients whose treatment included irradiation failed to demonstrate a statistically significant increased risk of second primary tumors in the same region [35,50,57–59].

While multiple screening programs have been designed to evaluate the risk of thyroid cancers in patients previously irradiated for benign conditions [60,61], no attempt has ever been made to screen for mucosal cancers in these patients. From the above evidence, it seems unlikely that a screening program will be particularly fruitful; however, it seems reasonable that all patients who have a history of radiation to the head and neck should have the mucosa of the upper aerodigestive tract, thyroid, and salivary glands carefully examined at regularly intervals.

It is therefore apparent that the only group truly worth screening is the patient who has already developed a mucosal upper aerodigestive tract cancer, particularly if there is a continued history of tobacco and alcohol abuse.

Timing considerations

Once it has been decided to institute a screening program for patients already diagnosed with an index cancer, a practical schedule for screening needs to be established. The optimum interval between screening tests is that which provides the highest degree of cancer detection at the least cost [1]. Many factors interact to determine this theoretical optimal frequency, including the sensitivity, complexity, and cost of the test and the length of the detectable preclinical phase. The high sensitivity of endoscopy theoretically lengthens the optimum interval, as does a cancer with a relatively long detectable preclinical phase. The more complex the test, the greater the cost, and this too will lengthen the optimal interval. Excessively long intervals will lead to failure in detecting preclinical cancer in many patients, while excessively short intervals will result in prohibitive expense.

Unfortunately, our lack of understanding of the natural history of cancer of the upper aerodigestive tract precludes the incorporation of these theoretical considerations. In the final analysis, the only way the optimal screening interval can be determined is to examine patient survival as a function of varied screening intervals. This has never been addressed in the head and neck literature and would be extremely difficult logistically to perform.

One absolute is that the initial screening should be performed when the person at risk is identified, that is, when the diagnosis of the index mucosal cancer is made. It is at this time that a large proportion of the multicentric cancers are identified [36,62], with several prospective studies identifying an incidence of simultaneously developing cancers of 9–16% [17,18,29,63–65], which was confirmed by a number of retrospective studies [19,20,38,66,67].

After the diagnosis and management of the index cancer, the majority of second aerodigestive tract malignancies will develop metachronously over the ensuing years, with 50% developing in the first 2 years [29,38,66,68] and approximately a further 3% per year for at least the next 7 years, although they may occur 20 years later.

Therefore, approximately 1 patient in 10 will have a second tumor diagnosed at the same time as the index and one half of the metachronous tumors will be identified within a 2-year period. The first 2 years consequently represents a window in time when screening efforts should be concentrated. The frequency of follow-up visits should therefore reflect this knowledge, being monthly for the first year, bimonthly for the second year, trimonthly for the third year, quarterly during the fourth year, and semiannually thereafter. The patient's mucosa should be carefully evaluated at this time.

The follow-up, looking for late developing cancers, should of course be lifelong, particularly if the patient should continue to smoke and drink. The concept of 5-year survival being equated with cure from the index cancer is valid, but long-term surveillance of these patients is essential.

Screening techniques

The mucosa of the upper aerodigestive tract, that is, the oral cavity, oropharynx, larynx, hypopharynx, and even nasopharynx, is easily visualized during routine clinical examination using contemporary diagnostic techniques, including mirrors and fiberoptic endoscopy. The lower aerodigestive tract, that is, the inferior hypopharynx, esophagus, trachea, and bronchi, is, however, not easily evaluated and usually requires more formal endoscopy for visualization. Even though second cancers at these inaccessible sites represent over 50% of the subsequent developing aerodigestive tract malignancies [29,66], endoscopy to visualize these lower areas is not usually routinely performed in follow-up. The rationalization is that this would logistically be extremely difficult and expensive to perform and compromise procedures, for example, x-ray chest and esophagograms, have been recommended which have been proven to be less effective than screening techniques.

Another source of concern is that endoscopy is only of value in detecting overt clinically apparent lesions, for example, leukoplakia, erythroplakia, ulcer, or mass, with the premalignant lesions being very subjective in their interpretation. In order to facilitate the diagnosis of these earlier cancers, in vivo staining techniques have been proposed. The best known of these is toluidine blue, which has been used in the oral cavity, oropharynx, and larynx and esophagus. Toluidine blue is a basic metachromatic nuclear stain that stains the nuclear material of malignant lesions but spares normal mucosa. It has an acceptable specificity rate for malignancy if used correctly, but because of a high false-positive rate due to staining of inflammatory lesions, it has not gained popular acceptance. A major reason may be because of poor technique. If a 1% toluidine blue solution mixed with acetic acid and alcohol, rather that a 1% aqueous solution, is used and all debris and saliva are removed before application, the false-positive rate declines to 6.8% [69,70]. Perhaps its most useful role is not to diagnose cancer but to guide the physician where to biopsy.

Devices to detect tumor autofluorescence and drug-induced fluorescence, for example, hematoporphyrin, are intriguing, particularly when combined with image enhancers and endoscopy, for example, fiberoptic bronchoscopy for the detection of early bronchial cancer [71,72], but these devices remain expensive, cumbersome, and experimental. Cytologic evaluation and DNA analysis of suspicious areas remain interesting, but how to incorporate these techniques in a screening program remains elusive. For these reasons, contemporary screening techniques remain somewhat unsatisfactory, particularly for cancer of the esophagus and bronchi.

148

Screening for esophageal cancer

The esophagus is a frequent site for the development of second cancers, either synchronously [19] or metachronously [66,73,74]. Likewise, there is a high incidence of second cancers in the upper aerodigestive tract associated with esophageal cancer, although the true incidence is difficult to determine as the long-term survival after treatment for esophageal cancer is less than 10% [75–77].

Esophageal carcinoma found subsequent to the identification of an index head and neck cancer has an extremely poor survival rate, reflecting their late diagnosis, usually because endoscopy or contrast study performed to establish the diagnosis is symptom directed and not the result of a formal screening process. Earlier diagnosis of these esophageal cancers through screening could potentially increase this dismal survival rate. Early diagnosis of esophageal carcinoma has proved distinctly possible. In northern China, where a high incidence of esophageal cancer is found with concomitant poor survival rates, mass screening has been employed over the past 20 years with the 5-year survival improving from 10% in the 1950s to 30% for advanced cancer and 90% for early cancers today [78]. This has been accomplished by examining cytologic specimens collected from a mesh-covered balloon pulled through the length of the esophagus. Positive screens are followed up with endoscopy and biopsy. The detection rate using this technique is extremely high, with 75% of those diagnosed being early cancer.

This screening program is an outstanding example of a screening program successfully accomplishing its objective, but the lessons learned are not applicable in the United State because of the relatively low incidence of esophageal cancer. However, similar cytologic screening programs have been instituted in other countries with high rates of esophageal cancer. The theory as to why this screening program is so successful is that cancer of the esophagus has a prolonged preclinical phase [79], and therefore if the disease is diagnosed at an early enough stage, the chances of cure are very high. Whether this applies to all esophageal cancers is unknown, and some may behave in a more aggressive manner and therefore not benefit from screening.

An esophagogram has been recommended as a compromise screening technique [17,64,76,80], but this is less sensitive than endoscopy and therefore not very effective in diagnosing early cancer [81–83]. As a screening tool it therefore has little value, and esophagoscopy remains the screening technique of choice, although timing and cost remain difficult issues.

The sensitivity and specificity (with biopsy) of esophagoscopy makes this a good but not infallible screening tool. It is important to note that up to 20% of patients with early cancer will have normal-appearing mucosa at endoscopy [78]. To enhance visualization of early lesions, the use of toluidine blue has been suggested, but as already stated, its value is marginal [84]. While its role during the initial evaluation of the index cancer is well accepted and routinely used, its role in routine follow-up remains controversial, particularly with regard to cost-effectiveness and patient convenience [18,19,85,86]. To be most effective, it should probably be performed at least semi-annually for the first 2 years, but there are few oncologists who follow this regimen.

The technique of esophagoscopy to be used is likewise fraught with controversy. Rigid esophagoscopy is regarded as the tried and trusted gold standard by head and neck surgeons, but it requires general anesthesia, with a concomitant increase in cost and potential complications. Fiberoptic esophagoscopy is equally effective in expert hands and, of course, can be performed under local anesthesia. The complication rates from both techniques are very low, but from the logistical and convenience perspective neither technique is acceptable. They are probably best combined with routine cytologic evaluations for the best results. Until head and neck oncologists can become convinced of the advantages of regular endoscopies in routine follow-up, esophagoscopy will continue to be confined to the initial evaluation of the index cancer and be performed only on a symptom-directed basis in follow-up.

Screening for cancer of the trachea and bronchi

The high incidence of second primary cancers developing in the bronchi is a significant problem and is associated with a very poor prognosis [66,87]. Survival rates for lung cancer as a second primary tumor are only slightly less than if the lung cancer presents as the index cancer [88], once again reflecting late diagnosis.

Screening for early detection of lung cancer has traditionally been performed using annual chest x-rays. Unfortunately, this has failed to improve the lung cancer mortality rates and has proved a failure as a screening technique. Sputum cytology to complement chest x-ray has been suggested, using the rationale that cytology is better able to detect endobronchial cancers, while chest x-ray is better at detecting peripheral lesions. Unfortunately, a number of large long-term, randomized, controlled trials of screening for early stage lung cancer using sputum cytology and chest x-ray under the auspices of the National Cancer Institute have failed to demonstrate a reduction in lung cancer mortality [88,89].

For this reason, it has been suggested that routine bronchoscopy be incorporated as a screening procedure to diagnose early lung cancer. While some believe this is redundant because of the low success rate in the presence of a normal chest x-ray, [85], others have demonstrated that this can be rewarding, particularly when combined with bronchial lavage and cytology of the washings [90]. False-positive cytology can, however, occur due to shedding of malignant cells from cancers in the upper aerodigestive tract [91].

While rigid or fiberoptic bronchoscopy can be performed, and there are proponents and detractors of each, fiberoptic bronchoscopy offers a more complete evaluation, while rigid is useful at the initial examination because of the ability to secure the airway with this scope. As with esophagoscopy, ideally screening fiberoptic bronchoscopy should be performed at semi-annual intervals in the follow-up period following identification of the index cancer. Cost, logistics, and convenience are all factors that detract from its role.

In an attempt to clarify the role of various techniques designed in Europe, the EUROSCAN program was developed for screening patients treated for oral cavity, laryngeal, or lung cancer with bronchoscopy, sputum cytology, and chest x-ray for 4 years with continued follow-up for 10 years [92]. This ambitious plan could potentially provide the first meaningful information on the effectiveness of bronchoscopic screening for second primary lung cancers.

Screening for nasopharyngeal cancer

Nasopharyngeal carcinoma is rarely associated with other cancers of the mucosa of the upper aerodigestive tract, and most investigators do not feel that routine nasopharyngoscopy should be included in the endoscopic evaluation of head and neck cancer patients [17,32,36,66,85], the rationale being that different carcinogenic agents are responsible for nasopharyngeal cancer. If, however, the patient falls into a high risk group for the development of nasopharyngeal cancer, for example, Chinese, Aleuts, etc., then the nasopharynx should be screened regularly using mirror, direct, or fiberoptic endoscopy.

An alternative screening tool to direct visualization is the use of serological tests looking for the presence of IgA anti-viral capsid antigen (VCA). This may be useful in screening relatives of patients with nasopharyngeal cancer or high-risk groups with a propensity for nasopharyngeal cancer.

Problems associated with screening for cancers of the upper aerodigestive tract

As already noted, the evaluation of screening programs must consider the merits, limitations, and cost. Since the concept of at-risk groups and field cancerization became understood, and the importance of early diagnosis as a means of improving survival became apparent, every attempt has been made to establish effective screening programs. Routine endoscopies occupy a pre-eminent role as screening procedures, but their use has not yet been demonstrated as being able to reduce the mortality of these cancers. In fact, the time, expense, and morbidity of these procedures may offset the benefits [62,93,94].

Financial considerations

The issue of the financial benefits of a screening program is difficult to evaluate, particularly in the United States, where costs are being critically appraised. If it is felt that endoscopic evaluation is overall the most effective method of detecting preclinical cancer, then this must be judged in terms of its cost-benefit ratio. Several investigators have attempted to address this issue. Parker and Hill felt that routine laryngoscopy is the only one of the three components of triple endoscopy that could be supported, citing low yield and high additional costs for esophagoscopy and bronchoscopy [94]. Shaha et al. questioned the role of routine triple endoscopy in every patient with head and neck cancer because of the high cost [62]. Others, however, have attempted to justify the cost of routine panendoscopy in head and neck cancer patients [95].

In the final analysis, if it is felt that panendoscopy to detect early cancer can be equated with the highest standard of care, cost should not enter into the equation when managing an individual patient. The overall cost-benefit ratio in evaluating a screening program, however, is a different matter and, at this stage, there is no evidence that these procedures constitute a successful screening program. As health-care dollars become increasingly scarce, some harsh decisions will have to be made. It is possible, therefore, that through necessity a compromise position will be reached in which non-invasive radiographic or cytologic screening will become the optimal screening measure.

Morbidity

Additional morbidity produced by screening techniques must also be examined closely. Good screening procedures should be relatively free of complications, and it does appear that multiple endoscopy is a safe procedure with low morbidity [17,18,21,64,93]. Therefore, the concern that patients undergoing panendoscopy are at significant additional risk is not valid and probably not a consideration.

Ability to influence survival

The major issue of concern is the ability of the screening programs, particularly those employing multiple endoscopy, to alter the ultimate outcome of the patient. It unfortunately remains unclear whether this objective can truly be accomplished, even in as focused a population as those with an index cancer already diagnosed. The only exception is the extremely successful program being utilized for managing esophageal cancer in China. This negative sentiment reflects our lack of understanding of cancer behavior and the inadequacy of the screening techniques currently being utilized.

Considerations for the future

At this moment in time, it is not clear if screening for head and neck cancer will improve mortality rates and even less clear whether they are cost-effective. However, even if the screening protocols should fail to fulfill these criteria, this does not mean that routine endoscopy, radiographic evaluation, and frequent clinical examinations should not be performed in individual patients, as this constitutes optimal patient care. It is only in the context of evaluating the efficacy of a screening program that this bears careful analysis. Hopefully, more sensitive low cost screening methods for patients at risk will ultimately lead to better survival rates. Perhaps further identification of particular subgroups among head and neck cancer patients with a higher risk of multiple cancers will improve the efficacy of the screening program, for example, immunologic anomalies or genetic influences [96,97].

References

1. Cole P, Morrison AS. Basic issues in population screening for cancer. J Natl Cancer Inst 64:1263–1272, 1980.
2. Miller AB. Principles of screening and the evaluation of screening programs. In: AB Miller, ed. Screening for Cancer. Academic Press, 1985, p 359.
3. Bailar JC III. Mammographic screening, a reappraisal of benefits and risks. Clin Obstet Gynecol 21:1–14, 1978.
4. Lund CC. Second primary cancer in cases of cancer of the buccal mucosa: A mathematical study of susceptibility to cancer. N Engl J Med 209:1144–1152, 1933.
5. Warren S, Gates O. Multiple primary malignant tumors: A survey of the literature and a statistical study. Am J Cancer 51:1358–1403, 1932.
6. Watson WL. Cancer of the esophagus, some etiologic considerations. Am J Roentgenol 41: 420–424, 1939.
7. Lombard HL, Doering CR. Cancer studies in Massachusetts. Habits, characteristics and environment of individuals with and without cancer. N Engl J Med 198:481–487, 1928.
8. Levin ML, Goldstein H, Gerhardt PR. Cancer and tobacco smoking: A preliminary report. JAMA 143:336–338, 1950.
9. Mills CA, Porter MM. Tobacco smoking habits and cancer of the mouth and respiratory system. Cancer Res 10:539–542, 1950.
10. Wynder EL, Graham EA. Tobacco smoking as a possible etiologic factor in bronchogenic carcinoma. A study of 684 proved cases. JAMA 143:329–336, 1950.
11. Hellendall H. Multiple carcinoma: The clinical picture, diagnosis and prognosis. Am J Surg 60:22–35, 1943.
12. Byars LT, Anderson R. Multiple cancers of the oral cavity. Am Surg 18:386–391, 1952.
13. Cahan WG. Lung cancer associated with primary cancer in other sites. Am J Surg 89:494–514, 1955.
14. Shedd DP, Kligerman MM, Gowen GF. Multifocal carcinogenesis in the oral cavity. Am J Surg 104:692–696, 1962.
15. Slaughter DP, Southwick HW, Smejkal W. 'Field cancerization' in oral stratified squamous epithelium. Cancer 6:963–968, 1953.
16. Atkinson D, Fleming S, Weaver A. Triple endoscopy: A valuable procedure in head and neck surgery. Am J Surg 144:416–419, 1982.
17. Leipzig B, Zellmer JE, Klug D. The panendoscopy study group: The role of endoscopy in

evaluating patients with head and neck cancer: A multi-institutional prospective study. Arch Otolaryngol 111:589–594, 1985.

18. McGuirt WF. Panendoscopy as a screening examination for simultaneous primary tumors in head and neck cancer: A prospective sequential study and review of the literature. Laryngoscope 92:569–576, 1982.

19. Shapshay SM, Hong WK, Fired MP, et al. Simultaneous carcinomas of the esophagus and upper aerodigestive tract. Otolaryngol Head Neck Surg 88:373–377, 1980.

20. Weaver A, Fleming SM, Knechtges TC, et al. Triple endoscopy: A neglected essential in head and neck cancer. Surgery 86:493–496, 1979.

21. Atkins JP, Keane WM, Young KA, et al. Value of panendoscopy in determination of second primary cancer: A study of 451 cases of head and neck cancer. Arch Otolaryngol 110:533–534, 1984.

22. Cole P, Goldman MB. Occupation. Persons at high risk of cancer. In: JF Fraumeni, ed. An Approach To Cancer Etiology and Control. New York: Academic Press, 1975, pp 167–184.

23. Harper PS, Garper RMJ, Howel-Evans AW. Carinoma of the esophagus with tylosis. Q J Med 39:317–333, 1970.

24. Carter R, Brewer LA III. Achalasia and esophageal carcinoma. Am J Surg 130:114–120, 1975.

25. Hopkins RA, Postlewait RW. Caustic burns and carcinoma of the esophagus. Ann Surg 194:146–148, 1981.

26. Ahlbom HE. Simple achlorhydric anemia, Plummer-Vinson syndrome and carcinoma of the mouth, pharynx and esophagus in women. Br Med J 2:331–333, 1936.

27. Swinson CM, Slavin G, Coles EC, et al. Coeliac disease and malignancy. Lancet 1(8316): 111–115, 1983.

28. Naef AP, Savary M, Ozello L. Columnar-lined lower esophagus: An acquired lesion with malignant predisposition. Report on 140 cases of Barrett's esophagus with 12 adeno-carcinomas. J Thorac Cardiovasc Surg 70:826–835, 1975.

29. Gluckman JL, Cissman JD, Donegan JO. Multicentric squamous cell carcinoma of the upper aerodigestive tract. Head Neck Surg 3:90–96, 1980.

30. Hordijk, GJ, DeJong JMA. Synchronous and metachronous tumors in patients with head and neck cancer. J Laryngol Otol 97:619–621, 1983.

31. Jesse RH, Sugarbaker EV. Squamous cell carcinoma of the oropharynx: Why we fail. Am J Surg 132:435–438, 1976.

32. Tepperman BS, Fitzpatrick PJ. Second respiratory and upper digestive tract cancers after oral cancer. Lancet 2:547–549, 1981.

33. Moore C. Cigarette smoking and cancer of the mouth, pharynx and larynx: A continuing study. JAMA 218:553–558, 1971.

34. Schantz SP, Byers RM, Geopfert H, et al. The implication of tobacco use in the young adult with head and neck cancer. Cancer 62:1374–1380, 1988.

35. Kogelnik, HD, Fletcher GH, Jesse RH. Clinical course of patients with squamous cell carcinoma of the upper respiratory and digestive tracts with no evidence of disease 5 years after initial treatment. Radiology 115:423–427, 1975.

36. Cohn AM, Peppard SM. Multiple primary malignant tumors of the head and neck. Am J Otolaryngol 1:411–417, 1980.

37. DeVries N, Snow GB. Multiple primary tumors in laryngeal cancer. J Laryngol Otol 100:915–918, 1986.

38. Vrabec DP. Multiple primary malignancies of the upper aerodigestive system. Ann Otol Rhinol Larynol 88:846–854, 1979.

39. Berg JW, Schottenfeld D, Ritter F. Incidence of multiple primary cancers. III. Cancers of the respiratory and upper digestive system as multiple primary cancers. J Natl Cancer Inst 44:263–274, 1976.

40. Martland HS. The occurrence of malignancy in radioactive persons. Am J Cancer 15:2435–3118, 1931.

41. Duffy BJ, Fitzgerald PJ. Cancer of the thyroid in children: A report of 28 cases. J Clin Endocrinol Metab 10:1296–1308, 1950.
42. De Groot L, Palyan E. Thyroid carcinoma and radiation. JAMA 225:487–491, 1973.
43. Schneider AB, Shore-Fredman E. Radiation-induced tumors of the head and neck following childhood irradiation. Medicine 64:1–5, 1985.
44. Scanlon EF. Head and neck tumors associated with irradiation for benign conditions. CA Cancer J Clin 31:177–182, 1981.
45. Scanlon EF, Sener SF. Head and neck neoplasia following irradiation for benign conditions. Head Neck Surg 4:139–145, 1981.
46. Schneider AB, Favus MJ, Stachura ME, et al. Salivary gland neoplasms as a late consequence of head and neck irradiation. Ann Intern Med 87:160–164, 1977.
47. Sirota DK, Eden AR, Biller HF. Multiple head and neck neoplasia following radiation for benign disease during childhood. J Surg Oncol 38:101–103, 1988.
48. Tisell LE, Hansson G, Lindberg S, et al. Hyperparathyroidism in persons treated with X-rays for tuberculous cervical adenitis. Cancer 40:846–854, 1977.
49. Schneider AB, Shore-Freedman E, Wenstein RA. Radiation-induced thyroid and other head and neck tumors: Occurrence of multiple tumors and analysis of risk factors. J Clin Endocrinol Metab 63:107–112, 1986.
50. Modan B, Baidaz D, Mart H, et al. Radiation-induced head and neck tumors. Lancet 1:277–279, 1974.
51. Mole RH. Ionizing radiation as a carcinogen: Practical questions and academic pursuits. Br J Radiol 48:157–169, 1975.
52. Cronin J. Radiation-induced cancer of the larynx and pharynx. J Laryngol Otol 25:621–622, 1971.
53. Goolden AWG. Radiation cancer: A review with special reference to radiation tumors in the pharynx, larynx and thyroid. Br J Radiol 30:626–640, 1957.
54. Sakamoto A, Sakamoto G, Sugano H. History of cervical radiation and incidence of carcinoma of the pharynx, larynx and thyroid. Cancer 44:718–723, 1979.
55. Schindel J, Castoriano IM. Late-appearing (radiation-induced) carcinoma. Arch Otolaryngol 95:205–210, 1972.
56. Southwick HW. Radiation-associated head and neck tumors. Am J Surg 134:438–443, 1977.
57. Jy DMC. Salivary gland tumors occurring after radiation of the head and neck area. Am J Surg 116:518–523, 1968.
58. Parker RG, Enstrom JE. Second primary cancers of the head and neck following treatment of initial primary head and neck cancer. Int J Radiat Oncol Biol Phys 14:561–564, 1988.
59. Seydel HG. The risk of tumor induction in man following medical irradiation for malignant neoplasm. Cancer 35:1641–1645, 1975.
60. Royce PC, MacKay BR, DiSabella PM. Value of postirradiation screening for thyroid nodules: A controlled study of recalled patients. JAMA 242:2675–2678, 1979.
61. Schneider AB, Pinsky S, Bekerman C, et al. Characteristics of 108 thyroid cancers detected by screening in a population with a history of head and neck irradiation. Cancer 46:1218–1227, 1980.
62. Shaha AR, Hoover EL, Mitrani M, et al. Synchronicity, multicentricity and metachronicity of head and neck cancer. Head Neck Surg 10:225–228, 1988.
63. Lau WF, Siu KF, Wei W, et al. Prospective screening for multiple tumors of the upper aerodigestive tract: A simple routine procedure. Laryngoscope 96:1149–1153, 1986.
64. Schuller DE, Fritsch MH. An assessment of the value of triple endoscopy in the evaluation of head and neck cancer patients. J Surg Oncol 32:156–158, 1986.
65. Shaha A, Hoover E, Marti J, et al. Is routine triple endoscopy cost-effective in head and neck cancer. Am J Surg 155:750–753, 1988.
66. Shons AR, McQuarrie DG. Multiple primary epidermoid carcinomas of the upper aerodigestive tract. Arch Surg 120:1007–1009, 1985.
67. Gluckman JL. Synchronous multiple primary lesions of the upper aerodigestive system.

Arch Otolaryngol 105:597–598, 1979.

68. Marchetta FC, Sako K, Camp F. Multiple malignancies in patients with head and neck cancer. Am J Surg 110:537–541, 1965.

69. Mahberg A. Re-evaluation of toluidine blue application as a diagnostic adjunct in the detection of asymptomatic oral squamous cell carcinoma: A continuing prospective study of oral cancer III. Cancer 46:758–763, 1980.

70. Strong MS, Vaughan CW, Incze JS. Toluidine blue in the management of carcinoma of the oral cavity. Arch Otolaryngol 87:101–105, 1968.

71. Hayat Y, Kato H, Ono J. Fluorescence fiberoptic bronchoscopy in the diagnosis of early stage lung cancer. Recent Results Cancer Res 82:121, 1982.

72. Balchum OF, Doiron DR, Profia AE, et al. Fluorescence bronchoscopy for localizing early bronchial cancer and carcinoma in situ. Recent Results Cancer Res 82:97–120, 1982.

73. Vikram B, Strong EW, Shah JP, et al. Second malignant neoplasms in patients successfully treated with multimodality treatment for advanced head and neck cancer. Head Neck Surg 6:734–737, 1984.

74. Odette J, Szymanowski RT, Nichols RD. Multiple head and neck malignancies. Trans Am Acad Ophthalmol Otol 84:805–813, 1977.

75. Fogel TD, Harrison LB, Son YN. Subsequent upper aerodigestive tract malignancies following treatment of esophageal cancer. Cancer 55:1882–1885, 1985.

76. Goldstein HM, Zornoza J. Association of squamous cell carcinoma of the head and neck with cancer of the esophagus. Am J Roentgenol 131:791–794, 1978.

77. Mantravadi RVP, Lad T, Briele H, et al. Carcinoma of the esophagus: Sites of failure. Int J Radiat Oncol Biol Phys 8:1897–1901, 1982.

78. Shu YJ. Cytopathology of the esophagus. An overview of cytopathology in China. Acta Cytol 27:7–16, 1983.

79. Guanrei Y, He H, Sungliang Q. Endoscopic diagnosis of 115 cases of early esophageal carcinoma. Endoscopy 14:157–161, 1982.

80. Bundrick TJ, Cho SR. Evaluation of the esophagus in patients with head and neck cancer. Am J Roentgenol 142:1082–1083, 1984.

81. Moss AA, Koehler RE, Margulis AR, Initial accuracy of esophagrams in detection of small esophageal carcinoma. Am J Roentgenol 127:909–913, 1976.

82. Zornoza J, Lindell MM, Jr. Radiographic evaluation of small esophageal carcinoma. Gastrointest Radiol 5:107–111, 1980.

83. Grossman TW, Kita MS, Toohill RJ. The diagnostic accuracy of pharyngoesophagram compared to esophagoscopy in patients with head and neck cancer. Laryngoscope 97:1030–1032, 1987.

84. Jessen K, Paolucci P, Classen M. Endoscopic vital staining of the esophagus in high risk patients: Detection of dysplasia and early carcinoma. In: P Sherlock, BC Morson, L Barbara, V Veronesi, eds. Precancerous Lesions of the Gastrointestinal Tract. New York: Raven Press, 1983, pp 65–70.

85. Maisel RH, Vermeersch H: Panendoscopy for second primaries in head and neck cancer. Ann Otol Rhinol Laryngol 90:460–464, 1981.

86. Abemayor E, Moore DM, Hanson DG. Identification of synchronous esophageal tumors in patients with head and neck cancer. J Surg Oncol 38:94–96, 1988.

87. Atabek U, Mirseyed AM, Suresh R, et al. Lung cancer in patients with head and neck cancer: Incidence and long-term survival. Am J Surg 154:434–437, 1987.

88. Fontana RS, Sanderson DR, Woolner LB, et al. Lung cancer screening: The Mayo program. J Occup Med 28:746–750, 1986.

89. Early Lung Cancer Cooperative Study. Early lung cancer detection: Summary and conclusions. Am Rev Resp Dis 130:554–570, 1984.

90. Leipzig B. Bronchoscopy in the staging and evaluation of head and neck carcinoma. Ann Otol Rhinol Laryngol 92:373–376, 1983.

91. Johnson JT, Turner J, Dekker A. The significance of positive bronchial cytology in the

156

presence of squamous cell carcinoma of the upper aerodigestive tract. Ann Otol Rhinol Laryngol 90:454–456, 1981.

92. DeVries N, Snow GB. Prevention of second primary cancers in head and neck cancer patients: New perspectives. Am J Otolaryngol 9:151–154, 1988.

93. Neew HB III. Routing panendoscopy—is it necessary every time? (commentary) Arch Otolaryngol 110:531–532, 1984.

94. Parker JT, Hill JH. Panendoscopy in screening for synchronous primary malignancies. Laryngoscope 98:147–149, 1988.

95. McGuirt WF. Panendoscopy (letter). Laryngoscope 98:688, 1988.

96. DeVries N, Delange G, Drexhage H, et al. Immunoglobulin allotypes in head and neck cancer patients with multiple primary cancers. Acta Otolaryngol 104:187–191, 1987.

97. DeVries N, Drexhage HA, Dewaal LP, et al. Human leukocyte antigens and immunoglobulin allotypes in head and neck cancer patients with and without multiple primary tumors. Cancer 60:957–961, 1987.

9. Photodynamic therapy for cancer of the head and neck

Jack L. Gluckman and Louis G. Portugal

Photodynamic therapy (PDT) is a therapeutic modality that utilizes a photo-sensitizing drug that selectively localizes in tumors and, on activation by exposure to light, results in preferential tumor necrosis. Like all new therapies directed to cancer, this modality was initially greeted with great enthusiasm and was heralded as an excellent therapy, not only for early superficial cancer but also the more advanced tumors. Time and experience have tempered this unrealistic expectation and, therefore, in spite of its initial promise, PDT remains for the present an investigational modality whose potential has yet to be realized. Much basic research and more clinical trials are required before its exact role in contemporary cancer therapy can be accurately defined, but one remains optimistic that this will soon occur. Two components are necessary for this therapy to be utilized, that is, a photosensitizer drug and a laser to activate the drug.

Photosensitizer

The first known use of phototherapy occurred when the ancient Egyptians over 6000 years ago used this technique to treat depigmented areas of the skin [1]. They applied crushed leaves from plants related to parsley (which contain the photosensitizer psoralens) to the depigmented areas and, on exposure to sunlight, a sunburn occurred on the affected area.

In 1903 Tappenier and Jesionek [2] were the first to utilize this process for the treatment of malignant disease when they treated skin cancers using topical eosin as the photosensitizer together with white light. Over the years, numerous substances have been used as photosensitizers, for example, tetracycline, berberine sulfate, acridine orange, fluorescein, rhodamine, various porphyrins, and more recently, sulphonated metallophthalocyanines, diaziquone, N,N'*bis* (2-ethyl-1,3-dioxolane)-kryptocyaine (EDKC), Nile blue A (NBA), tetra-(4-sulfonatophenyl) porphine (TPPS), silicon naph-

Hong, Waun Ki and Weber, Randal S., (eds.), Head and Neck Cancer. © *1995 Kluwer Academic Publishers. ISBN 0-7923-3015-3. All rights reserved.*

thalocyanine, hypocrellin A, and prophycenes, amongst many others. Porphyrins, however, have attracted the most interest and have been the drug of choice for all the clinical work in the head and neck. Initially hematoporphyrin derivative (HPD) was the drug of choice, but a more purified active component, porfimer sodium (Photofrin; Quadralogic Technologies, Vancouver, Canada), is now used and seems to have an increase in potency.

Photofrin fulfills most of the criteria for a satisfactory photosensitizer for use in humans. These include the absence of systemic toxicity apart from temporary generalized photosensitivity, which may last 4–6 weeks, activation by light at wavelengths that are transmitted by human tissue, and the fact that generally the drug is concentrated in malignant tumors at a higher level than the surrounding tissues, with the exception of the kidney, spleen, and liver.

The serum half-life following injection is 3 hours, and during this period the hematoporphyrin is evenly distributed throughout the stroma and parenchyma of normal tissues. Once the serum level begins to fall, normal parenchymal cells and stroma begin to clear hematoporphyrin, but it is retained in tumor and the cells of the reticuloendothelial system (liver and spleen) for longer periods of time.

The retention in tumor remains relatively high for several days. The reasons for preferential retention in tumors is not clear, but it has been theorized that tumors have a high vascular permeability with an inefficient lymphatic clearance. Therefore, protein-bound substances such as hematoporphyrin are trapped by these tumors. Tumors appear to concentrate Photofrin predominantly in the vascular stroma, with the ratio of stroma to tumor cells being approximately 5:1. After 5–7 days, tumor cells demonstrate reduced amounts of hematoporphyrin, whereas the vascular stroma continues to demonstrate high levels [3].

Shortcomings of hematoporphyrin as a photosensitizer include a less than ideal absorption spectrum, with the most ideal wavelength (±400 nM) only penetrating human tissue to 1 mm, thereby rendering it unsatisfactory for treatment of human tumors. As a compromise, light at 630 nM is used that can penetrate tissue to 5–10 mm.

Lasers

The other essential component used in this technology is the light source, which consists of a laser channeled down a fiber for delivery by surface illumination (which is the technique of choice for superficial cancers) or implanted into the substance of the tumor (which is the technique of choice for more bulky tumors). The laser most commonly used in North America consists of a 5–20 watt argon ion laser, which pumps a dye laser to produce light at 630 nM. This is the longest wavelength capable of activating the hematoporphyrin and permits the deepest tissue penetration (5–10 mm). The dyes used in the dye laser include Rhodamine B or Kiton Red. The dye laser converts the wavelength of the blue-green beam (454–514.5 nM) from the argon laser to the red-orange range (630 nM). This produces 1–4 watts when tuned to 630 nM, depending on the power emitted by the argon tube. The light is then coupled to single or multiple optical fibers for delivery.

The pulsed output lasers, for example, gold vapor and pulsed vapor lasers, have been used in Europe and Australia; these produce a pulsed beam at 627.8 nM, which may be advantageous in enhancing tumor necrosis, or possibly deleterious in causing damage to surrounding normal tissue. The use of pulsed lasers is being actively investigated with a view to improving the effectiveness of tumor ablation [4]. In Japan, the eximer laser-pumped dye system has been used. This has a high power output and possibly, along with metal vapor laser systems, represents the future of lasers in PDT [5].

Delivery systems

A fiberoptic system is used for delivery of the laser energy during photodynamic therapy. The optical fibers are long, flexible rods made of silicone quartz covered with a protective coating. The distal end of the optical quartz fiber may be modified in several ways to obtain optimal light delivery. These applicators direct the light to the lesion in a pattern, depending on the configuration of the tip. The microlens tipped applicator delivers a spot field of light and is used for surface application, while various cylinder diffusers can be used to treat a hollow viscus, for example, the esophagus or trachea, or can be inserted into the substance of a tumor for interstitial delivery. A spherical diffuser may be used for bladder and oral cavity cancers.

The calculation of the optimal amount of light to be delivered to a particular cancer is referred to as dosimetry. The required exposure time for tumor ablation is dependent on laser *power output* in watts and *dose rate* measured in watts/cm^2, and is expressed as a *light dose* in Joules/cm^2.

At this stage in the development of this technology, the calculated optimal light dosage is inexact and dependent on many variables, particularly the anatomy of the structure being treated. This is generally less complicated for treating skin cancer, but can be most difficult in treating complex anatomical sites, for example, the oral cavity, esophagus, and pharynx.

Mode of action

While the mode of action of PDT is not clear, some understanding of the mechanism at a cellular and subcellular level has resulted from numerous in vitro and in vivo animal experiments. The mechanism generally accepted for

161

causing cell necrosis after light exposure is an energy transfer process from the excited triplet state of the hematoporphyrin to oxygen producing singlet oxygen, which causes irreversible oxidation of some essential cellular components [6]. Oxygen is necessary for this reaction to occur, although there may be a non-oxygen-dependent process that results in cell necrosis.

Another mechanism of tumor necrosis is ischemia secondary to the effect on tumor vasculature that has a high uptake of hematoporphyrin [7]. This has been confirmed in animal experiments [3] and is thought to be at least partially mediated by thromboxane [8]. The reasons for preferential tumor necrosis as compared to surrounding normal tissues are not well understood but are at least partially explained by the phenomenon of photobleaching, which is the permanent loss of the photosensitizing effect of the drug after being exposed to light, that is, the greater the uptake of drug in tissue, the greater the cytotoxic effect. If there is significant uptake of drug, the photochemical effect will cause necrosis, but if there is only minimal drug in the tissue, no necrosis will occur [6,9].

There is a striking similarity between the effects produced by PDT and those produced by hyperthermia; however, at the low power produced by the laser, thermal damage should not be a factor. Of interest is that in animal work both the curability and depth of necrosis produced by PDT can be enhanced by combining heat with PDT [10].

Technique

There are two basic approaches to the administration of PDT: (1) surface illumination and (2) interstitial implantation, with surface illumination sufficing for superficial lesions and implantation being used on its own or to complement surface illumination for larger tumors. The following regimen is the approach used by the authors for treatment of upper aerodigestive tract and cutaneous cancers. The reader should appreciate that this does not necessarily represent the standard of care, but what works well for the authors. Drug doses and light dosage may vary from investigator to investigator, from patient to patient, and from lesion to lesion, although every attempt is now being made to standardize therapy.

The drug of choice, Photofrin (2.0 mg/kg body wt), is given by intravenous bolus over 10 minutes, 72 hours prior to the therapy. Precautions against exposure to light are immediately instituted. The procedure is usually performed without anesthesia, with the laser fiber being held in position by a mechanical holder or manually. If the area is inaccessible, surface illumination is administered via a fiberoptic or rigid endoscope under general anesthesia, if necessary. A light dose of $50-100 \text{J/cm}^2$ is usually used. In treating a bulky lesion, the fiber may be implanted directly into the tumor using a sharp-tipped cylinder diffuser or through a hollow needle. This will result in circumferential tumor necrosis of approximately 2 cm. Within a few hours there will develop significant edema and ulceration, with eschar formation within a few days. In the trachea, esophagus, or larynx, this may need to be debrided. The size of the tumor and depth of infiltration will dictate which approach to use. If the tumor should prove refractory, the treatment can be repeated. Postoperatively, precautions should be taken to avoid skin photosensitivity, that is, avoiding sunlight and bright artificial light, and using protective clothing and sunscreen preparations. This should be continued for 4–6 weeks post-therapy, although in some cases photosensitivity may last months.

As already stated, the major thrust in PDT today is an attempt not only to standardize the technology, but also to maximize its effectiveness. At this moment in time, hematoporphyrin and the argon dye–pumped lasers remain the gold standard, while other drugs and lasers are being evaluated. To minimize the photosensitivity and maintain effectiveness, it has been suggested that the dosage of Photofrin be dropped to 1 mg/kg and the light dose increased to 250 J/cm [4,11,12]. Others have, however, noted that as the drug dosage is decreased, the efficacy diminishes [13].

Clinical application of PDT

The efficacy of PDT in the treatment of cancer has long been demonstrated in both animal experiments and the clinical setting. Phase III studies are at present underway for treatment of cancer of the lung, esophagus, and bladder [9]; however, significant experience with tumors in other areas of the body has been obtained with variable results. In discussing the role of PDT in head and neck cancers, its role in cutaneous cancers, cancer of the mucosa of the upper aerodigestive tract, and Kaposi's sarcoma and other assorted malignancies will be presented.

Role in cutaneous and subcutaneous malignancies

Review of the literature devoted to the use of PDT in skin malignancies reveals that initially this treatment was used predominantly for palliation of advanced cancer, for example, recurrent breast carcinomas that had proved refractory to standard therapies. Most series revealed a dramatic initial response in many patients, but long-term follow-up was rarely possible because of the advanced nature of these cancers [14–17]. Overall, the results of PDT in these patients were quite variable, and not only was the response unpredictable, but severe pain and skin necrosis were common findings. Our personal experience with five such cases confirmed these results, and we abandoned this treatment for this disease as satisfactory palliation was not obtained and the pain and necrosis frequently impaired the quality of life.

Basal cell and squamous cell carcinoma. Initial reports describing PDT for basal cell and squamous cell carcinoma were quite enthusiastic and demonstrated significant effectiveness [14–19]. Subsequent reports have been somewhat inconclusive, and the exact role of PDT for these lesions has as yet not been established. A major problem in evaluating the literature is the tremendous variability in technique, drug, and light dosage in the various series. In one study, Pennington et al. [20], using HPD 5 mg/kg, obtained a 52% complete response rate for basal cell cancers and 81% for squamous cell carcinoma, but almost all of the basal cell and more than half of the squamous cell cancers had recurred by 6 months. Total light dose was low ($30 J/cm^2$). No attempt was made to determine the possible causes of failure, for example, inadequate light or drug dose. McCaughan et al. [15], on the other hand, in treating a variety of skin cancers, noted an excellent complete response rate with 50% of complete responses at 1 month persisting at 1 year. They suggested that tumors thicker than 2 cm should be debulked before using PDT to improve efficacy.

Wilson et al. [21], using higher light doses ($180-233 J/cm^2$) and lower drug doses (Photofrin 1 mg/kg) to treat large and multiple basal cell cancers, had dramatic results. Of 151 tumors treated, 133 responded completely and 18 partially. Of those partial responders that were retreated, all had a complete response. At 1 year follow-up only 13 of 133 complete responders had recurred. The morpheoform type tended to recur, and the authors suggested that these be treated with higher light doses or interstitial implants. Equally good results were noted in treating the multiple basal cell cancers seen in basal cell nevus syndrome using HPD 3 mg/kg and light doses of $38-180 J/cm^2$ [22]. Keller et al. have also reported excellent results using low drug dose and high laser dose [11,23].

Presently it appears PDT may become an option where surgical excision of large basal cell cancers is undesirable for medical reasons and where the lesions are multiple. It is this latter indication that is potentially so attractive for PDT, as multiple lesions can be treated at one sitting.

Malignant melanoma. Metastatic pigmented malignant melanoma has been treated with PDT by a number of investigators [12,14,15,24]. In general, it has been noted that the highly pigmented lesions are poorly responsive to PDT, whereas lightly pigmented lesions responded in a more dramatic fashion. This is probably due to the pigment absorbing the light and preventing the photochemical reaction from occurring. After increasing the light dose, McCaughan et al. [15] noted improved responses in the pigmented lesions, but recurrence was frequent. For practical purposes, therefore, there is no real role for PDT in treating malignant melanoma.

Role in cancer of the mucosa of the upper aerodigestive tract

Review of the literature devoted to the role of PDT in cancer of the mucosa of the upper aerodigestive tract reveals that initially this modality was used to palliate advanced cancer, particularly in those tumors that were not treatable by, or were refractory to, conventional therapy [25–27]. Palliation was successfully accomplished in a high percentage of cases and, while many of these responses were transient, a major potential advantage was that this therapy could be administered repeatedly. Because of the poor tissue penetration accomplished by surface illumination, the preferred technique to debulk these large tumors was interstitial implantation together with surface illumination as needed. Probably the best example of such therapy is the treatment of obstructive dysphagia due to advanced esophageal cancer [28,29].

A personal experience in using PDT to treat advanced recurrent head and neck cancer has been unrewarding [30]. Essentially, the purpose of the treatment was to achieve tumor debulking in order to relieve pain, airway obstruction, etc. While tumor shrinkage could be obtained, it was usually unpredictable in its extent and could just as easily be obtained by more conventional and less complicated techniques, for example, surgical debulking with CO_2 laser and electrocautery. In fact, in some patients the added photosensitivity due to the hematoporphyrin further impaired the quality of life. For this reason, it is our opinion that this therapy has little role for debulking, except in the most unusual circumstance.

Other workers, however, continue to use this therapy in advanced cancers, sometimes achieving the desired palliative effect [27,31,32]. Others have combined PDT with radiation therapy with excellent responses [33], although this work has, to the best of our knowledge, not been duplicated elsewhere.

A more appropriate role for PDT appears to be the treatment of early superficial cancers of the mucosa of the upper aerodigestive tract for the following reasons:

1. The anatomy of the upper aerodigestive tract usually permits adequate visualization of the cancer but renders endoscopic excision or ablation cumbersome and difficult. A technique that requires visualization but a 'no touch' technique to attain ablation is a significant advantage over more conventional means.
2. Potentially, if performed correctly, selective necrosis of the tumor occurs, and therefore frozen section histologic control, which is somewhat unsatisfactory, becomes redundant.
3. In most circumstances, this technique requires no anesthesia and can be performed in an office setting. Access to other sites may be obtained using fiberoptic endoscopy, and only in certain situations will general anesthesia be necessary to achieve access to the tumor. Very rarely, tracheostomy may be necessary to safeguard the airway, at least until the acute reactive phase has passed.
4. Field cancerization, with large areas of superficial premalignant and malignant change and multicentric early malignancies, is ideal for this therapy. This 'condemned mucosa' is extremely difficult to treat using

conventional therapies, that is, excision or CO_2 laser ablation. This technique allows relatively large affected areas to be treated with preservation of normal tissue and, in addition, can be repeated as often as necessary.

5. Finally, these superficial cancers can easily be treated using surface illumination because they are rarely deeper than 1 cm, thereby avoiding the use of interstitial implantation, which is more difficult, cumbersome, and less predictable in its response.

Treatment of early cancers, however, has had mixed results, with the literature being somewhat difficult to evaluate because of differences in technique, particularly in the light dose and drug dose. We experienced excellent results for cancers of the oral cavity and oropharynx, with a 85% complete response rate with a follow-up of 1–4 years but with a high recurrence rate of almost 30% at 1 year [30]. Results with small numbers of T_1 cancers elsewhere in the upper aerodigestive tract were somewhat disappointing. It was, however, appreciated that while some of these failures could be attributed to the inadequacy of the technology, some of these tumors were probably understaged, especially as many were radiation failures. Some of the failures may in fact have been due to the development of second cancers. If one combines this failure rate with the lengthy photosensitivity that the treated patient has to endure, it can be concluded that if the tumor is amenable to simpler therapies, PDT should not be recommended.

Wenig et al. [31], using more sophisticated dosimetry to determine whether surface illumination or interstitial implantation should be used, achieved excellent results for superficial mucosal cancers. Likewise, Freche and DeCorbiere [34] achieved excellent results with early vocal cord cancers with long-lasting results. They concluded that early cancers may well be ideal to be treated with photodynamic therapy once the dosimetry has been refined and the skin photosensitivity minimized.

The one condition for which PDT unequivocally appears tailormade is the 'condemned mucosa,' which in essence is multicentric areas of premalignant and early malignancy involving the mucosa of the upper aerodigestive tract. This is refractory to alternate methods, mainly because of the diffuse nature of the disease and the difficulty in defining the extent of the condition. Excellent results have been obtained using PDT by a number of workers [27,30,31], and a major advantage is that the treatment can be repeated if necessary. Overall the advantages of this technology far outweigh its disadvantages in dealing with 'condemned mucosa.'

Role in Kaposi's sarcoma

Mucocutaneous Kaposi's sarcoma involving the head and neck is not an uncommon finding in patients with acquired immunodeficiency syndrome (AIDS). Involvement of the upper airway may cause cosmetic and functional disorders, particularly dysphagia and airway obstruction. While most respond to radiotherapy, some may prove refractory and have been found responsive to PDT [35]. The five reported cases in this series required either surface illumination or interstitial implantation. All patients obtained symptomatic relief and some obtained a complete response with a relatively short follow-up. The future role of PDT in this condition is yet to be determined.

There exist intrinsic limitations in the technology that have to be addressed before this technology will gain universal acceptance, and these relate to the drug, laser, and delivery system.

1. Unpredictable Uptake of Hematoporphyrin by the Tumor

The intratumoral distribution of hematoporphyrin has not yet been well determined. While uptake has been demonstrated in the perivascular stroma [3], it is still unclear to what extent the tumor cells themselves take up the hematoporphyrin. In addition, whether these animal findings occur in spontaneous tumors in humans has not yet been established. It appears that an anoxic necrotic tumor may not take up hematoporphyrin, and this may be a factor in the unpredictable effectiveness of this therapy.

Initially, hematoporphyrin was thought to be taken up selectively by neoplastic tissue; however, it is now recognized as being taken up by all tissues, particularly liver, spleen, kidney, lung, skin, and muscle, but is preferentially retained in tumors for several days. There is, at present, no absolute means of determining in any given patient when the tumor to background tissue levels of hematoporphyrin are maximal, and thereby knowing the optimal moment to treat with the laser. This inexactness in the timing of treatment may account for a number of failures.

2. Unpredictable Depth of Laser Light Penetration

This is dependent on multiple factors, including the wavelength of light used, which, in turn, is dependent on the absorption spectrum of the hematoporphyrin, the power output of the laser, and the effectiveness of the delivery system. All these factors are at present in the process of being standardized. If any question exists as to whether the tumor is thicker than 1 cm, the treatment should be augmented with interstitial implantation.

3. Ability to Expose the Entire Malignancy to the Laser

In the upper aerodigestive tract, the complex nature of the anatomy may render adequate exposure of the tumor to the laser extremely difficult. In addition, it is frequently difficult to define the extent of the cancer. Of great concern is the difficulty in estimating the depth of the tumor infiltration, making the decision whether to use surface illumination or interstitial implantation very difficult.

4. Problems with the Technology

The inconveniences of the technology, that is, expense, specialized instrumentation, and special training, need to be weighed against the potential advantages, particularly when dealing with superficial solitary lesions, which could perfectly reasonably be treated by more simple alternative therapies.

As has already been mentioned, hematoporphyrin, even in the purified form, is a less than ideal photosensitizing drug in humans. The unsatisfactory absorption spectrum and the nonspecific tissue uptake impair the effectiveness of this photosensitizer. In an attempt to minimize the prolonged skin photosensitivity, with all its inconveniences, it has been recommended that the dosage of Photofrin be reduced from 2 mg/kg to 1 mg/kg [9,11,12], but in our experience [30], like that of others [13], it was noted that while the skin photosensitivity was significantly diminished, the results appeared less satisfactory.

In addition, the argon ion pumped dye laser, which is the laser most commonly used, is cumbersome, temperamental, and only capable of a low power output. For this reason, the search continues for a more ideal laser. Finally, calculating the ideal dosimetry required, particularly in an area like the upper aerodigestive tract, is extremely difficult and remains unsatisfactory.

5. *Complications*

Complications that have been encountered include edema, local pain, and skin photosensitivity. *Edema* has not been a major problem in our own experience; however, if an extensive area is treated, or if too high a power is used, this may occur. If it is suspected that this might develop, for example, in treating the larynx, trachea, and hypopharynx, a prophylactic tracheostomy may be indicated. *Local pain* has not been highlighted in the literature, but has been an occasional severe problem in our experience. The reasons for this are obscure, but it may be due to local fat necrosis or even tumor necrosis.

By far the most common problem, however, is *skin photosensitivity*. This may last from 4 to 6 weeks following the administration of hematoporphyrin. This reaction is usually mild and easily managed by taking appropriate protective precautions, as already described. Occasionally, however, it may be severe and cause considerable discomfort.

Considerable research is currently being devoted to developing a more satisfactory photosensitizer. Rhodamine-123 has particularly attracted a great deal of attention. The potential of rhodamine-123 as a photosensitizer combined with the argon laser at 514.5 nM was initially reported in 1936 [37]. Castro et al. [37] demonstrated complete eradication of human squamous cell carcinoma transplanted to nude mice without regrowth using rhodamine-123 photodynamic therapy. To this date, however, no work in humans has been reported. Other promising photochemosensitizers with a potential for clinical use are sulfonated metallophthalocyanines, diaziquone [38], berberine [39], N,n'-*bis* (2-ethyl-1,3-dioxolane)-kryptocyanine (EDCK) [40], Nile blue A (NBA) [41], tetra-(4-sulfonatophenyl) porphine (TPPS) [42], silicon naphthalocyanine, hypocrellin A, and prophycenes. Metals which have been complexed to form sulfonated metallophthalocyaines possessing photochemosensitizing characteristics are zinc, gallium, cerium, and aluminum [43,44].

None of these newer photosensitizers has had extensive evaluation in either animals or humans to date. It is hoped, however, that some of these agents will exhibit better tumor specificity and, consequently, more complete and selective tumor eradication with less side effects than are currently available with the hematoporphyrins.

While this work is progressing, equal attention is being directed to improving lasers and delivery systems [45] so that, after a relatively stagnant period, the future will indeed be bright for PDT in managing head and neck malignancies.

References

1. Castro DJ, Saxton ER, Fetterman H. New concepts in photodynamic therapy with lasers. In: W Fee, H Geopfert, M Johns, eds. Head and Neck Cancer, Vol. 2. Philadelphia: B.C. Decker, 1988, pp 400–408.
2. Tappenier H, Jesionek A. Theropeutische reosuche met floureszierenden stoff. Muench Med Wochsder 1:2042, 1903.
3. Wieman TJ, Mang TS, Fingar UH. Effect of photodynamic therapy on blood flow in normal and tumor blood vessels. Surgery 104:512–517, 1990.
4. Bellnier DA, Lin LW, Parrish JA. Hematoporphyrin derivative and pulse laser photoradiation, porphyrin localization and treatment of tumors. In: Photodynamic Therapy. New York: Alan R. Liss, 1984, pp 533–540.
5. Ainsworth MD, Piper JA. Laser systems for photodynamic therapy. In: G Morstyn, A Kaye, eds. Phototherapy of Cancer. New York: Harwood Academic, 1990, pp 37–72.
6. Dougherty TJ, Potter WR, Belhier D. Photodynamic therapy for the treatment of cancer: Current status and advances. In: D Kessel, ed. Photodynamic Therapy of Neoplastic Disease. Boca Raton, FC: CRC Press, 1990, pp 1–19.
7. Gomer CJ. Photodynamic therapy in the treatment of malignancies. Semin Hematol 26:27–34, 1989.
8. Fingar UH, Wieman KW. Role of thromboxane and prostacyclin release on photodynamic therapy–induced tumor destruction. Cancer Res 50:2599–2603, 1990.
9. Marcus S. Photodynamic therapy of human cancer. Proc IEEE 80:1–21, 1992.
10. Waldow SM, Henderson BW, Dougherty TJ. Potentiation of phototherapy by heat. Lasers Surg Med 5:83–99, 1985.
11. Keller G. Photodynamic laser therapy. Arch Otolaryngol Head Neck Surg 118:15–16, 1992.
12. Gilson D, Asl D, Drirer J, et al. Therapeutic ratio of photodynamic therapy in the treatment of superficial tumors of skin and subcutaneous tissues in man. Br J Cancer 58:665–669, 1988.
13. Robinson PJ, Carruth JAS, Fairris GM. Photodynamic therapy: A better treatment for widespread Bowen's disease. Br J Dermatol 199:59–61, 1988.
14. Dougherty T. Photoradiation therapy for cutaneous and subcutaneous malignancies. J Invest Dermatol 77:122–123, 1981.
15. McCaughan JS Jr, Guy JT, Hicks WM, et al. Photodynamic therapy for cutaneous and subcutaneous malignant neoplasms. Arch Surg 124:211–116, 1989.
16. Schuh M, Nseyo UO, Potter W, et al. Photodynamic therapy for palliation of locally recurrent breast carcinoma. J Clin Oncol 5:1766–1770, 1987.
17. Waldow SM, Lobraico RV, Kohler IK, et al. Photodynamic therapy for treatment of malignant cutaneous lesions. Lasers Surg Med 7:451–456, 1987.
18. Carruth JAS, McKenzie AL. Preliminary report of a pilot study of photoradiation therapy for the treatment of superficial malignancies of the skin, head, and neck. Eur J Surg Oncol 11:47–50.
19. Tokuda Y. Primary skin cancer. In: Y Hayata, TJ Dougherty, Igaku-Sloin, eds. Lasers and Hematoporphyrin Derivative In Cancer. Tokyo: New York: Igaku-Shoin, 1983, pp 88–96.

20. Pennington DJ, Waner M, Knox A. Photodynamic therapy for multiple skin cancers. Plast Reconst Surg 82:1067–1071, 1987.
21. Wilson BD, Mang TS, Cooper MC, et al. Use of photodynamic therapy for the treatment of extensive basal cell carcinomas. Facial Plastic Surg 6:185–189, 1989.
22. Tse DT, Kersten RC, Anderson RL. Hematoporphyrin derivative photoradiation therapy in managing nevoid basal cell carcinoma syndrome. Arch Ophthalmol 102:990–994, 1984.
23. Keller GS, Razum NJ, Dorion D. Photodynamic therapy for non-melanoma skin cancer. Fac Plast Surg 6:180–184, 1989.
24. Forbes I, Cowled A, Leong AS-Y, et al. Phototherapy of human tumors using hematoporphyrin derivative. Med J Aust 2:489–493, 1980.
25. Schuller DE, McCaughan JS, Rock RP. Photoradiation in head and neck cancer. Arch Otolaryngol 3:351–355, 1985.
26. Wile AG, Novotny J, Mason GR. Photoradiation therapy of head and neck cancer. Am J Clin Oncol 6:39–63, 1984.
27. Schweitzer VG. Photodynamic therapy for treatment of head and neck cancer. Otolaryngol Head Neck Surg 102:255–232, 1990.
28. McCaughan JS, Nims TA, Guy JT. Photodynamic therapy for esophageal tumors. Arch Surg 124:74–80, 1989.
29. Likier HM, Levine JG, Lightdale C. Photodynamic therapy for completely obstructing esophageal carcinoma. Gastrointest Endosc 37:75–78, 1991.
30. Gluckman JL. Hematoporphyrin photodynamic therapy: Is there truly a future in head and neck oncology? Reflections on a five year experience. Laryngoscope 101:36–42, 1991.
31. Wenig BL, Kurtzman DM, Grossweiner L, et al. Photodynamic therapy in the treatment of squamous cell carcinoma of the head and neck. Arch Otolaryngol Head Neck Surg 116:1267–1270, 1990.
32. Grossweiner L, Hill J, Lobraico R. Photodynamic therapy for head and neck squamous cell carcinoma: Optical dosimetry and clinical trial. Photochem Photobiol 46:911–917, 1987.
33. Zhao F, Zhang K, Huang H, et al. Use of hematoporphyrin derivative as a sensitizer for radiotherapy of oral and maxillofacial tumors. Lasers Med Sci 1:253–256, 1986.
34. Freche C, DeCorbiere S. Use of photodynamic therapy in the treatment of vocal cord carcinoma. J Photochem Photobiol 6:291–296, 1990.
35. Schweitzer VG, Visscher D. Photodynamic therapy for treatment of AIDS-related Kaposi's sarcoma. Otolaryngol Head Neck Surg 102:639–649, 1990.
36. Marchesini R, Melloni E, Dasdia T, et al. Photosensitizing properties of rhodamine-123 on different human tumor cell lines. Laser Surg Med 6:163, 1986.
37. Castro DJ, Saxton RE, Fetterman HR. Rhodamine-123 as a new photochemosensitizing agent with the argon laser: 'Non-thermal' and thermal effects on human squamous carcinoma cells in vitro. Laryngoscope 97:554–561, 1987.
38. Kessel D, Thompson P. Photosensitization of leukemia L1210 cells with diaziquone. Cancer Res 46:5587–5588, 1986.
39. Wang MX, Huo LM, Yang HC, et al. An experimental study of the photodynamic activity of berberine in vitro on cancer cells. J Trad Chin Med 6:125–127, 1986.
40. Oseroff AR, Ohuoha D, Ara G, et al. Intramitochrondrial dyes allow selective in vitro photolysis of carcinoma cells. Proc Natl Acad Sci USA 83:9729–9733, 1986.
41. Oseroff AR, Ohuoha D, Ara G, et al. Selective photochemotherapy of melanoma and human squamous cell carcinoma using cationic photosensitizers (abstr). J Invest Dermatol 88:510, 1987.
42. Sacchini V, Melloni E, Marchesini R, et al. Topical administration of tetrasodium-meso-tetraphenyl-porphinesulfonate (TPPS) and red light irradiation for the treatment of superficial neoplastic lesions. Tumori 73:19–23, 1987.
43. Van Lier JE, Brasseur N, Ali H, et al. Sulfonated metallophthalocyanines: New agents for photodynamic therapy. Lasers Surg Med 6:230–231, 1986.

44. Straight RC, Spikes JD, et al. Phthalocyanine dyes as photodynamic sensitizers in-vivo: Localization, retention and photoxicity in a mouse tumor model. Photochem Photobiol 43(Suppl):638 (abstract), 1986.
45. Dorion DR. Future directions in photodynamic therapy. Fac Plast Surg 6:190–192, 1989.

10. Timing and sequencing of chemoradiotherapy

Daniel J. Haraf, Ralph R. Weichselbaum, and Everett E. Vokes

There are three main objectives in the treatment of cancer: (1) curing disease, (2) keeping the morbidity of treatment to a minimum, and (3) preserving function and cosmesis. It may be difficult to achieve all three of these objectives in all cases. However, cure may be the most important single goal. Thus, a more aggressive treatment regimen with an increase in treatment morbidity or loss of function/cosmesis may be tolerated in order to increase cure rates. Current treatments for cancers of the head and neck can be used to illustrate these principles. Standard treatments for carcinomas of the head and neck include surgery and radiation therapy. Both methods of treatment have been shown to have high cure rates with minimum morbidity when the disease is detected early. For example, radiation therapy alone is curative in the majority of patients with stage I and II glottic carcinoma with preservation of voice. Those few patients who fail radiotherapy are usually salvaged by surgery [1]. Also, newer surgical techniques, such as hemilaryngectomy or laser surgery, have been shown to be curative with voice preservation in selected early glottic cancers, although voice quality is diminished [1]. Cure rates and functional results are also generally good with single modality therapy in early stage tumors located in other head and neck sites. In these favorable cases standard therapy is appropriate, and combined modality therapy should not be considered.

Unfortunately, only one third of patients present with these early favorable stage T1 and T2 lesions. The remaining two thirds of patients present with locally advanced (T3 or T4) lesions and/or regional lymph node involvement (N1–N3). In those patients with locally advanced disease, more aggressive surgery or radiotherapy has been used in an attempt to increase the cure rates while sacrificing functional or cosmetic results. Nevertheless, survival results after single modality therapy in patients with locally advanced disease are poor, even though distant metastases are detected in less than 10% of patients at the time of diagnosis. Local and regional tumor control remain difficult problems with single modality therapy in locally advanced disease, and thus, single modality treatment is not commonly used. Fre-

Hong, Waun Ki and Weber, Randal S., (eds.), Head and Neck Cancer. © *1995 Kluwer Academic Publishers. ISBN 0-7923-3015-3. All rights reserved.*

quently, combined modality therapy, consisting of surgery with preoperative or postoperative radiation therapy, has been employed in an effort to improve local control. In most advanced head and neck cancers local control appears to improve with a combination of surgery and radiotherapy compared to either treatment alone. However, local recurrences continue to occur in up to 60% of patients, and overall survival is poor [2]. Those few patients who survive long term are usually left with severe functional deficits from treatment.

The risk of distant metastases in head and neck tumors usually receives little attention, since local failure continues to be the major cause of morbidity and mortality. Only 20–30% of patients develop distant disease [3]. While a low incidence of metastatic disease may be true clinically, some series suggest that more patients are at risk to develop distant metastases. Autopsy series detected micrometastases in over 50% of patients treated for head and neck cancers. Most of these patients had persistent or locoregionally recurrent disease at the time of death [4,5]. Therefore, one cannot determine whether systemic micrometastases were present at the time of diagnosis or developed at the time of regional progression. A recent retrospective analysis of 2648 patients with head and neck cancer reported that locoregional control was the most significant variable affecting the development of distant metastases [6]. Nevertheless, the 5-year time-adjusted incidence of distant metastases was 21% for patients with continuous local control at 6 months after treatment and 38% for patients with locoregional failure. The reduction in distant metastases with increasing local control was seen in all head and neck sites except the hypopharynx and nasopharynx, suggesting a high rate of micrometastatic dissemination at the time of diagnosis.

Rationale for multimodal therapy

It is obvious that standard treatment methods are inadequate to cure the majority of patients with locally advanced head and neck cancer, since local and regional failure remain the leading causes of death. A secondary consideration in the treatment of advanced disease is to reduce the functional deficits patients must cope with after treatment. These deficits must frequently be endured without the benefit of cure. Nevertheless, one must be aware of the potentially high incidence of distant metastases in these patients. If locoregional control is increased by more effective radiation and/or surgery, systemic failure will potentially become an increasingly important problem. However, it is unlikely that further improvements in surgical or radiotherapeutic techniques will result in significant gains in regional control. Normal tissue tolerance and the potential for severe complications continue to limit the dose of radiation that can be delivered to cancer-bearing areas. Similar anatomic factors also limit the ability to completely resect disease-bearing tissues in advanced cases. Also, surgery and radiotherapy are local treatments that do not address the possibility of metastatic disease.

The traditional role of chemotherapy in this disease has been limited to the treatment of patients with recurrent or metastatic disease [7,8]. Several active single agents have been identified in this setting, including methotrexate, cisplatin, carboplatin, 5-fluorouracil (5-FU), bleomycin, hydroxyurea, ifosfamide, edetrexate, cyclophosphamide, and probably taxol. Nevertheless, response rates with these agents have been low (approximately 30%), and the duration of response has ranged from 3 to 6 months. One randomized study compared symptomatic care to cisplatin, bleomycin, or a combination of cisplatin and bleomycin, and found the cisplatin-containing regimens significantly prolonged survival over symptomatic care or bleomycin alone [9]. Nine randomized trials have compared single-agent to combination chemotherapy in patients with advanced or recurrent head and neck cancer [10–18]. While four of these trials were able to demonstrate an increase in response rates in favor of combination chemotherapy, they did not report any survival benefit [10,13,15,16]. Only one randomized study reported a survival benefit for combination chemotherapy [17].

The results of single-agent or combination chemotherapy in advanced or recurrent head and neck cancers are not impressive, and new more active therapies need to be identified. However, it would be premature to conclude that there is no role for chemotherapy in the treatment of head and neck cancer. An alternative conclusion is that the role of chemotherapy needs to be better defined and integrated into a multimodal treatment approach for patients with less advanced disease. Both single-agent and combination chemotherapy have exhibited limited curative potential as a single treatment modality in solid tumors. In non-small cell lung cancer, colorectal cancer, and breast cancer, adjuvant chemotherapy appears to be effective in reducing the incidence of metastases in patients at risk but has been largely ineffective in controlling sites with known disease. Thus the effective integration of chemotherapy into standard treatment regimens of radiotherapy and/or surgery, which address sites of gross disease, will most likely be necessary for significant progress in treatment.

The integration of chemotherapy in advanced head and neck cancer continues to be attractive for many reasons [19]. Since chemotherapy by itself has reproducible activity but is not curative, it may be more effective if used earlier in the course of the disease and in conjunction with standard local therapy as sequential or simultaneous treatment. One proposed mechanism of interaction between radiotherapy and chemotherapy is spatial cooperation. This is a belief that chemotherapy can eliminate distant metastases, while local therapy eliminates regional disease. Although important, spatial cooperation should not be the main consideration in head and neck cancer since the majority of patients die from local progression or recurrence before distant disease can become manifest. However, spatial cooperation may assume more importance if local control improves.

A potentially more important result from the combination of chemotherapy and radiotherapy would be a direct local interaction, resulting in improved locoregional control and cure rates. Several mechanisms have been proposed by which a direct interaction could increase regional control [20]. Chemotherapy and radiation may be active against different tumor populations and eliminate cells that could develop resistance to either chemotherapy or radiation. Also, chemotherapy may increase tumor cell recruitment from G_0 into a more radiation-therapy–responsive phase of the cell cycle. Thus, a locoregional interaction could be beneficial for two reasons.

While the integration of chemotherapy and radiation are theoretically appealing, the optimal sequencing remains obscure. Thus far studies have investigated chemotherapy combined with radiation in one of two main settings: (1) sequential administration as adjuvant or neoadjuvant therapy, or (2) concomitant chemoradiotherapy. There are advocates for each method but data conclusively supporting one schema over the other are lacking. The remainder of this chapter will discuss the advantages and disadvantages of each method along with the results of important studies.

Sequential chemoradiotherapy

There is a strong rationale to support the use of neoadjuvant chemotherapy. It is probably the simplest way to integrate chemotherapy into a multimodal treatment, since overlapping toxicities will be minimized and the efficacy of each therapy can be monitored. Also, the concept of spatial cooperation applies since distant micrometastases are addressed early. Local control with radiation therapy may improve through a reduction in tumor bulk or improved vascularization, resulting in fewer hypoxic cells and/or cells in inactive phases of the cell cycle. Theoretically a reduction in tumor bulk from chemotherapy might allow for less radical surgical procedures and improve functional results. Early administration of chemotherapy may result in improved drug delivery to the tumor, since radiation fibrosis or surgical scarring would not be present. The sequential use of chemotherapy permits the administration of adequate drug doses, as the potential for the increased toxicity seen with concomitant therapy is reduced. However, the increase in overall treatment time required for neoadjuvant therapy could adversely affect outcome. The use of neoadjuvant therapy could prolong the overall treatment time by months, depending upon the number of treatment cycles. Recently, evidence has been presented suggesting that any prolongation of treatment time during radiation therapy will adversely affect local control in head and neck cancers [21,22]. The inferior outcome has been attributed to accelerated repopulation of clonogenic cells once the tumor population has been perturbed. Whether the prolongation of treatment time applies to neoadjuvant chemotherapy in combined modality treatment is unknown. An important factor could be the induction of radiation-resistant cells by chemotherapy or inherent cross-resistance between both modalities [23]. If this is the case, any potential benefit of chemotherapy could be lost.

Induction chemotherapy in advanced head and neck cancer has been intensely investigated over the past 15 years. The initial experience in nonrandomized trials used one cycle of single-agent therapy. However, Clark et al. presented evidence to suggest that more than one cycle may be necessary for maximum response [24]. In their studies a progressive increase in the number of complete responses was observed from cycles 1–3 but no change after cycle 4. Similar results have been reported from our institution [25,26] and by other investigators [27,28]. Dreyfus et al., utilizing a regimen of cisplatin, 5-FU, and leucovorin, reported a complete response rate of 26% following two cycles, which increased to 66% with the addition of a third cycle [27]. Thus, the current trend is to administer three cycles of combination chemotherapy prior to local treatment. Whether additional cycles improve response rates or survival remains unknown. One study that employed five cycles of chemotherapy reported complete response rates that were inferior to trials using three cycles [29]. This suggests that the gain from additional chemotherapy may be small or potentially become harmful by delaying local therapy after a certain point. Nevertheless, phase II trials of neoadjuvant chemotherapy have shown that high response rates (70–100%) can be consistently achieved, with complete response rates of 20–66%. Nearly all of these studies show that a complete response to induction therapy predicts a longer survival and better prognosis [30]. However, phase II trials prevent the conclusion that chemotherapy improves survival. Responders to chemotherapy may simply be a subgroup of patients with a more favorable prognosis that is not related to the administration of chemotherapy. The notion that chemotherapy identifies a subset of patients with a more favorable prognosis is supported by the fact that the overall survival for all patients receiving chemotherapy is no better than that expected following standard therapy [31].

Proof of treatment efficacy requires well-designed phase III trials incorporating the lessons learned from phase II studies. Trial design is critical in head and neck cancer, since outcome can be influenced by many variables. Adequate treatment regimens should include multiagent chemotherapy with an established high overall and complete response rate. Other factors have been shown to influence prognosis, including (1) stage of disease, (2) primary site, (3) resectability, and (4) weight loss [32–34]. Thus, the study population should be stratified for these and other prognostic factors known to influence outcome. Since an optimistic assessment of differential survival benefit might be only 10–20%, a sufficient number of patients necessary to detect such a difference must be entered on each trial.

Table 1 summarizes the results of selected neoadjuvant randomized trials [35–45]. None of the trials to date have been successful at decreasing the local failure rate or prolonging survival. Yet, the results of these trials do

Table 1. Neoadjuvant trials

Ref.	Chemotherapy	Stage	Local treatment	Stratification	RT dose (Gy)	Response rate% (CR %)	Local failure	Survival	Comments
35	MTX	III–IV	RT	No	50–60	NR	NR	ND	
36	MTX	III–IV	RT ± S	Yes	55–80	NR	NR	ND	
37	MTX	II–IV	S or RT	Yes	NR	34 (6)	ND	ND	
38	VCR, B, FU, MTX, CORT, 6-MP, CPA	III–IV	RT	No	40–60	NR	ND	ND	
39	B, CPA, MTX, FU	II–IV	Preop RT	No	NR	67 (5)	ND	ND	
40	CP, FU	I–IV	RT, S, or both	Yes	55–70	46 (22)	ND	ND	
41	CP, FU	II–IV	Preop RT or RT alone	No	50–70	67 (19)	NR	ND	
42	CP, MTX, B, VCR	III–IV	S + postop RT	No	NR	51 (19)	ND	ND	Fewer metastases with chemo
43,44	CP, B, MTX	II–IV	S + RT	Yes	50–60	34 (3)	ND	ND	Fewer metastases with chemo Subgroup survival benefit
45	CP, FU	III–IV	RT	Yes	66–76	98 (49)	Increased	ND	Larynx preserved in 64% Fewer metastases with chemo

MTX = methotrexate; VCR = vincristine; B = bleomycin; FU = 5-flourouracil; CORT = hydrocortisone; S = surgery; 6-MP = 6-mercaptopurine; CPA = cyclophosphamide; CP = cisplatin; NR = not reported; ND = no difference; RT = radiotherapy.

not prove that chemotherapy is ineffective, since major flaws are present in many of these studies. Many of these trials failed to use effective chemotherapy, and criticisms include (1) the number of cycles administered were inadequate, (2) drug dosages were too low, or (3) multiagent chemotherapy was not employed. Some of these studies used radiation therapy alone as definitive local treatment. A frequently overlooked criticism is that a total dose of radiation less than 66 Gy given with 180–200 cGy/day fractions should not be considered curative if gross disease is present. Finally, few studies have entered a patient cohort sufficiently large enough to detect small differences in survival.

Although all the trials are flawed and largely disappointing, a few provide some valuable insights and deserve closer analysis. The study by Schuller et al. used an active regimen of combination chemotherapy for three cycles [42]. While this trial failed to demonstrate an improvement in survival or local control, distant metastases were noted to occur twice as frequently in the standard therapy group as in the group receiving chemotherapy (28% vs. 49%, respectively). Unfortunately, the poor compliance rate and the reluctance of patients to complete the assigned treatment may have affected the overall survival results.

The Head and Neck Contracts study employed a single cycle of induction chemotherapy with or without maintenance single-agent chemotherapy [43]. This study also suffers from problems with poor patient compliance. Again there was no difference in survival or local control. However, a statistically significant decrease in the number of patients developing distant metastases as a first site of failure was observed with maintenance cisplatin compared to patients receiving induction therapy alone or standard treatment. A subset analysis of this trial published in 1990 provided some interesting observations [44]. Statistically significant differences in disease-free survival were noted for patients with T1–2 primary lesions or N1–2 nodal disease in favor of maintenance chemotherapy. However, a significant overall survival advantage was only found in patients with N2 disease receiving maintenance chemotherapy. No advantages for chemotherapy were seen in T3–4 or N3 disease. A final subset of patients that benefitted from maintenance chemotherapy were patients with carcinoma of the oral cavity. This study supports the idea that a single cycle of chemotherapy is inadequate in head and neck cancer.

The Veterans Administration trial deserves special discussion [45]. This study randomized patients with advanced laryngeal cancer into one of two arms. Patients in the control arm underwent standard surgery followed by postoperative radiotherapy. Patients in the chemotherapy arm received three cycles of chemotherapy with cisplatin and 5-FU followed by radiation therapy alone for patients responding to chemotherapy. Patients in this series received adequate doses of radiation. Surgery was reserved for those patients who did not respond to chemotherapy and salvage of radiation failures. The study posed two questions. First, could chemotherapy combined with radiation substitute for surgery and result in preservation of the larynx? This goal was achieved in 64% of the patients treated on this study. Second, could multi-agent chemotherapy followed by radiotherapy result in a longer survival compared to standard treatment of surgery and postoperative radiation? Clearly the results of this trial indicate that chemotherapy and radiation can successfully substitute for routine laryngectomy without jeopardizing survival. The 3-year results of this trial suggested that the incidence of distant metastases was reduced in the group receiving chemotherapy. With longer follow-up this difference is no longer statistically significant, and it appears chemotherapy simply delayed the time to the development of metastatic disease [46]. These results confirm those reported in pilot trials [47–49].

Finally, the RTOG activated a trial in 1985 that was incorporated into a randomized Head and Neck Intergroup study [50]. The goal of the trial was to test the efficacy of adjuvant chemotherapy in patients with resectable squamous cell carcinoma of the head and neck. Between 1985 and 1989, 442 patients were randomized to receive standard fractionation postoperative radiotherapy or chemotherapy with 5-FU and cisplatin followed by standard fractionation postoperative radiotherapy. At a median time-at-risk of 37.2 months, there was no significant difference in locoregional control, survival, or disease-free survival between the two groups. However, the group receiving chemotherapy had a reduced incidence of distant metastases overall ($p = 0.03$) and as a first site of failure ($p = 0.02$).

In conclusion, the neoadjuvant trials show high response rates with modern regimens. These response rates have not resulted in improved local control or survival when compared to standard therapy. Recent trials appear to show a beneficial reduction in the number of patients developing distant metastases, suggesting that current drugs and regimens may be effective in sites containing minimal disease. However, this illustrates the point that the majority of failures remain locoregional, and it is unlikely that survival will improve until more effective local therapy becomes available. While the primary goal of increased survival remains unaffected by neoadjuvant chemotherapy, significant progress has been made. The results of the Veterans Administration study show organ preservation can be achieved with sequential chemotherapy and radiation in most patients with advanced laryngeal cancer. Thus, quality of life after treatment is improved. A new randomized study by the Veterans Administration Cooperative Group will be activated to investigate organ preservation in sites other than the larynx. Also, the study will include a radiation alone arm to address the question of whether chemotherapy is an essential component of the treatment regimen. Finally, more aggressive chemotherapy may be necessary to improve survival and is under investigation [51].

Concomitant chemoradiotherapy

The use of chemotherapy in the neoadjuvant setting is one method to integrate chemotherapy into the multimodal treatment of head and neck cancer. In essence it is the addition of another independent treatment modality in sequence with other standard treatments. Thus, the most one could hope for in improving outcome is an additive effect from each independent treatment. While sequential treatments might help reduce the risk for toxicity during treatment, overall prolongation in treatment time may offset any potential gains of the added treatment. This may help explain why an improvement in locoregional control has not been demonstrated in randomized neoadjuvant trials to date. Unlike sequential multimodal therapy, concomitant chemoradiotherapy specifically aims at enhancing one modality through the simultaneous use of another. Thus concomitant therapy may have a synergistic effect. This would be highly desirable in control of locoregional disease, but the risk of increased toxicity tends to limit potential gains.

Chemotherapy and radiation therapy can be integrated into a concomitant treatment in a wide range of schema. Examples of potential concomitant schema are shown in Table 2. Example 1 illustrates rapid alternating modalities where chemotherapy incorporated into a standard split-course radiotherapy plan. The examples in Table 2 illustrate a progressively more complete integration of chemotherapy and radiation from examples 1–5. In example 2 radiotherapy and chemotherapy are given together on some weeks of treatment. As can be seen, concomitant therapy can be used to reduce the breaks employed for hematologic recovery present with induction chemotherapy since the patient continuously receives some type of therapy. Also, the overall treatment time could be reduced. Examples 4 and 5 in Table 2 illustrate complete integration of chemotherapy with radiation when patients receive both treatments together on all treatment days. In theory, a complete integration of chemotherapy and radiation would be optimal if toxicity did not become prohibitive. Such an approach would address potentially micrometastatic disease early in the course of

Table 2. Examples of schema for chemoradiotherapy

	Week							
	1	2	3	4	5	6	7	8
Example 1	RT	RT	C	RT	RT	C	RT	RT
Example 2	RT/C	RT	RT	C	RT	RT	RTC	—
Example 3	RT/C	RT	RT	—	RT/C	RT	RT	—
Example 4	RT/C	—	RT/C	—	RT/C	—	RT/C	—
Example 5	RT/C	RT/C	RT/C	RT/C	RT/C	RT/C	RT/C	—

RT = radiation therapy; C = chemotherapy.

therapy, as in neoadjuvant treatment. In contrast to neoadjuvant treatment, definitive treatment of locoregional disease would not be delayed and could be enhanced through the use of radiosensitizing agents.

If one considers the number of drugs available, drug dosages, potential variations on radiotherapy dosage, and amount of overlap between chemotherapy and radiation, the number of potential treatment schema is infinite. These variables complicate any analysis of concomitant therapy, unlike neoadjuvant treatment. Current treatment designs have evolved using two approaches. One method employs standard radiation therapy doses and fractionation schemes (i.e., 180–200 cGy per fraction, five fractions per week, total dose 65–70 Gy) as local therapy. Single-agent chemotherapy is intermittently added to the radiation schedule. In this schema the dose and schedule of chemotherapy is usually suboptimal, since doses are less than those used to obtain maximum response if the chemotherapy was given alone. In these regimens the chemotherapy is intended to act more as a radiation-enhancing agent. The second approach attempts to integrate combination chemotherapy in active doses and schedules with radiation therapy. Thus, toxicity may be more severe and require interruptions in radiation therapy to allow for at least partial recovery of normal tissues. In some respects this approach requires cycles of chemoradiotherapy analogous to standard chemotherapy. This protraction of therapy could be more risky, since chemotherapy will need to more than compensate for the loss of activity resulting from a prolonged radiation schedule. In order to be worthwhile, the results of concomitant therapy cannot merely compensate for radiation delays but must increase the activity of radiation therapy beyond that point if an advantage in locoregional control is to be seen.

Most concomitant studies in head and neck cancer have elected to use standard radiation therapy with the addition of single-agent chemotherapy at suboptimal doses. This approach is justified, since a small but reproducible proportion of patients are cured with radiation therapy alone. This cannot be said for chemotherapy. Most single-chemotherapy agents have been studied in this context. Even though single-agent chemotherapy has limited theoretical benefit, positive randomized clinical trials have been published and are summarized in Table 3.

One of the first large randomized trials to compare concomitant chemoradiotherapy to radiation therapy alone was conducted more than 20 years ago by Ansfield and coworkers [52]. In this trial 134 patients with stage II–IV squamous cell cancer of the head and neck were randomized to receive standard radiation therapy alone or radiation therapy plus 5-FU. The 5-FU was administered as an intravenous bolus of 10 mg/kg on the first 3 days of radiation and at 5 mg/kg on day 4. Thereafter, patients randomized to 5-FU were given 5 mg/kg three times each week throughout the entire course of radiation unless unequivocal toxicity appeared. Those patients who underwent concomitant treatment had a superior median survival (27 months) compared to those treated with radiation alone (14 months). Subset analysis

182

Table 3. Randomized trials of concomitant chemotherapy and radiation

Ref	Treatment	Stage	Patient number	Stratification	RT dose (Gy)	5-year DFS	5-year survival	Comments
52	5-FU + RT	I-IV	66	No	65	NR	36%	Significant increase for oral cavity, tonsil, and T3 tumors
	RT		68		65	NR	15%	
53	5-FU + RT	III-IV	68	No	60–70	49%	32%	Significant increase in DFS and survival
	RT		68		60–70	18%	13%	
54	B + RT	III-IV	84	No	55–60	72%	66%	Significant increase in DFS and survival
	RT		73		55–60	17%	26%	Suboptimal treatment for RT alone
55	B + RT	II-IV	111	Yes	Variable	53%	38	No differences with chemotherapy
	RT		111		Variable	58%	45	
56	B + RT	II-IV	107	No	70	22%	22%	No difference with chemotherapy
	RT		92		70	22%	23%	
57	B + RT	III-IV	43	Yes	70	31% (3 yr)	43% (3 yr)	Significant increase in DFS but not survival
	RT		48		70	15% (3 yr)	24% (3 yr)	
58	MC + RT	II-IV	56	Yes	50–70	75%	48%	Significant increase in DFS but not survival
	RT		61		50–70	49%	40%	
59	MTX + RT	I-IV	156	Yes	40–55	NR	43%[a]	Trend toward improved survival with chemotherapy
	RT		157		40–55	NR	35%[a]	

DFS = disease-free survival; MTX = methotrexate; MC = mitomycin C; B = bleomycin; NR = not reported; RT = radiotherapy.
[a] = Estimated from data.

revealed a significant survival benefit in those patients with intra-oral cancers, tonsilar cancers, and T3 lesions. While this trial reports favorable results for combined treatment, it also illustrates the need for stratification in trial design. The results of this trial were updated by Lo et al. [53]. Again, both local control and survival were better in the combined modality group, but only in the oral cavity population was this difference statistically significant. No additional trials have investigated the use of 5-FU as in this trial.

Three prospective randomized trials have investigated the use of bleomycin and concomitant radiotherapy. The first study was reported by Shanta and Krishnamurthi in 1980 [54]. Patients in this trial were randomized to radiation therapy or concomitant therapy with bleomycin. All head and neck sites were eligible and no stratification was employed. Bleomycin was given by intra-arterial, intramuscular, or intravenous routes in heterogenous doses two to three times per week, depending upon the mucosal reaction and route of administration, to a total dose of 150–250 mg. Chemotherapy was not given on the days patients were scheduled to receive radiation. The radiation therapy was also nonstandard, given in three fractions per week (300 cGy per fraction) to a total dose of 55–60 Gy over 7 weeks, which would be considered suboptimal for radiation alone by current standards. Survival, disease-free survival, and local control were reported to be statistically significantly improved in this series with the use of bleomycin. However, survival curves were not presented, and a large number of patients remained unaccounted for in the analysis. The use of suboptimal radiation therapy in the control arm, lack of complete data in the analysis, and lack of stratification indicate the results of this study must be interpreted with caution.

Although the trial above reported favorable results with concomitant bleomycin, three other trials failed to show any consistent improvement in treatment outcome [55–57]. Vermund et al. [55] reported their results on 222 patients in 1985. The 222 patients in this trial were stratified according to site, stage, and age. All patients in this study received a standard course of radiation therapy (180–200 cGy per fraction, five fractions per week) to a total dose of 65–70 cGy. Thus the radiation therapy employed in this study can be considered adequate for the radiation-alone arm of treatment. Patients in the concomitant arm received 5 mg of bleomycin intramuscularly on each day of radiotherapy until they developed 'excessive mucositis.' Thus the dose of bleomycin in this study varied from 10 to 175 mg. The concomitant therapy group experienced more acute toxic reactions during treatment without any improvement in outcome. The survival, disease-free survival, and local control were equivalent for both groups at 2 and 5 years. Also, no benefit could be found in patients who received higher doses of bleomycin (>100 mg) over the course of treatment.

In 1988 the European Organization for Research and Treatment of Cancer reported the 10-year results of a similar trial [56]. This trial used a standard fractionation scheme and adequate radiation doses in both arms of the study. The plan was to administer 15 mg of bleomycin twice each week for the first 5 weeks of radiotherapy. Only 64% of the patients in this trial received the entire planned dose of bleomycin because of toxic reactions. Also, patients in the concomitant group experienced more frequent delays in therapy. The results of the study found no difference in response rate, survival, or disease-free survival between the groups. This lack of a difference could be attributed to the delays in radiation experienced in the concomitant group or the large number of patients who did not complete the entire course of bleomycin therapy. Also, a lack of patient stratification in the trial design could have biased results.

The only other randomized trial to investigate bleomycin and concomitant radiotherapy was conducted by the Northern California Oncology Group [57]. Patients with stage III or IV disease without metastases were included in the study and appropriate stratification was used. Again, both arms included radiotherapy with a standard fractionation scheme to a dose considered adequate for cure. Patients in the concomitant arm received bleomycin 5 U twice weekly during the entire course of radiotherapy. The exact number of patients who did not receive the entire planned course of bleomycin during treatment was not stated, but toxicity was noted to be greater in the concomitant group. However, this trial differed from the other concomitant bleomycin trials by including planned maintenance chemotherapy, consisting of bleomycin and methotrexate for 16 weeks after concomitant treatment. Compliance during maintenance chemotherapy was poor. Only 31% of patients received 50% or more of the planned maintenance dose, and 33% received no maintenance chemotherapy. Nevertheless, this trial reported some positive results. While a superior survival was noted for the concomitant group, it was not statistically significant. The concomitant group did have a statistically significant improvement in disease-free survival and locoregional control as failure patterns were changed. Distant metastases were the most frequently seen site of failure in the concomitant group, while local failure was the primary site in the radiotherapy alone group.

Another agent investigated in randomized trial of concomitant chemoradiotherapy is mitomycin-C. This drug has been successfully incorporated into the concomitant treatment of squamous cell carcinoma of the anus, and it is understandable that mitomycin would be tested in concomitant therapy of head and neck carcinoma. Weissberg et al. studied the use of concomitant mitomycin-C in a heterogenous cohort of patients that included those patients receiving pre-operative, postoperative, or definitive radiation therapy [58]. Patients in this study were stratified by tumor site and type of surgery if any. The patients randomized to receive mitomycin received a maximum of two doses at 15 mg/m^2 during radiation therapy. These patients were compared to the group randomized to radiotherapy alone. The authors concluded that concomitant therapy with mitomycin-C results in an improvement in disease-free survival and local control but no change in the overall survival. Whether this is a valid conclusion can be questioned. Subset analysis showed that the only groups to have a local control benefit from concomitant therapy were those in the pre-operative or postoperative radiation group. Thus, concomitant therapy did not improve local or regional control in those patients who underwent radiation alone with curative intent. These results should not be surprising. It is unlikely that one or two doses of chemotherapy during a 5–7 week course of radiotherapy will significantly alter the failure pattern in patients with gross disease. The group of patients most in need of improved treatment, those with inoperable disease, did not benefit at all in this trial.

Very few other single agents active in head and neck cancer have been tested in randomized trials. While methotrexate has been extensively studied in neoadjuvant trials, its use in concomitant chemoradiotherapy has been investigated in only one randomized trial [59]. In this trial patients in the concomitant arm received two doses of $100 \, mg/m^2$ of methotrexate during the course of radiation therapy. Analysis of the entire group demonstrated a trend for increased survival and local control. However, only in patients with oropharyngeal primary tumors was this difference statistically significant. The radiation therapy plan was unusual in this study. Patients in both arms received treatment in 300 cGy fractions, and the entire 5000 cGy treatment was completed in 3 weeks. This fractionation scheme would be anticipated to increase both acute and late reactions from treatment. Approximately 10% of patients in both groups developed bone or soft-tissue necrosis in this study. While this trial employed adequate doses of an active agent, the results were equivocal. Again, one must conclude that two doses of chemotherapy during radiation are unlikely to significantly alter outcome.

Cisplatin is another agent widely used in head and neck cancer as a single agent and in combination therapy. This drug has been reported to act as a radiation enhancer in experimental settings, making it attractive to clinical investigators using concomitant chemoradiotherapy [60,61]. The Radiation Therapy Oncology Group reported the results of a large phase II trial of conventional radiation therapy with concomitant cisplatin [62]. Patients received intermittent cisplatin at high doses ($100 \, mg/m^2$) every 3 weeks during radiation therapy for a total of two to three doses. Of 124 patients with locoregionally advanced unresectable disease, 71% achieved a complete response (CR) and 34% were alive at 4 years. The survival rate was superior to that of historical controls, and toxicity was similar to that seen with radiation therapy alone.

Only one randomized trial studying cisplatin and concomitant radiation therapy has been completed [63]. Patients were treated with standard radiation therapy alone or weekly doses of cisplatin at $20 \, mg/m^2$ in addition to radiotherapy. The dose of cisplatin in this study is much lower than that commonly used when this drug is given as part of combination chemotherapy ($100 \, mg/m^2$ every 3–4 weeks). Thus, this drug dosage may have been insufficient for significant single-agent activity, and it is unknown whether doses in this range enhance radiotherapy. It may not be surprising that a preliminary analysis of this study reported no difference in complete response rate or survival between the two groups.

At this point the potential for concomitant chemoradiotherapy is only beginning to be realized. Other potentially useful agents in concomitant therapy have been studied in phase I–II trials but have not been tested in randomized trials. One such agent is carboplatin, which could be an attractive substitute for cisplatin. Eisenberger et al. conducted a phase I study and identified $100 \, mg/m^2$/week of radiotherapy as the recommended dose [64]. Mucositis was not increased over historical controls but myelosuppression was dose limiting. Fifty-two percent of the 25 patients in this study achieved a complete response, suggesting that further investigation is warranted.

Another drug studied with concomitant radiotherapy in head and neck cancer is hydroxyurea [65]. No recent single-agent trials with this agent have been published in head and neck cancer. However, positive randomized trials with this drug have been published in cancer of the cervix [66].

The single-agent concomitant studies have shown limited benefit in randomized trials. While a few of these trials have demonstrated superior survival or disease-free survival compared to standard therapy, the benefit has frequently been modest, while the side effects of therapy were almost always increased. However, these are the results that should be anticipated. Trials that attempted to give drug more frequently than once or twice during the course of radiation therapy administered low doses that may not have been effective. Those studies that administered drug at active doses gave one or two doses during the entire duration of radiation therapy. Although each dose may have been active, dosing was too infrequent to exploit any radiation-enhancing properties of the drug. While these trials do not justify the widespread use of concomitant therapy in the community, they do support continued investigation in well-controlled trials. The trials described thus far seem to suggest that more active radiation enhancers, drug combinations, or dosing schedules are needed to further improve survival at the cost of acceptable toxicity.

A more recent approach has been to combine multiagent chemotherapy with radiation in clinical studies. While several drug combinations have been tested, results from randomized trials are not yet available. However, response rates with multiagent regimens have been high, often exceeding 90%, and the proportion of complete responses has ranged between 40% and 80%. The toxicity with polychemotherapy tends to be greater. Therefore, investigators have used nonstandard radiation therapy schedules and incorporated rest periods in the treatment schema in order to keep toxicity within acceptable levels.

Taylor et al. adopted a 2-week treatment schedule [67]. Cisplatin at $60 \, mg/m^2$ was given on day 1 along with a 5-day continuous infusion of 5-FU at $800 \, mg/m^2$/day. Patients received radiotherapy on each day of chemotherapy. The 5 days of treatment were followed by a 9-day rest period and constituted one cycle. These cycles were repeated until the end of radiation therapy. Fifty-three patients were treated with this regimen; mucositis was the dominant toxicity. The complete response rate of 55% is similar to that seen in other concomitant trials. However, the freedom from progression (73%) and median survival (37 months) were superior to those reported in the literature.

We added hydroxyurea to the combination of 5-FU and radiation therapy in a phase I trial [68]. Hydroxyurea was chosen due to its activity in head and neck cancer, radiation-enhancing properties, and ability to modulate the activity of 5-FU. Treatment was given 5 out of every 14 days, as in the Taylor et al. study. The study cohort was heterogeneous and included patients with metastatic or recurrent disease after radiation and or surgery. The response rate was 100% (71% CR) in previously untreated patients and 93% (40% CR) in those with recurrent disease. We recently published the long-term follow-up of the patients on this study [69]. Long-term local control in the untreated group was 84%, and most patients died from distant metastases. A later trial attempted to add infusional cisplatin to the concomitant regimen in a similar group of patients. Again, high response and local control rates were observed, as patients continued to fail at distant sites [70].

Wendt et al. investigated the use of cisplatin, infusional 5-FU, and leucovorin with radiation therapy using a complex treatment schedule [71]. Patients received chemotherapy over 4 days with hyperfractionated concomitant radiotherapy during 3 of those days and 4 days of the subsequent week. This was followed by a 1-week rest and repeated for two more cycles. Sixty-two patients were entered in this trial. The response rate was 100%, with 77% of patients achieving a complete response. The 2-year actuarial survival rate reported was 52%. Acute toxicity was considered acceptable, although 34% of patients developed grade II mucositis during treatment.

Adelstein et al. reported the results of a pilot trial with cisplatin and a 4-day infusion of 5-FU ($1000 \, mg/m^2$/day) with radiation therapy during and after chemotherapy (30 Gy over 3 weeks) [72]. This cycle of treatment was followed by break-in therapy of at least 2 weeks. Surgery or additional chemoradiotherapy followed the break. At a minimum follow-up of 42 months, the actuarial disease-free survival was 70% and the overall survival 52%.

The results of the reported trials using multi-agent chemotherapy with concomitant radiation are suggestive that this approach is more effective than the single-agent trials. Although the results are promising, it is necessary to compare them in randomized studies to standard therapy in order to determine the ultimate impact on survival and disease-free survival. To date only one such trial comparing concomitant therapy to standard radiotherapy has been presented in abstract form [73]. Chemotherapy consisted of cisplatin ($20 \, mg/m^2$/day) and 5-FU ($200 \, mg/m^2$/day) for 5 days during a 2-

week cycle of radiation therapy. This treatment cycle was repeated after a 1-week break for a total of three cycles. Concomitant therapy was compared to standard radiotherapy. In a preliminary analysis, patients in the concomitant arm were reported to have a higher complete response rate of 46% versus 28% with radiotherapy alone. The authors also reported a survival and progression-free survival benefit for concomitant therapy. The main benefit noted with combined modality therapy was an improvement in the probability of local control. The probability of a local relapse was twofold greater in complete responders treated with radiotherapy alone [74].

Although trials comparing concomitant therapy to standard treatment are lacking, there are three randomized trials that have compared concomitant (or rapidly alternating) chemoradiotherapy to neoadjuvant chemotherapy with the same drugs followed by radiotherapy [75–77]. A European trial by the South-East Cooperative Oncology Group studied the combination of vincristine, bleomycin, and methotrexate with or without 5-FU [75]. A total of 267 patients were randomized to receive sequential or concomitant therapy. A trend toward improved survival and disease-free survival in favor of concomitant therapy was noted, but this did not reach statistical significance.

A similar design was used in a small randomized trial by Adelstein et al. [76]. Patients randomized to the sequential arm received three cycles of cisplatin and 5-FU followed by surgery and/or radiation therapy. The concomitant arm received two cycles of the same drugs prior to surgical evaluation. This was followed by a second cycle of chemoradiotherapy. Patients in the concomitant group had statistically superior relapse-free survival (60% vs. 39%; p = 0.03) and complete response rates (67% vs. 32%; p = 0.02). However, the survival advantage with concomitant therapy was not statistically significant.

A third randomized trial comparing rapidly alternating therapy to sequential therapy was reported by Merlano et al. [77]. This trial differed from the two trials above in that none of the combination chemotherapy was given concomitantly with radiation. Instead, the authors chose to rapidly alternate treatment modalities. Patients in this trial were randomly assigned to one of two arms. The chemotherapy in both arms consisted of vinblastine, bleomycin, methotrexate, and leucovorin. Patients assigned to the sequential therapy arm received four cycles of chemotherapy followed by continuous course radiation therapy for a dose of 65–70 Gy. Those patients randomized to alternating therapy received four cycles of identical chemotherapy as the sequential group. Radiation therapy in the alternating therapy group was divided into three 2-week cycles of 20 Gy and was given after the second, third, and fourth cycle of chemotherapy. Thus the overall treatment time was compressed, since patients received radiation therapy during the standard rest periods incorporated in cyclical chemotherapy. Patients in the alternating therapy arm had significantly more mucosal toxicity than those receiving sequential treatment. Rapidly alternating therapy compared to sequential treatment also resulted in improved 4-year progression-free survival (12% vs. 4%; p = 0.02) and overall survival (22% vs. 10%; p = 0.02).

Finally, it should be noted that other radiation therapy schedules are being investigated in an attempt to improve disease-free and overall survival without the use of chemotherapy. The main thrust in this area has been to administer more than one radiation treatment per day. Standard radiation fractionation has been 180–200 cGy per day in a single dose given 5 days per week. Some investigators have begun to use hyperfractionated radiotherapy where patients receive two treatments of 120–160 cGy or more each day. One large randomized trial reported that hyperfractionated radiotherapy resulted in superior disease-free survival but not overall survival compared to single fraction radiotherapy [78]. A more recent randomized study of hyperfractionated radiation therapy compared to standard fractionation in oropharyngeal carcinoma found a survival benefit for hyperfractionation in all lesions other than those involving the base of the tongue [79].

Highly interesting preliminary results have been published by Saunders et al. for a regimen of continuous hyperfractionated accelerated radiotherapy called CHART [80]. In this regimen, patients receive 150 cGy every 8 hours for 12 consecutive days for a total dose of 54 Gy. This accelerated treatment resulted in a 90% complete response rate. While acute reactions tended to be more severe, late reactions tended to be less marked with CHART therapy than with conventional radiation. However, four patients have developed unexpected radiation myelitis [81].

Since acute reactions are more intense, hyperfractionated radiotherapy trials have rarely incorporated concomitant radiotherapy. Choi et al. have reported one such trial in 12 patients with paranasal and nasopharyngeal tumors [82]. Patients received 120 cGy twice each day in a split course and an infusion of cisplatin at $5-7 \, mg/m^2/day$. The complete response rate was 92% (11/12) and 58% were alive up to 72 months after treatment.

One randomized study has attempted to compare standard radiotherapy to hyperfractionation and concomitant therapy [83]. In this study 859 patients with advanced head and neck cancer were randomized to one of three groups. Patients in the standard radiotherapy group received a total dose of 60 Gy in 200 cGy fractions. Patients in the hyperfractionated radio-therapy arm received 220 cGy per day in two fractions to a total dose of 70.4 Gy. Those patients randomized to concomitant therapy were given 200 cGy per day to a total dose of 60 Gy and 5-FU at $250 \, mg/m^2$ every other day for the entire course of treatment. Patients who received hyperfrac-tionated radiotherapy or concomitant therapy had statistically superior response, progression-free survival, and overall survival rates compared to standard radiotherapy. There were no differences between hyperfractionated and concomitant arms. However, the total dose of radiation delivered in the standard radiation and concomitant arms would not be considered adequate in most centers.

190

Conclusions

Clearly, the results of clinical studies thus far illustrate the difficulty in treating squamous cell carcinoma of the head and neck. In spite of aggressive surgery and radiation therapy, local failure remains a significant problem in advanced cases. Also, the functional results after treatment in those few patients who are cured of their disease are less than optimal. Current studies have shown that the majority of failures in advanced head and neck cancer continue to occur locally and regionally after standard therapy. Additional evidence has been presented to suggest that an improvement in locoregional control in itself may not result in an improvement in the cure rates, since a large number of patients with advanced head and neck cancer may have micrometastases at the time of diagnosis. Therefore, it is likely that both of these issues will need to be addressed in future treatment strategies if a significant improvement in outcome can be expected.

The results of neoadjuvant chemotherapy trials thus far have been largely disappointing, as none have been able to demonstrate a survival benefit. Although the design of these trials can be criticized, it is unlikely that sequential treatment with neoadjuvant chemotherapy will significantly alter the outcome in most patients. Patients with advanced head and neck cancers have a large locoregional disease burden and tend to fail in these areas. Even trials using an adequate number of cycles and dosage of multi-agent chemotherapy have shown that local failures frequently occur, even with high complete response rates to chemotherapy. Although many reasons have been put forth to explain this observation, including the induction of resistant cells, the most likely cause may be tumor repopulation. Multiple reports in the radiotherapy literature have shown that any delay in standard radiation therapy for head and neck cancer results in a decrease in local control [84]. This decrease in local control has been attributed to accelerated tumor clonogen repopulation during treatment [85]. Although the size of the tumor may be decreasing during neoadjuvant chemotherapy, the number of clonogenic cells may be increasing during the periods between chemotherapy cycles, limiting any gain in local control.

Though disappointing, the neoadjuvant trials are not without merit. There is ample evidence that sequential neoadjuvant chemotherapy can decrease the incidence of distant metastases. Another important result of these studies is that neoadjuvant chemotherapy may identify patients with a more favorable prognosis, and those patients with a favorable response may be eligible for more conservative surgical treatment, including organ preservation.

While the lack of randomized data from well-designed trials prevents conclusions regarding the efficacy of concomitant chemoradiotherapy, the treatment approach to head and neck cancer remains attractive. The simultaneous administration of chemotherapy with radiation can shorten the overall treatment time and limit tumor repopulation. The use of chemotherapeutic agents known to be active in head and neck cancer that have the potential of enhancing the effects of radiotherapy remains attractive. In theory this would address locoregional and distant failure simultaneously.

To date, phase II–III trials have shown that concomitant therapy results in improved local control and disease-free survival. These results are highly encouraging for the following reasons. Most of the concomitant trials to date have used doses of chemotherapy that would be considered ineffective if administered as single agents. Other studies have attempted to give higher doses but at infrequent intervals during radiation therapy. In some studies the dose of radiotherapy was reduced to less than curative doses when concomitant chemotherapy was added. The fact that even suboptimal chemotherapy and or radiotherapy, when incorporated into a concomitant regimen, impacts on the major site of failure justifies additional investigation.

Future directions

Concomitant trials remain a promising area for future investigation, since randomized trials have shown an improvement in disease-free survival and local control. However, the optimal regimen and best method to integrate chemotherapy with radiation into a concomitant program must be determined. In theory the optimal regimen would integrate active doses of multi-agent chemotherapy with full-course radiotherapy. Unfortunately, the toxicity of such a regimen would be prohibitive. Therefore, adjustments in the dose, number of agents, or sequencing of therapy must be made in order to keep toxicity within acceptable limits. One option that has shown some promise is to completely integrate chemotherapy with radiosensitizing properties with radiation and impose scheduled breaks in treatment to limit toxicity. A second option to limit toxicity would be to rapidly alternate cycles of radiotherapy with high-dose combination chemotherapy. The superior method of concomitant therapy should be determined in future trials. Whether the enhancement in the effectiveness of radiation can compensate for delays in treatment is unknown but has been suggested in some studies. Similarly, whether the loss of radiation enhancement by rapidly alternating cycles of chemotherapy and radiation affects outcome deserves further investigation.

Consideration should also be given to the use of concomitant chemoradiotherapy in earlier stage disease with the goal of organ preservation. The local control results with concomitant therapy suggest this type of treatment may be used to substitute for surgery and achieve the same good survival without loss of function. Neoadjuvant chemotherapy may be necessary to reduce the incidence of distant metastases, followed by concomitant therapy for improved locoregional control. In those patients who are successfully treated, chemoprevention with retinoids should be considered to decrease the incidence of second malignancies.

Acknowledgments

We wish to thank the Geraldi Norton Memorial Corporation and the Center for Radiation Therapy for their continued support. This work was also supported by American Cancer Society Clinical Oncology Career Development Award #92-252 to DJH.

References

1. Haraf DJ, Weichselbaum RR. Treatment selection in T1 and T2 vocal cord carcinoma. Oncology 2:41–47, 1988.
2. Cachin Y, Eschwege F. Combination of radiotherapy and surgery in the treatment of head and neck cancers. Cancer Treat Rev 2:177–191, 1975.
3. Probert JC, Thompson RW, Bagshaw MA. Pattern of spread of distant metastases in head and neck cancer. Cancer 33:127–133, 1974.
4. Zbaeren P, Lehmann W. Frequency and sites of distant metastases in head and neck squamous cell carcinoma. Arch Otolarygol Head and Neck Surg 113:762–764, 1987.
5. Takagi M, Kayano T, Yamamoto H, Shibuya H, Hoshina M, Shioda S, Enomoto S. Causes of oral tongue cancer treatment failures. Analysis of autopsy cases. Cancer 69:1081–1087, 1992.
6. Leibel SA, Scott CB, Mohiuddin M, Marcial VA, Coia LR, Davis LW, Fuks Z. The effect of local-regional control on distant metastatic dissemination in carcinoma of the head and neck: Results of an analysis from the RTOG head and neck database. Int J Radiat Oncol Biol Phys 21:549–556, 1991.
7. Pinto HA, Jacobs C. Chemotherapy for recurrent and metastatic head and neck cancer. Hematol Oncol Clin North Am 5:667–686, 1991.
8. Clark JR, Fallon BG, Dreyfuss AI, Norris CM Jr, Anderson JW, Ervin TJ, Anderson RF, Chaffey JT, Mille D, Frei E III. Chemotherapeutic strategies in the multidisciplinary treatment of head and neck cancer. Semin Oncol 15(Suppl 3):35–44, 1988.
9. Morton RP, Rugman F, Dorman EB, Stoney PJ, Wilson JA, McCormick M, Veevers A, Stell PM. Cisplatinum and bleomycin for advanced or recurrent squamous cell carcinoma of the head and neck: A randomized factorial phase III controlled trial. Cancer Chemother Pharmacol 15:283–289, 1985.
10. DeConti RC, Schoenfeld D. A randomized prospective comparison of intermittent methotrexate, methotrexate with leucovorin, and a methotrexate combination in head and neck cancer. Cancer 48:1061–1072, 1981.
11. Kaplan BH, Schoenfeld D, Vogl SE. Treatment of recurrent (REC) or metastatic (MET) squamous cancer of the head and neck (SCH&N) with methotrexate (M), M plus *Corynebacterium parvum* (CP) or M plus bleomycin (B) plus diamminedichloroplatinum (D): A prospective randomized trial of the Eastern Cooperative Oncology Group. Proc Am Assoc Cancer Res 22:532, 1981.
12. Jacobs C, Meyers F, Hendrickson C, Kohler M, Carter S. A randomized phase III study of cisplatin with or without methotrexate for recurrent squamous cell carcinoma of the head and neck. A Northern California Oncology Group Study. Cancer 52:1563–1569, 1983.
13. Drelichman A, Cummings G, Al-Sarraf M. A randomized trial of the combination of cis-platinum, oncovin, and bleomycin (COB) versus methotrexate in patients with advanced squamous cell carcinoma of the head and neck. Cancer 52:399–403, 1983.
14. Vogl SE, Schoenfeld DA, Kaplan BH, Lerner HJ, Engstrom PF, Horton J. A randomized prospective comparison of methotrexate with a combination of methotrexate, bleomycin, and cisplatin in head and neck cancer. Cancer 56:432–442, 1985.
15. Williams SD, Velez-Garcia E, Essessee I, Ratkin G, Birch R, Einhorn LH. Chemotherapy

for head and neck cancer: A combination of cisplatin + vinblastine + bleomycin versus methotrexate. Cancer 57:18–23, 1986.

16. Jacobs C, Lyman G, Velez-Garcia E, Sridhar KS, Knight W, Hochster H, Goodnough LT, Mortimer JE, Einhorn LH, Schacter L, et al. A phase III study comparing cisplatin and fluorouracil as single agents and in combination for advanced squamous cell carcinoma of the head and neck. J Clin Oncol 10:257–263, 1992.

17. Forastiere A, Metchy B, Keppen M, Schuller D, Ensley J, Coltmann C Jr. Randomized comparison of cisplatin + 5-fluorouracil (5-FU) vs. carboplatin + 5-FU vs. methotrexate in advanced squamous cell carcinoma of the head and neck. Proc Am Soc Clin Oncol 8:168, 1989.

18. The Liverpool Head and Neck Oncology Group. A phase III randomized trial of cis-platinum, methotrexate, cisplatinum + methotrexate and cisplatinum + 5-FU in end stage squamous carcinoma of the head and neck. Br J Cancer 61:311–315, 1990.

19. Steele GG, Peckham MJ. Exploitable mechanisms in combined radiotherapy-chemo-therapy: The concept of additivity. Int J Radiat Oncol Biol Phys 5:85–91, 1979.

20. Vokes EE, Weichselbaum RR. Concomitant chemoradiotherapy: Rationale and clinical experience in patients with solid tumors. J Clin Oncol 8:911–934, 1990.

21. Bentzen SM, Johansen LV, Overgaard J, Thames HD. Clinical radiobiology of squamous cell carcinoma of the oropharynx. Int J Radiat Oncol Biol Phys 20:1197–1206, 1991.

22. Taylor JMG, Whithers HR, Mendenhall WM. Dose-time considerations of head and neck squamous cell carcinomas treated with irradiation. Radiother Oncol 17:95–102, 1990.

23. Ensley J, Jacobs J, Weaver A, Kinzie J, Crissman J, Kish J, Cummings G, Al-Sarraf M. Correlation between response to cisplatinum-combination chemotherapy and subsequent radiotherapy in previously untreated patients with advanced squamous cancers of the head and neck. Cancer 54:811–814, 1984.

24. Clark JR, Fallon BG, Dreyfuss AI, Norris CM Jr, Anderson JW, Ervin TJ, Anderson RF, Chaffey JT, Miller D, Frei E 3d. Chemotherapeutic strategies in the multidisciplinary treatment of head and neck cancer. Semin Oncol 15(Suppl 3):35–44, 1988.

25. Vokes EE, Moran WJ, Mick R, Weichselbaum RR, Panje WR. Neoadjuvant and adjuvant methotrexate, cisplatin and flourouracil in multimodal therapy of head and neck cancer. J Clin Oncol 7:838–845, 1989.

26. Vokes EE, Panje WR, Mick R, Kozloff MF, Moran WJ, Sutton HS, Goldman MD, Tybor AG, Weichselbaum RR. A randomized study comparing two regimens of neoadjuvant chemotherapy in multimodal therapy for locally advanced head and neck cancer. Cancer 66:206–213, 1990.

27. Dreyfus AI, Clark JR, Wright JE, Norris CM Jr, Busse PM, Lucarini JW, Fallon BG, Casey D, Andersen JW, Klein R, et al. Continuous infusion high-dose leucovorin with 5-fluorouracil and cisplatin for untreated stage IV carcinoma of the head and neck. Ann Intern Med 112:167–172, 1990.

28. Rooney M, Kish J, Jacobs J, Kinzie J, Weaver A, Crissman J, Al-Sarraf M. Improved complete response rate and survival in advanced head and neck cancer after three-course induction therapy with 120-hour 5-FU infusion and cisplatin. Cancer 55:1123–1128, 1985.

29. Ensley J, Kish J, Tapazoglou E, Jacobs J, Weaver A, Atkinson D, Ahmed K, Mathog R, Al-Sarraf M. An intensive, five course, alternating combination chemotherapy induction regimen used in patients with advanced, unresectable head and neck cancer. J Clin Oncol 6:1147–1153, 1988.

30. Kies MS, Gordon LI, Hauck WW, Krespi Y, Ossoff RH, Pecaro BC, Yuska C, Lamut CH, Brand WN, Chang SK, et al. Analysis of complete responders after initial treatment with chemotherapy in head and neck cancer. Otolaryngol Head Neck Surg 93:199–205, 1985.

31. Vokes EE, Mick R, Lester EP, Panje WR, Weichselbaum RR. Cisplatin and flourouracil chemotherapy does not yield long-term benefit in locally advanced head and neck cancer: Results from a single institution. J Clin Oncol 9:1376–1384, 1991.

32. Dreyfuss AI, Clark JR. Analysis of prognostic factors in squamous cell carcinomas of the head and neck. Hematol Oncol Clin North Am 5:701–712, 1991.

33. Hill BT, Price LA, MacRae K. Importance of site in addressing chemotherapy response and 7 year survival data in advanced squamous-cell carcinomas of the head and neck treated with initial combination chemotherapy without cisplatin. J Clin Oncol 4:1340–1347, 1986.

34. Mick R, Vokes EE, Weichselbaum RR, Panje WR. Prognostic factors in advanced head and neck cancer patients undergoing multimodal therapy. Otolaryngol Head Neck Surg 105:62–73, 1991.

35. Knowlton AH, Percarpio B, Bobrow S, Fischer JJ. Methotrexate and radiation in the treatment of advanced head and neck tumors. Radiology 116:709–712, 1975.

36. Fazekas JT, Sommer C, Kramer S. Adjuvant intravenous methotrexate or definitive radiotherapy alone for advanced squamous cancers of the oral cavity, oropharynx, supraglottic larynx or hypopharynx. Int J Radiat Oncol Biol Phys 6:533–541, 1980.

37. Taylor SG, Applebaum E, Showel JL, Norusis M, Holinger LD, Hutchinson JC Jr, Murthy AK, Caldarelli DD. A randomized trial of adjuvant chemotherapy in head and neck cancer. J Clin Oncol 3:672–679, 1985.

38. Stell PM, Dalby JE, Strickland P, Fraser JG, Bradley PJ, Flood LM. Sequential chemotherapy and radiotherapy in advanced head and neck cancer. Clin Radiol 34:463–467, 1983.

39. Holoye PY, Grossman TW, Toohill RJ, Kun LE, Byhardt RW, Duncavage JA, Byhardt RW, Ritch PS, Grossman TW, Hoffmann RG, Cox JD, Malin T. Randomized study of adjuvant chemotherapy for head and neck cancer. Otolaryngol Head Neck Surg 93:712–717, 1985.

40. Martin M, Hazan A, Vegnes L, Peytral C, Mazeron JJ, Senechaut JP, Lelievre G, Peynegre R. Randomized study of 5-fluorouracil and cisplatin as neoadjuvant therapy in head and neck cancer: A preliminary report. Int J Radiat Oncol Biol Phys 19:973–975, 1990.

41. Toohill RJ, Anderson T, Byhardt RW, Cox JD, Duncavage JA, Grossman TW, Haas CD, Haas JS, Hartz AJ, Libnoch JA, et al. Cisplatin and fluorouracil as neoadjuvant therapy in head and neck cancer. Arch Otolaryngol Head Neck Surg 113:758–761, 1987.

42. Schuller DE, Metch B, Mattox D, Stein DW, McCracken JD. Preoperative chemotherapy in advanced resectable head and neck cancer: Final report of the Southwest Oncology Group. Laryngoscope 98:1205–1211, 1988.

43. Final Report of the Head and Neck Contracts Program. Adjuvant chemotherapy for advanced head and neck squamous carcinoma. Cancer 60:301–311, 1987.

44. Jacobs C, Mauch R. Efficacy of adjuvant chemotherapy for patients with resectable head and neck cancer: A subset analysis of the head and neck contracts program. J Clin Oncol 8:838–847, 1990.

45. The Department of Veteran Affairs Laryngeal Cancer Study Group. Induction chemotherapy plus radiation compared with surgery plus radiation in patients with advanced laryngeal cancer. N Engl J Med 324:1685–1690, 1991.

46. Laramore GE, Wolf GT, Fisher SG, et al. Surgery and postoperative radiotherapy vs. induction chemotherapy and definitive radiotherapy for advanced laryngeal cancer: Control of neck disease and distant metastases as a function of nodal staging (abstr). Proc Am Radium Soc 74:14, 1992.

47. Jacobs C, Goffinet DR, Goffinet L, Kohler M, Fee WE. Chemotherapy as a substitute for surgery in the treatment of advanced resectable head and neck cancer. A report from the Northern California Oncology Group. Cancer 60:1178–1183, 1987.

48. Pfister DG, Strong E, Harrison L, Haines IE, Pfister DA, Sessions R, Spiro R, Shah J, Gerold F, McLure T, et al. Larynx preservation with combined chemotherapy and radiation therapy in advanced but resectable head and neck cancer. J Clin Oncol 9:850–859, 1991.

49. Karp DD, Vaughan CW, Carter R, Willett B, Heeren T, Calarese P, Zeitels S, Strong MS, Hong WK. Larynx preservation using induction chemotherapy plus radiation therapy as an alternative to laryngectomy in advanced head and neck cancer. A long-term follow-up

report. Am J Clin Oncol 14:273–279, 1991.

50. Laramore GE, Scott CB, Al-Sarraf M, Haselow RE, Ervin TJ, Wheeler R, Jacobs R. Adjuvant chemotherapy for resectable squamous cell carcinomas of the head and neck: Report on intergroup study 0034 (abstr). Int J Radiat Oncol Biol Phys 21(Suppl 1):190, 1991.

51. Vokes EE, Weichselbaum RR, Mick R, McEvilly JM, Haraf DJ, Panje WR. Favorable long-term survival following induction chemotherapy with cisplatin, flourouracil, and leucovorin and concomitant chemoradiotherapy for locally advanced head and neck cancer. J Natl Cancer Inst 84:877–882, 1992.

52. Ansfield FJ, Ramirez G, Davis HL, Korbitz BC, Vermund H, Gollin FF. Treatment of advanced cancer of the head and neck. Cancer 25:78–82, 1970.

53. Lo TC, Wiley AL Jr, Ansfield FJ, Brandenburg JH, Davis HL Jr, Gollin FF, Johnson RO, Ramirez G, Vermund H. Combined radiation therapy and 5-fluorouracil for advanced squamous cell carcinoma of the oral cavity and oropharynx: A randomized study. Am J Roentgenol 126:229–235, 1976.

54. Shanta V, Krishnamurthi S. Combined bleomycin and radiotherapy in oral cancer. Clin Radiol 31:617–620, 1980.

55. Vermund H, Kaalhus O, Winther F, Trausjo J, Thorud E, Harang R. Bleomycin and radiation therapy in squamous cell carcinoma of the upper aero-digestive tract: A phase III clinical trial. Int J Radiat Oncol Biol Phys 11:1877–1886, 1985.

56. Eschwege F, Sancho-Garnier H, Gerard JP, Madelain M, DeSaulty A, Jortay A, Canchin Y. Ten-year results of randomized trial comparing radiotherapy and concomitant bleomycin to radiotherapy alone in epidermoid carcinomas of the oropharynx: Experience of the European Organization for Research and Treatment of Cancer. Monogr Natl Cancer Inst 6:275–278, 1988.

57. Fu KK, Phillips TL, Silverberg KJ, Jacobs C, Goffinet DR, Chun C, Friedman MA, Kohler M, McWhirter K, Carter SK. Combined radiotherapy and chemotherapy with bleomycin and methotrexate for advanced inoperable head and neck cancer: Update of a Northern California Oncology Group Randomized Trial. J Clin Oncol 5:1410–1418, 1987.

58. Weissberg JB, Son YH, Papac RJ, Sasaki C, Fischer DB, Lawrence R, Rockwell S, Sartorelli AC, Fischer JJ. Randomized clinical trial of mitomycin C as an adjunct to radiotherapy in head and neck cancer. Int J Radiat Oncol Biol Phys 17:3–9, 1989.

59. Gupta NK, Pointon RCS, Wilkinson PM. A randomized trial to contrast radiotherapy with radiotherapy and methotrexate given synchronously in head and neck cancer. Clin Radiol 38:575–581, 1987.

60. Coughlin CT, Richmond RC. Biologic and clinical developments of cisplatin combined with radiation: Concepts, utility, projections for new trials, and emergence of carboplatin. Semin Oncol 16(Suppl 6):31–43, 1989.

61. Douple EB. Keynote address: Platinum-radiation interactions. Monogr Natl Cancer Inst 6:315–319, 1988.

62. Al-Sarraf M, Pajak TF, Marcial VA, Mowry P, Cooper JS, Stetz J, Ensley JF, Velez-Garcia E. Concurrent radiotherapy and chemotherapy with cisplatin in inoperable squamous cell carcinoma of the head and neck. Cancer 59:259–265, 1987.

63. Haselow RE, Warshaw MG, Oken MM, Adams GL, Aughey JL, Cooper JS, Schuller DE, Jacobs CD. Radiation alone versus radiation with weekly low dose cisplatinum in unresectable cancer of the head and neck. In: Fee WE, Goepfert H, Johns ME, Strong E, Ward PH, eds. Head and Neck Cancer. Toronto: B.C. Decker, 1990, pp 279–281.

64. Eisenberger M, Van Echo D, Aisner J. Carboplatin: The experience in head and neck cancer. Semin Oncol 16:34–41, 1989.

65. Richards GJ, Chambers RG. Hydroxyurea: A radiosensitizer in the treatment of neoplasms of the head and neck. Am J Roengenol Radium Nucl Med 55:555–565, 1969.

66. Piver MS, Barlow JJ, Vongtama V, Blumenson L. A radiation potentiator in carcinoma of the uterine cervix. A randomized double-blind study. Am J Obstet Gynecol 147:803–808, 1983.

67. Taylor SG, Murthy AK, Caldarelli DD, Showel JL, Kiel K, Griem KL, Mittal BB, Kies M, Hutchinson JC Jr, Holinger LD, Campanella R, Witt TR, Hoover S. Combined simultaneous cisplatin/fluorouracil chemotherapy and split course radiation in head and neck cancer. J Clin Oncol 7:846–856, 1989.

68. Vokes EE, Panje WR, Schilsky RL, Mick R, Awan AM, Moran WJ, Goldman MD, Tybor AG, Weichselbaum RR. Hydroxyurea, fluorouracil, and concomitant radiotherapy in poor-prognosis head and neck cancer. J Clin Oncol 7:761–768, 1989.

69. Haraf DJ, Vokes EE, Panje WR, Weichselbaum RR. Survival and analysis of failure following hydroxyurea, 5-fluorouracil and concomitant radiation therapy in poor prognosis head and neck cancer. Am J Clin Oncol 14:419–426, 1991.

70. Haraf DJ, Vokes EE, Weichselbaum RR, Panje WR. Concomitant chemoradiotherapy with cisplatin, 5-fluorouracil and hydroxyurea in poor prognosis head and neck cancer. Laryngoscope 102:630–636, 1992.

71. Wendt TG, Hartenstein RC, Wustrow TPU, Lissner J. Cisplatin, fluorouracil with leucovorin calcium enhancement, and synchronous accelerated radiotherapy in the management of locally advanced head and neck cancer: A phase II study. J Clin Oncol 7:471–476, 1989.

72. Adelstein DJ, Sharan VM, Earle AS, Shah AC, Vlastou C, Haria CD, Carter SG, Damm C, Hines JD: Long-term results after chemoradiotherapy for locally confined squamous-cell head and neck cancer. Am J Clin Oncol 13:440–447, 1990.

73. Merlano M, Rosso R, Benasso M, Corvo R, Margarino G, Rubagotti A, Zarrilli D, Toma S, Brema F, Grimaldi A, Luzi G, Vitale V. Alternating chemotherapy (CT) and radiotherapy (RT) vs RT in advanced inoperable SCC-HN: A cooperative randomized trial (abstr). Proc Am Soc Clin Oncol 10:198, 1991.

74. Merlano M, Benasso M, Blengio F. The integration of chemotherapy and radiotherapy in the management of advanced squamous cell carcinoma of the head and neck. J Infusional Chemother 2:16–20, 1992.

75. South-East Co-operative Oncology Group. A randomized trial of combined multidrug chemotherapy and radiotherapy in advanced squamous cell carcinoma of the head and neck. An interim report. Eur J Surg Oncol 12:289–295, 1986.

76. Adelstein DJ, Sharan VM, Earle AS, Shah AC, Vlastou C, Haria CD, Damm C, Carter SG, Hines JD. Simultaneous versus sequential combined technique therapy for squamous cell head and neck cancer. Cancer 65:1685–1691, 1990.

77. Merlano M, Corvo R, Margarino G, Benasso M, Rosso R, Sertoli MR, Cavallari M, Scala M, Guenzi M, Siragusa A, Brema F, Luzi G, Bottero G, Bioni G, Scasso F, Garaventa G, Accomando E, Santelli A, Cordone G, Comella G, Vitriolo S, Santi L. Combined chemotherapy and radiation therapy in advanced inoperable squamous cell carcinoma of the head and neck. The final report of a randomized trial. Cancer 67:915–921, 1991.

78. Horiot JC, Le Fur R, N'Guyen T, Chenal C, Schraub S, Alfonsi S, Gardani G, Van den Bogaert W, Danczak S, Bolla M, et al. Hyperfractionated compared with conventional radiotherapy in oropharyngeal carcinoma: An EORTC randomized trial. Eur J Cancer 26:779–780, 1990.

79. Pinto LHJ, Canary PCV, Araujo CMM, Bacelar SC, Souhami L. Prospective randomized trial comparing hyperfractionated versus conventional radiotherapy in stages III and IV oropharyngeal carcinoma. Int J Radiat Oncol Biol Phys 21:557–562, 1991.

80. Saunders MI, Dische S, Hong A, Grosch EJ, Fermont DC, Ashford RFU, Maher EJ. Continuous hyperfractionated accelerated radiotherapy in locally advanced carcinoma of the head and neck region. Int J Radiat Oncol Biol Phys 17:1287–1293, 1989.

81. Saunders MI, Dische S, Grosch EJ, Fermont DC, Ashford RFU, Maher EJ, Makepeace AR. Experience with CHART. Int J Radiat Oncol Biol Phys 21:871–878, 1991.

82. Choi KN, Rotman M, Aziz H, et al. Locally advanced paranasal sinus and nasopharynx tumors treated with hyperfractionated radiation and concurrent infusion cisplatin. Cancer 67:2748–2752, 1991.

83. Sanchiz F, Milla A, Torner J, Bonet F, Artola N, Carreno L, Moya LM, Riera D, Ripol S,

Cirera L. Single fraction per day versus two fractions per day versus radiochemotherapy in the treatment of head and neck cancer. Int J Radiat Oncol Biol Phys 19:1347–1350, 1990.

84. Lindstrom MJ, Fowler JF. Analysis of the time factor in local control by radiotherapy of T_3T_4 squamous cell carcinoma of the larynx. Int J Radiat Oncol Biol Phys 21:813–817, 1991.

85. Whithers HR, Taylor JMG, Maciejewski B. The hazard of accelerated tumor clonogen repopulation during radiotherapy. Acta Oncol 27:131–146, 1988.

11. Organ preservation in advanced head and neck cancer

Charles R. Dibb, Susan Urba, and Gregory T. Wolf

Cancers of the upper aerodigestive tract represent a major medical problem. In the United States, 42,800 new diagnoses of malignancies of the oral cavity, oropharynx, and larynx are anticipated in 1992, resulting in 11,600 deaths. The death rate from laryngeal cancer has remained unchanged in U.S. men (at approximately 2.5/100,000 population) for the last 30 years [1]. The problem is global: Countries in the Far East (Singapore, Hong Kong) and Europe (France, Hungary) have age-adjusted death rates from oral cancer that are triple that of the United States [2].

Current therapy of advanced head and neck cancer remains unsatisfactory. Patients presenting with advanced local-regional disease (T3–4 or N1–3) have less than one-third likelihood of 2-year disease-free survival despite definitive therapy. Additionally, local treatment of upper aerodigestive tract tumors is associated with substantial morbidity. Total laryngectomy remains part of the traditional treatment regimen for advanced laryngeal and hypopharyngeal tumors, as well as some advanced tumors of the oropharynx and tongue [3]. Clearly, improved therapies that serve to decrease treatment-related morbidity, as well as to increase disease-free and overall survival, are needed.

Psychosocial considerations

The psychosocial problems associated with laryngectomy can be severe. Esophageal speech is acquired only by approximately two thirds of laryngectomees, with only 15% achieving excellent intelligibility [4,5]. Studies have reported vocational difficulties [6], depression [7], social isolation [8,9], embarrassment [4], and sexual dysfunction [10] related to the postlaryngectomy state. One group of investigators sought to document attitudes regarding laryngectomy in a group of normal volunteers: They reported that an average 40-year-old, faced with a choice between laryngectomy or a

Hong, Waun Ki and Weber, Randal S., (eds.), Head and Neck Cancer. © *1995 Kluwer Academic Publishers. ISBN 0-7923-3015-3. All rights reserved.*

voice-sparing procedure with a substantially lower cure rate, would accept a 14% loss from an average life span in order to preserve his speech [11].

Postoperative psychological and functional difficulties in head and neck cancer patients are not restricted to postlaryngectomy patients. Most patients undergoing radical resections of oral cavity or oropharynx cancer will experience significant problems in deglutition, dysphagia, aspiration, and articulation. Resection of the mandible or maxilla also often result in cosmetic disability. These problems continue to be important despite ever improving methods of surgical reconstruction. Further, a substantial portion of patients undergoing radical neck dissection or modified radical neck dissection report dissatisfaction with their appearance (24–41%), difficulty lifting an arm (30–70%), or neck numbness (30–40%) postoperatively [9]. Clearly, when measuring potential benefits of therapy in patients presenting with advanced head and neck cancer, consideration must be given to quality of life as well as to traditional criteria of response rate, disease-free survival, and overall survival. This chapter will focus on progress reported to date in organ-sparing treatment regimens for advanced, resectable head and neck cancer.

Radiation therapy alone in advanced head and neck cancer

Substantial controversy exists over the role of primary radiation therapy in the treatment of advanced laryngeal cancer. Studies done prior to 1980 [12–16] show a persistent 20–30% decrease in 3-year survival in patients with T3 laryngeal cancer compared with patients treated surgically. However, the statistics in these reports may be misleading. While several of these studies contained large numbers of patients, few patients had advanced disease, so that the reported 20–30% decreased survival is based on comparatively few patients [13–16]. All data are retrospective from single institutions, and no randomized study has been reported. Some of the radiation therapy studies included a sizable number of poorer prognosis patients 'rejected . . . by reasons of age or infirmity' [14], who had tumors judged inoperable [14], or who had refused surgery [12,14,15,16]. Additionally, studies reported prior to the A.J.C. classification system (1972) [17] used unspecified tumor staging criteria. Finally, not all trials included contemporary megavoltage radiation. Still, the results from these early studies seemed to favor surgery over primary radiation therapy in the treatment of advanced laryngeal cancer.

In 1955, C.C. Wang retrospectively compared patients with fixed vocal cords and clinically negative neck nodes treated with either radiation or surgery, with a minimum of 5 years follow-up [5]. He reported 24% (14/58) 5-year survival with primary radiation, compared with 53% (25/47) 5-year survival in those patients treated with surgery. In a 1970 review of the literature, Vermund reported that absolute 5-year survival for patients with

Table 1. Larynx preservation in advanced larynx cancer with primary radiation and surgical salvage

Author [ref.]	Site	Stage	No. patients	RX	% survival (5 years)	% organ preservation in survivors
Goepfert et al. [20]	Supraglottic	III, IV	59	RTSS	55[a]	64[b]
Harwood [21]	Glottic	T_3N_0	68	RTSS	49	65
		T_4N_0	39	RTSS	49	90
Harwood et al. [22]	Supraglottic	$T_{3,4}\,N_0$	265	RTSS	51	64
		N_+	145	RTSS	24	39
Mittal et al. [23]	Transglottic	$T_{2,3,4}$	98	TL	50	—
			24	RTSS	8	67
			30	VCS	67	60
Meredith et al. [24]	Glottic/ supraglottic	$T_{3,4}$	150	RTSS	40	55[b]
Croll et al. [25]	Glottic/ supraglottic	$T_{3,4}$	55	RTSS	51	73
Viani et al. [27]	Glottic	T_3N_0	60	RTSS	28	82

[a] Determinate NED survival rate.
[b] Percent of total alive and dead.
RTSS = radiation therapy with surgical salvage; TL = total laryngectomy; VCS = voice conservation surgery.

T3N0 glottic cancer treated with radiation was 50%, and with surgery it was 61% [18]. For T4 glottic tumors, survival was 8% and 32%, respectively. Similarly, Skolnik et al. (1975) concluded in their 5-year end results report for glottic carcinoma: 'Surgery is the treatment of choice for Stage III glottic cancer' [19].

However, several recent retrospective studies have reported more favorable survival results with definitive radiation therapy (Table 1). In 1975, Goepfert et al. reported a chart review of 431 patients with squamous cell carcinoma of the supraglottic larynx treated at the M. D. Anderson Cancer Cencer over a period of 17 years [20]. Fifty-nine of these patients had stage III or IV disease treated with primary irradiation. At 5 years, the determinate disease-free survival rate was 55%, and 64% of patients maintained their larynx until death or the time of most recent follow-up. In 1979, Harwood reported a retrospective study of 358 patients with glottic cancer treated with radical irradiation [21]. Sixty-eight patients had T3N0 tumors, and 39 had T4N0 disease. Actuarial 5-year survival for these patients was 49%. The number of node-positive patients was small, but actuarial survival for these patients at 5 years approximated 40% overall. The same author also later reported a retrospective analysis of patients with T3 or T4 supraglottic laryngeal carcinoma treated with radiation alone [22]. Two hundred and sixty-five patients had node-negative disease and 145 were node positive. The patients without neck disease had better survival (51% vs. 24% at 5 years) and a higher rate of organ preservation (64% vs. 39%).

Mittal and colleagues reviewed their experience with transglottic carcinoma [23]. All patients had T2, T3, or T4 disease. Ninety-eight were treated with total laryngectomy, 24 were treated with primary radiation and surgical salvage, and 30 patients were treated with voice conservation surgery. Sixty percent of the patients treated with voice conservation surgery and 67% of those treated with radiation alone did not require laryngectomy. However, patients treated with radiation alone had a worse 5-year survival rate (8%) than either those treated with voice conservation surgery (67%) or total laryngectomy (50%). The authors stated that the marked difference in survival was attributable to death from intercurrent disease, because of the older age and the poorer physical condition of the patients selected for radiation. The death rate due to laryngeal cancer was nearly the same in the radiation and voice conservation surgery groups (45–50%), but was even higher in the total laryngectomy group (78%) because larger lesions were treated with this procedure. This report illustrates clearly the effect of patient selection on the outcome of any therapy.

Meredith et al. reviewed 150 cases of T3 and T4 larynx carcinoma treated with radiation and surgical salvage at the Royal Marsden Hospital in London [24]. Absolute survival at 5 years was 40%, but, as expected, patients with nodal disease did more poorly. Croll reported a 1989 retrospective analysis of 58 patients with T3 or T4 squamous cell carcinoma treated with radiation therapy, with a minimum of 3 years follow-up [25]. Actuarial survival at 5 years was 51% for all patients. More specifically, it was 83% for the T3N0 group, 75% for the T4N0 group, and 29% for the T4N1 group. This author also commented on laryngeal preservation: 36% of the T3 group and 39% of the T4 group had not recurred (thus never requiring salvage laryngectomy) at the time of publication.

For comparison, in 1984 DeSanto reported approximately 80% 5 year survival in patients with previously untreated T3N0 glottic carcinoma who were treated surgically [26]. Most recently, Viani treated 60 patients with T3N0 glottic carcinoma with definitive radiation therapy [27]. At 5 years, survival was poor. Only 17 patients (28%) were alive, 14 with the larynx intact and 3 who required laryngectomy. In summary, these studies show laryngeal irradiation to be most successful in patients with node-negative disease, but most of the reports were retrospective, with patient selection influencing the resultant data.

Preservation of the larynx, even at the price of slight decrease in survival, may be preferable to some people, according to the results of a study of normal volunteers [11]. Healthy 40-year-old volunteers were presented with a hypothetical choice between a laryngectomy, with an associated 60% 3-year survial, and voice-sparing therapy with a 30% 3-year survival. Three percent chose the latter. However, when volunteers were given a scenario in

202

which the voice-sparing procedure was associated with a 40% 3-year survival (thought by the investigators to represent the 'best results' of T3 vocal cord irradiation), 19% chose this alternative. In light of recent reports of up to 83% actuarial survival at 5 years in patients with T3 laryngeal cancers, it would appear that radiation therapy alone (with careful followup) as an alternative to surgery in T3 and T4 laryngeal cancers is not entirely discredited.

Induction (neoadjuvant) chemotherapy

Head and neck cancer is a relatively chemosensitive tumor. Effective antineoplastic drugs include cisplatin, carboplatin, methotrexate, 5-fluorouracil (5-FU), and bleomycin. The overall response to these drugs when used singly ranges from 24–36% [28,29].

Results are somewhat better with combination chemotherapy, and previously untreated patients have a better tumor response than patients with recurrent disease. One of the first encouraging studies in previously untreated patients was conducted by Randolph et al. in 1978 [30]. They reported a 71% major (complete plus partial) response rate when a combination of cisplatin and bleomycin was given to patients with unresectable disease. Other early single-arm studies had comparable results: Using similar drug regimens, the overall response was approximately 70–90% [31–33], with an approximately 20% complete response.

The ability of chemotherapy to induce significant tumor shrinkage in patients presenting with advanced head and neck cancer gave credence to the intuitively attractive concept of neoadjuvant chemotherapy administered prior to surgery or radiation. Investigators postulated that preoperative chemotherapy would allow drug delivery via a fairly normal vascular system and would permit the earliest possible therapy for occult micrometastatic disease, and that patients would be treated at a time when they presumably had their best performance status [34,35].

The goal of the first induction chemotherapy trials was improved survival, not organ preservation. This was measured in a prospective randomized fashion by the Head and Neck Contracts Program between 1978 and 1982 [36,37]. A total of 462 patients with resectable stage III or IV cancers were randomized to either surgery and radiation, a single course of induction chemotherapy (cisplatinum and bleomycin) followed by standard therapy, or induction therapy followed by standard therapy with subsequent maintenance chemotherapy. There was no difference in disease-free survival or overall survival between treatment groups, although there was an increased time to distant relapse in the group treated with induction and maintenance chemotherapy. These results were difficult to interpret because it was felt that inadequate chemotherapy had been utilized, both as induction and maintenance regimens. However, the study did show that delivery of traditional adjuvant chemotherapy is very difficult in the population of patients with head and neck cancer.

Subsequently, a large randomized study was conducted by the Southwest Oncology Group, using a more aggressive regimen of three cycles of cisplatin, methotrexate, bleomycin, and vincristine for induction chemotherapy, versus standard therapy with surgery and radiation [38]. Overall response to chemotherapy was a promising 70%, but this did not translate into improved disease-free survival or overall survival. In fact, there was a trend toward decreased survival in the chemotherapy arm, although this was not statisti-

Table 2. Randomized trials of induction chemotherapy versus surgery/radiation

Author [ref.]	No. patients	Regimen	Response rate (%)	Complete response (%)	Survival (%)
Head/neck contracts [36]	443	CDDP/bleo + S/RT vs. Induct + S/RT + Maint vs. S/RT	37	3	5 yr 37 vs. 45 vs. 35
Schuller et al. [38]	158	CDDP/bleo/MTX/VCR + S/RT vs. S/RT	70	19	Median 18 mos vs. 30 mos
Holoye et al. [39]	83	Bleo/cytoxan/MTX/5-FU + S/RT vs. S/RT	72	5	2 yr 35 vs. 41
Taylor et al. [40]	82	MTX + S/RT vs. S/RT	40	6	Median 22 mos vs. 23 mos
Toohil et al. [41]	60	CDDP/5-FU + S/RT vs. S/RT	85	18	2 yr 56 vs. 70
Martin et al. [42]	107	CDDP/5-FU/bleo/MTX + S/RT vs. S/RT	49	6	DFS, 2 yr 39 vs. 42
Martin et al. [43]	75	CDDP/5-FU + S/RT vs. S/RT	68	46	1 yr 73 vs. 61

CDDP = cisplatin; Bleo = bleomycin; MTX = methotrexate; VCR = vincristine; S = surgery; RT = radiation; Induct = induction chemotherapy; Maint = maintenance chemotherapy; DFS = disease-free survival.

cally significant. Despite this, there was a suggestion that the frequency of distant metastasis was reduced. The authors noted that there was no increase in incidence of radiation or surgical complications when administered after induction chemotherapy.

Other randomized studies have used a variety of induction regimens in an effort to try to achieve significant increases in complete response rates (see Table 2) [36,38–43]. To date, the combination of cisplatin and 5-fluorouracil appears the most promising.

An important goal of induction chemotherapy has been achievement of a complete response rate. Investigators from Wayne State [44] reported that patients who are histologically complete responders to induction chemotherapy have superior survival. Thirty-two clinical complete responders to cisplatin/5-fluorouracil therapy underwent surgery after chemotherapy at Wayne State. Thirteen had no histologic evidence of tumor in their surgical specimens. All of these patients were alive at 4 years, whereas median survival was 2 years for those patients with residual disease. In other trials of induction chemotherapy, improved survival has been consistently demonstrated for responders to chemotherapy when compared to nonresponders. In most studies, response to chemotherapy is also associated with tumor extent [45–47].

It is possible that response to induction chemotherapy may only serve to select a group of patients destined to do well because of favorable tumor characteristics [48]. However, in studies done for organ preservation these are precisely the 'good prognosis' chemotherapy-responsive patients who are identified, because they may represent a favorable subgroup of advanced head and neck cancer patients who will do well with radiation alone rather than surgery. Whether the toxicities of chemotherapy (which is of yet unproven benefit) outweigh the additional morbidity of salvage surgery in previously irradiated tissue is an unresolved issue.

Organ preservation studies

Investigators conducting induction chemotherapy trials observed that a considerable number (28–31%) of patients enrolled in a protocol of preoperative chemotherapy refused surgery if they had a complete response to chemotherapy [44,49]. Some of these patients did quite well when subsequently treated only with radiation: Long-term follow-up showed some with durable remissions. Therefore, trials and reviews began to emerge in which surgery was not planned for patients who achieved complete response to chemotherapy.

Thyss et al. treated 108 patients with squamous cell tumors of the upper aerodigestive tract (predominately stage III) with neoadjuvant cisplatin and 5-fluorouracil [50]. It was unclear how the investigators decided whether to treat a patient with surgery or radiation after the induction chemotherapy.

However, ultimately 63% of the patients were treated with definitive radiation after chemotherapy, without surgery. The local control rate for this group was 80%, and the authors concluded that 'a marked reduction in the use of major surgical procedures' was possible, as treatment strategies may be changed in favor of radiation in selected patients.

Vikram et al. reported a series of 19 patients with advanced carcinoma of the hypopharynx or upper esophagus, seven of whom had disease that was judged resectable but who refused surgery [51]. They were treated with cisplatin $100 \, mg/m^2$ on day 1 and 5-fluorouracil $900 \, mg/m^2$ on days 1–4 every 3 weeks × 3 cycles. This was rapidly alternated with accelerated radiation $200 \, cGy$ twice a day on days 8–12 × 3 cycles, for a total dose of $6000 \, cGy$. Overall response rate was 100%, complete response rate was 83%, and the 1-year survival rate was 80%. Toxicity of this intensive regimen was substantial, and included one death due to nadir-associated sepsis, one episode of grade IV hematologic toxicity, and a 21% late complication rate, including laryngeal necrosis, pneumonitis, tracheoesophageal fistula, and esophageal stricture.

Pfister et al. reported on 40 patients with resectable squamous cell cancer of the larynx, oropharynx, or hypopharynx whose surgery would have required total laryngectomy [52]. They were assigned to three cycles of a cisplatin-containing regimen with the intent of organ preservation. All patients who had a major response at the primary tumor site went immediately to radiation therapy. Neck dissection was performed for any residual neck disease. Patients who experienced progression of disease or less than a major response to chemotherapy had surgical resection of the primary site. Sixty-five percent of patients experienced a major response to chemotherapy, with 37.5% complete responders. Complete responses were documented in patients with cancer of the oropharynx, hypopharynx, and larynx. Actuarial survival rate was 58% and disease-free survival was 42% at 2 years. The actual larynx preservation rate was 85%, but if seven patients who refused total laryngectomy were included, the anticipated preservation rate was 68%. This study was complicated by variations in chemotherapy doses and regimen (cisplatin/vinblastine vs. cisplatin/bleomycin) and poor patient compliance (7 of 40 patients refused salvage laryngectomy). However, the authors concluded that this study demonstrated the feasibility of an organ-sparing approach in the treatment of advanced head and neck cancer. They emphasized that this innovative therapy required a motivated patient, careful patient monitoring, and close interdisciplinary cooperation between oncologists, surgeons, and radiation therapists.

This group also later reported independent analysis of 33 patients with advanced oropharyngeal cancer who would have required partial glossectomy, total laryngectomy, and neck dissection [53]. Utilizing a cisplatinum-based regimen followed by radiation therapy, they reported a 2-year survival rate of 56%, with a laryngeal preservation rate of 94% and avoidance of tongue surgery in 76%.

Hirsch et al. did a retrospective analysis of 29 patients with advanced tongue, hypopharyngeal, or laryngeal tumors who would have required either a total laryngectomy or more than a hemiglossectomy for surgical control of the primary disease [54]. The intent was to determine if concomitant chemotherapy and radiation could substitute for surgery and radiation in this group of patients who would suffer substantial speech and swallowing difficulties from surgical resection. The regimen used was cisplatin $60 \, mg/m^2$ on day 1, 5-fluorouracil $800 \, mg/m^2$ on days 1–5, and radiation 200 cGy on days 1–5 every other week for seven cycles. Sixty-two percent of the patients received the full seven cycles, and 86% received at least six cycles. The response to chemotherapy was 97%, with 59% complete responses. Following completion of treatment, three patients required laryngectomies, one for suspected residual disease, one for repeated aspiration, and one due to local recurrence at 18 months. One patient required a partial glossectomy. Twenty-five (86%) of the patients in the series had preservation of speech/swallowing function. With a median follow-up of 5 years, median survival was 48%. Poorer outcome was associated with N3 disease and fewer cycles of chemotherapy.

Several pilot studies testing chemotherapy/radiation regimens for the purpose of organ preservation are listed in Table 3. In 1987, the Northern California Oncology Group (Jacobs et al.) reported the results of a study done to determine whether chemotherapy could substitute for surgery in patients with advanced squamous cell carcinoma who achieved a complete response to induction chemotherapy [55]. Thirty patients with previously untreated, resectable stage III or IV squamous cell cancer of the oral cavity, oropharynx, hypopharynx, or larynx were treated with three cycles of cisplatin $100 \, mg/m^2$ and either bleomycin $15 \, mg/m^2 \times 5$ days or 5-fluorouracil $1000 \, mg/m^2 \times 5$ days. Complete clinical responders underwent endoscopy

Table 3. Nonrandomized trials of chemo/radiation for organ preservation

Author [ref.]	No. patients	Site	Regimen	CR	Organ pres.	Survival (F/U)
Jacobs et al. [55]	30	All	CDDP/5FU	43%	40%	53% (2 yr)
Karp et al. [56]	35	Larynx, hypo	CDDP/Bleo, CDDP/5FU	26%	94%	44% (3 yr)
Urba [57]	43	All	CDDP/5FU + MG BG	46%	71%	48% (3 yr)
Demard et al. [59]	71	Larynx, hypo	CDDP/5FU	52%	27%	42% (?)
Grégoire et al. [60]	79	All	CBDCA/5FU	14%	41%	—

CR = complete response; F/U = follow-up; Hypo = hypopharynx; CDDP = cisplatin; 5FU = 5-fluorouracil; Bleo = bleomycin; MGBG = mitoguazone; CBDCA = carboplatin; Pres. = preservation.

with multiple biopsies; if these biopsies were negative, the patient underwent primary radiotherapy for cure. Patients with persistent microscopic disease at the primary site were treated with the originally planned surgery, with no modification for tumor response.

Forty-three percent of patients achieved a complete clinical response at both primary and nodal sites: 33% (10 of 30) achieved a complete pathologic response and were thus spared any surgery; two additional patients underwent neck dissection only (having a complete histologic response at the primary site but persistent nodal disease). For this group of 12 patients who were spared surgery, 2-year overall survival was 70% and disease-free survival was 60%. These statistics were slightly better than those for the group as a whole. While the improved results seen in the 12 complete responders may only reflect selection of patients already destined to have a good outcome, the investigators noted that if chemotherapy could select such a group, then those patients could have surgery safely eliminated from their treatment regimen.

Karp et al. reported long-term follow-up of a pilot study conducted from 1977 to 1987 [56]. Thirty-five patients with advanced laryngeal or hypopharyngeal cancer (who declined advised laryngectomy) were treated with chemotherapy, consisting of cisplatin and bleomycin for the earlier patients, and then cisplatin and 5-fluorouracil for the patients entered later into the study. Radiation therapy to a total dose of 6500–7500 cGy was administered in lieu of laryngectomy, with curative intent. They reported a 77% overall response rate, and 26% complete response after chemotherapy alone. With a median 7-year follow-up, the failure-free survival rate was 35%. The 3-year survival rate of 44% for these patients was considered promising, in view of the fact that 3-year survival for patients treated historically with surgery and postoperative radiation is 30%, plus 94% of the patients treated with chemotherapy/radiation retained their larynx for the remainder of their lives. It appeared that the larynx could be preserved without compromise of survival in patients treated with the combination of chemotherapy and radiation. Data from this study and others served as the basis for the randomized prospective study of organ preservation eventually reported by the Department of Veterans Affairs Laryngeal Cancer Study Group [49].

In 1985, an aggressive protocol for organ preservation was conducted at the University of Michigan [57]. Forty-three patients with advanced cancer of the oral cavity, pharynx, larynx, or sinuses were treated with mitoguazone $400-500 \, mg/m^2$ on days 1 and 8, cisplatin $30 \, mg/m^2/day$ as a continuous infusion on days 8–12, and 5-FU $100 \, mg/m^2/day$ as a continuous infusion on days 8–12. Three cycles of chemotherapy were given every 28 days. The overall response was 86%, with a 46% complete response and a 68% complete response at the primary site. Seventy-one percent of patients were initially spared surgery at the primary site, although 19% required neck dissection. Sixteen percent of patients required late salvage surgery to the primary. At a median follow-up of 32 months, 52% of all patients were still alive. This was not significantly different from the estimated 2-year survival of 50% for a similar historical control group of 152 patients with Stage III or IV disease treated with surgery and radiation. Encouraged that organ preservation may be possible at a variety of head and neck sites, and yet interested in reducing the toxicity of the cisplatin-containing regimen, the same group of investigators has recently completed a protocol of neoadjuvant chemotherapy consisting of carboplatin and 5-fluorouracil [58]. The complete response rate at the primary site was 50%. Seventy percent were initially spared surgery to the primary; however, follow-up is too short for conclusions about the duration of response or survival.

Demard et al. treated 71 evaluable patients with laryngeal or hypopharyngeal cancr with induction chemotherapy [59]. However, 25% of the patients had stage II disease. Chemotherapy with standard doses of cisplatin and 5-fluorouracil were given at 15-day intervals. Nine deaths occurred during the chemotherapy, although only three were attributed to toxicity. The complete response rate was 52%, and as expected, the earlier stage tumors did very well. Nine patients were spared total laryngectomy, and 10 were spared pharyngolaryngectomy. Patients with laryngeal cancer did better than those with hypopharyngeal disease during follow-up. The authors concluded that it is justifiable to forego surgery in some complete clinical responders to chemotherapy.

Grégoire et al. recently reported the results of a phase I–II trial in which 83 patients were treated with carboplatin and 5-FU [60]. After three cycles of therapy, patients who were nonresponders or partial responders underwent surgical resection of the primary tumor. Radiotherapy alone was proposed for patients considered inoperable, complete responders, or partial responders with tumors in the oral cavity or oropharynx whose surgery would be potentially 'mutilating.' The maximum tolerated dose of carboplatin was $420 \, mg/m^2$. A fifty-seven percent overall response and 32% complete response rate at the primary tumor site was noted. At a median follow-up of 12 months, there was no recurrence at the primary for those patients treated with chemotherapy and radiation alone. The authors concluded that carboplatin and 5-FU followed by radiation is a tolerable regimen, and some patients can benefit from this method of conservative local treatment and avoid surgery. However, a longer follow-up is obviously needed to determine the ultimate outcome of these patients.

Organ preservation in advanced laryngeal cancer

In 1991, the Department of Veterans Affairs Laryngeal Cancer Study Group reported the results of a large randomized trial designed specifically to test the feasibility and safety of laryngeal preservation in treatment of advanced cancer of the larynx [61]. In this trial, 332 patients with stage III or stage IV laryngeal squamous cell cancer were randomly assigned to initially undergo either three cycles of chemotherapy (CDDP 100mg/m^2 day 1 and 5-FU 1000mg/m^2 days 1–5 continuous infusion every 21 days) or surgery. Those patients in the chemotherapy arm who had at least a partial response after two cycles of chemotherapy underwent a third cycle, followed by definitive radiation therapy (RT). Nonresponders underwent surgery (as dictated by the original evaluation), followed by RT; those randomized to the surgery arm also received postoperative RT.

One hundred sixty-six patients were randomly assigned to each arm. The two arms were well matched in terms of patient characteristics and stage of disease. Forty-six percent were node positive; of these, two thirds had N2 or N3 disease. Approximately two thirds had supraglottic cancers. Over 30% of the patients assigned to chemotherapy required pretreatment tracheostomy for airway obstruction due to the size of the primary tumor. Median follow-up of all patients was 33 months. Seven patients (2%) were lost to follow-up.

Of those patients who received chemotherapy, 85% were partial or complete responders after two cycles of chemotherapy. One hundred and seventeen patients went on to receive a third cycle of chemotherapy: 49% of these had a complete response at the primary, and another 49% had a partial response. Of the 166 patients assigned to the chemotherapy group, 101 were alive at the time of the publication, 65 of whom had a functioning larynx, and 36 of whom had a total laryngectomy. Therefore, 64% of the surviving patients treated successfully retained a functioning larynx. Altogether, 59 patients underwent laryngectomy, 30 of whom had the surgery before radiation. Twenty-nine patients had a laryngectomy after radiation therapy; 18 of these were within the first 3 months after completion of radiation, and the remaining 11 patients underwent late salvage laryngectomy for recurrences 5–40 months after radiation. The great majority of recurrences happened in the first post-treatment year. In summary, 29% of patients treated with chemotherapy required salvage laryngectomy for persistent disease before radiation or 3 months afterwards, and another 7% required late salvage surgery.

Toxicity was not excessive: One patient died of septicemia during a period of neutropenia, and 12 patients (7%) had toxicity necessitating the discontinuation of chemotherapy. There were three deaths due to surgical complications in the surgery arm.

There was a trend toward better disease-free survival in the surgery group. At 36 months, 70% of the surgery group and 60% of the chemotherapy group were disease free, but the difference was not statistically significant ($p = 0.1195$). There was no difference in 2-year survival between the two arms; this was 68% for both groups. No survival differences were found between treatment arms when patients were analyzed according to tumor stage or site. Of the 107 patients who retained their larynx, 61% were alive at the time of publication. Of the 59 patients who required salvage laryngectomy, 61% were also still alive, implying that laryngeal preservation could be achieved without compromise of survival.

While the principal cause of death in both treatment arms was cancer (23% of patients in the surgery arm and 25% in the chemotherapy arm), the pattern of tumor recurrence as a site of first relapse varied. Recurrences at the primary tumor site were more frequent in the chemotherapy group (12%) than in the surgery group (2%; p = 0.001). Regional neck node recurrences were similar for both groups. Distant metastases occurred less frequently in the chemotherapy group (11%) compared to the surgery group (17%; p = 0.001). The rates of second primary tumors were also lower in the chemotherapy group (2%) versus the surgery group (6%; p = 0.048).

One criticism that has been raised of this study is the lack of a radiation-only arm. Similar rates of survival and laryngeal preservation have been reported using radiation therapy alone (with surgical salvage) for patients with T3 glottic or supraglottic cancers, with negative neck nodes [21,62]. Primary radiation is commonly used in Canada and Europe as initial therapy for such patients. However, 5-year survival of patients with supraglottic primaries decreases from 50% to less than 30% when regional nodes are involved [22,63]. One quarter of the patients in the Veterans Administration (VA) study had T4 primaries, and nearly half had regional disease, two thirds of which was N2 or N3. Two thirds of patients had supraglottic primaries. While a conclusion cannot be drawn without a direct comparison of radiation versus chemotherapy/radiation in a randomized trial, the high rate of laryngeal preservation and survival in these patients in the VA study with more advanced cancer suggests that chemotherapy may add to the effectiveness of radiation.

Other randomized trials

Preliminary results have been reported for a prospective, randomized trial in which patients with advanced head and neck cancers were treated with either primary radiation therapy or two courses of chemotherapy consisting of cisplatin, bleomycin, vindesine, and mitomycin-C followed by radiation therapy [64]. Patients were assessed after 50–55 Gy; if there was < 50% regression, salvage surgery was performed. One hundred patients were enrolled. Two deaths due to therapy were reported in the RT arm and none in the chemotherapy/RT arm. Major toxicities were identical in the two groups. Unfortunately, the response rate to chemotherapy was only 50%, with 10% of patients achieving a complete response. The overall tumor response rate after completion of all therapy was 77% for the combined modality group and 79% for the radiation arm. There was no significant difference in survival at 1 or 2 years between treatment groups. Both groups continued to experience local and distant recurrences past 1 year. Thirty-three percent of the combined modality arm and 38% of the radiation arm ultimately required salvage surgery. The authors concluded that they found no benefit to the addition of induction chemotherapy to radiation therapy. However, they noted that their overall response rate to chemotherapy (50% at primary site, 27% at nodal metastases) was lower than numerous other studies using more optimal regimens. Therefore, their new randomized trial utilizes the more effective regimen of cisplatin, 5-fluorouracil, and vindesine.

Future directions

It is clear from the foregoing that although some advances have been made in the treatment of advanced head and neck cancer, there is need for improvement and innovation of existing treatment regimens. Importantly, none of the recent clinical trials have demonstrated improvement in survival. Survival benefit is the appropriate primary goal of this frequently fatal malignancy, with quality of life issues of somewhat lesser importance. What are some of these future directions?

Larynx preservation

The success of the VA Cooperative Studies Program for larynx preservation is encouraging, but further questions remain regarding the optimal treatment of larynx cancer. Is sequential chemotherapy/radiation therapy better than concomitant administration of the two modalities? Is chemotherapy needed or is radiation therapy alone sufficient? An intergroup study for larynx preservation has recently been initiated to address these questions. This study is a phase III randomized trial for patients with resectable laryngeal

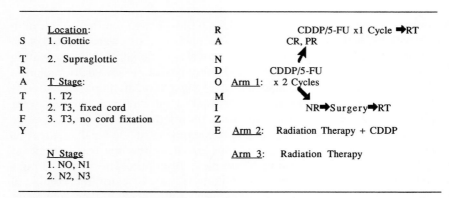

CDDP= Cisplatin
5-FU= 5-Fluorouracil

Figure 1.

212

cancer, stage III and IV (excluding T1 or T4 tumors). The schema is shown in Figure 1. All patients will be stratified for tumor location and T stage and N stage, and then randomized to 1 of 3 treatment arms. Arm 1 consists of two cycles of standard dose cisplatin and 5-fluorouracil, followed by a third cycle for responders or salvage surgery for nonresponders. Those patients who complete three cycles of chemotherapy will undergo definitive radiation therapy. Arm 2 of the study consists of full-course radiation therapy administered concomitantly with cisplatin at 3 week intervals during the treatment. Arm 3 consists of radiation therapy alone. Radiation for all arms of treatment is delivered in 2.0 Gy fractions 5 days a week for 7 weeks, to a total dose of 70 Gy. The trial will enroll 546 patients and will therefore take several years to complete.

New drugs

Carboplatin is a platinum analogue with activity in head and neck cancer that appears to be similar to cisplatin, with significantly less toxicity [65,66]. Side effects of carboplatin include moderate myelosuppression and mild nausea and vomiting. The drug can be easily administered in the outpatient setting [67].

Currently, carboplatin is most often used in combination with 5-fluorouracil. The Southwest Oncology Group conducted a randomized study comparing cisplatin/5-FU versus carboplatin/5-FU versus methotrexate in recurrent head and neck cancer [68]. Overall response rates were 32% for cisplatin + 5-FU and 21% for carboplatin + 5-FU, and this difference was not significant. Volling et al. treated 55 previously untreated patients with carboplatin and 5-FU and obtained a response rate of 88%, with 33% complete response [69]. This was nearly identical to the 80% overall response rate and 28% complete response achieved in a group of historical controls treated with cisplatin and 5-FU at the same institution. Toxicity was milder in the patients treated with carboplatin.

As trials utilizing carboplatin consistently show similar efficacy, less toxicity, and greater ease of administration than cisplatin, some investigators have started to substitute it for cisplatin in induction chemotherapy protocols. Lelièvre et al. have recently reported on 240 patients with carcinoma of the oropharynx or pharyngolarynx randomized to induction chemotherapy with carboplatinum and 5-FU followed by radiation therapy (with surgery reserved for patients achieving less than a complete response), or to 'locoregional therapy' (radiation therapy with or without surgery) alone. Of the 108 patients evaluable in the chemotherapy arm, the 2-year survival rate was 60%, which was not significantly different from that in the control arm (64%). 'Nonconservative surgery' was required in only 38% of the patients in the chemotherapy arm [70].

Another small trial (20 patients) has reported a 41% complete response rate with three cycles of carboplatinum and 5-FU; however, an additional

35% of patients had progression of disease while on study [71]. While this raises some concern regarding the efficacy of this regimen, larger studies are needed to confirm these results.

Other new approaches include the modulation of 5-FU with leucovorin, hydroxyurea, or interferon. Trials involving these drug combinations are underway across the country. However, there is increased toxicity with most of these combinations; therefore, determining the ideal doses for maximum drug intensity with tolerable side effects is the subject of ongoing investigation.

Organ preservation in nonlaryngeal sites

Another active research direction is organ preservation in nonlaryngeal sites of head and neck cancer. Several single arm trials have suggested that some sites of head and neck cancer, particularly the oropharynx, may be treatable with chemotherapy and radiation alone [55,72]. In these studies, it is important that different tumor sites and stages are analyzed separately, because it appears that organ preservation treatment may only be ideal for some select subsets of head and neck cancer patients.

Prognostic factors

Induction chemotherapy regimens have substantial toxicity, and so it would be invaluable to predict which patients would benefit from such therapy and who should go immediately to surgery. Tumor flow cytometry data for patients undergoing chemotherapy have shown that DNA content may be one of the most significant predictors of response to chemotherapy, relapse, and survival [73,74]. Ensley et al. have reported results of flow cytometry from 237 patients and concluded that diploid DNA content indicates poor responsiveness to cytotoxic agents and that chemotherapy response correlates with the percentage of tumor composed of aneuploid tumor cells [75,76]. Preliminary prospective data from the VA Laryngeal Cancer Study Group indicate that DNA content measured by image analysis of pretreatment biopsies correlates with disease-free survival and may predict those patients who will be complete responders to induction chemotherapy [77,78]. Further evaluation of this concept is underway on a national level.

Conclusions

Better therapy of advanced head and neck cancer includes reduction of morbidity as well as mortality. To date, trials evaluating organ preservation of the larynx have yielded encouraging results. Laryngeal preservation appears to be possible in approximately two thirds of patients with current induction chemotherapy regimens. While it is reasonable to offer patients

214

with advanced larynx cancer the option of chemotherapy followed by radiation as an alternative to surgery, it is still important to continue treating these patients on experimental protocols if available. Current areas of investigation include identification of more effective chemotherapy regimens that achieve higher complete response rates and innovative radiation therapy with altered fractionation schemes designed to try to reduce local recurrence. Also, the question of whether induction chemotherapy in fact increases the effectiveness of definitive radiation alone should be tested in a randomized trial.

Induction chemotherapy for organ preservation in patients with non-laryngeal head and neck cancers should be confined to the experimental protocol setting. While pilot studies appear promising, no major randomized trial has yet tested this issue. Finally, any discussion of the possibility of organ preservation in head and neck cancer should include a comment about cancer prevention. The VA study group reported that in its population of 332 patients, 85% used alcohol and 99% used tobacco [61]. Patient education regarding avoidance of these potential carcinogens may be as important as finding better treatment regimens for patients with advanced head and neck carcinoma.

References

1. Boring CC, Squires TS, Heath CW. Cancer statistics for African Americans. CA Cancer J Clin 42:7–17, 1992.
2. Boring CC, Squires TS, Tong T. Cancer statistics, 1992. CA Cancer J Clin 42:19–38,1992.
3. Million RR, Cassisi NJ, Clark JR. Cancer of the Head and Neck. In: VT DeVita, S Hellman, SA Rosenberg, eds. Cancer Principles and Practice of Oncology, 3rd ed. Philadelphia: JB Lippincott, 1989, pp 488–590.
4. Mathieson CM, Henderikus JS, Scott JP. Psychosocial adjustment after laryngectomy: A review of the literature. J Otolaryngol 19:331–336, 1990.
5. Wang CC, O'Donnell AR. Cancer of the larynx: Five-year results, with emphasis on radiotherapy. N Engl J Med 252:743–747, 1955.
6. Richardson JL. Vocational adjustment after total laryngectomy. Arch Phys Med Rehabil 64:172–175, 1983.
7. David DJ, Baritt JA. Psychosocial implications of surgery for head and neck cancer. Clin Plastic Surg 9:327–336, 1982.
8. Pruyn JF, De Jong PC, Bosman LJ, et al. Psychosocial aspects of head and neck cancer — a review of the literature. Clin Otolaryngol II:469–474, 1986.
9. Schuller DE, Reiches NA, Hamaker RC, et al. Analysis of disability resulting from treatment including radical neck dissection or modified neck dissection. Head Neck Surg 6:551–558, 1983.
10. Dhilion RS, Palmer BV, Pittam MR, et al. Rehabilitation after major head and neck surgery: The patient's view. Clin Otolaryngol 7:319–324, 1982.
11. McNeil BJ, Weichselbaum R, Pauker SG. Speech and survival. N Engl J Med 305:982–987, 1981.
12. Ennuyer A, Bataini P. Laryngeal carcinomas. Laryngoscope 85:1467–1476, 1975.
13. Stewart JG, Brown JR, Palmer MK, et al. The management of glottic carcinoma by primary irradiation with surgery in reserve. Laryngoscope 85:1477–1484, 1975.

14. Hawkins NV. The treatment of glottic carcinoma: An analysis of 800 cases. Laryngoscope 85:1485–1493, 1975.
15. Van Den Bogaert W, Ostyn F, Van Der Schueren E. The primary treatment of advanced vocal cord cancer: Laryngectomy or radiotherapy? Int J Radiat Oncol Biol Phys 9:329–334, 1983.
16. Constable WC, White RL, El-Mahdi AM, et al. Radiotherapeutic management of cancer of the glottis, University of Virginia. Laryngoscope 85:1494–1503, 1975.
17. American Joint Committee on Cancer. Manual for Staging of Cancer, 2nd ed. Philadelphia: JB Lippincott, 1983, pp 25–54.
18. Vermund H. Role of radiotherapy in cancer of the larynx as related to the TNM system of staging. Cancer 25:485–504, 1970.
19. Skolnik EM, Yee DF, Wheatley MA, et al. Carcinoma of the laryngeal glottis therapy and end results. Laryngoscope 85:1453–1466, 1975.
20. Goepfert H, Jesse R, Fletcher G, et al. Optimal treatment for the technically resectable squamous cell carcinoma of the supraglottic larynx. Laryngoscope 85:14–32, 1975.
21. Harwood AR. Management of advanced glottic cancer: A 10 year review of the Toronto experience. Int J Radiat Oncol Biol Phys 5:899–904, 1979.
22. Harwood AR, Beale FA, Cummings BJ, et al. Supraglottic laryngeal carcinoma: An analysis of dose-time-volume factors in 410 patients. Int J Radiation Oncology Biol Phys 9:311–319, 1983.
23. Mittal B, Marks J, Ogura J. Transglottic carcinoma. Cancer 53:151–161, 1984.
24. Meredith AP, Randall CJ, Show HJ. Advanced laryngeal cancer: A management perspective. J Laryngol Otol 101:1046–1054, 1987.
25. Croll GA, Gerritsen GJ, Tiwari RM, et al. Primary radiotherapy with surgery in reserve for advanced laryngeal carcinoma. Eur J Surg Oncol 15:350–356, 1989.
26. DeSanto LW. T_3 glottic cancer: Options and consequences of the options. Laryngoscope 94:1311–1315, 1984.
27. Viani L, Stell PM, Dalby JE. Recurrence after radiotherapy for glottic carcinoma. Cancer 67:577–584, 1991.
28. Million RR, Cassisi NJ, Clark JR. Cancer of the head and neck. In: VT DeVita, S Hellman, SA Rosenberg, eds. Cancer: Principles and Practice of Oncology, 3rd ed. Philadelphia: JB Lippincott, 1989, p 496.
29. Al-Sarraf. Platinum analogs in recurrent and advanced head and neck cancer: A Southwest Oncology Group and Wayne State University study. Cancer Treat Rep 71:723–72, 1987.
30. Randolph VL, Vallego A, Spiro RH, et al. Combination therapy of advanced head and neck cancer: Induction of remissions with diamminedichloroplatinum (II), bleomycin and radiation therapy. Cancer 41:460–467, 1978.
31. Ervin TJ, Weichselbaum RR, Fabian RL, et al. Advanced squamous carcinoma of the head and neck. Arch Otolaryngol 110:241–245, 1984.
32. Spaulding M, Klotch D, Lore J. Preoperative chemotherapy in advanced cancer of the head and neck. Proc Am Soc Clin Oncol 21:403, 1980.
33. Hong W, Shapshay S, Bhutani R, et al. Induction chemotherapy in advanced squamous head and neck carcinoma with high dose cisplatinum and bleomycin infusion. Cancer 44:19–25, 1979.
34. Hong WK, Popkin JD, Shapshay SM. Preoperative adjuvant induction chemotherapy in head and neck cancer. In: GT Wolf, ed. Head and Neck Oncology. Boston: Martinus Nijhoff, 1984, pp 287–300.
35. Urba S, Wolf GT. Organ preservation in multimodality therapy of head and neck cancer. Hematol Oncol Clin North Am 5:713–723, 1991.
36. Head and Neck Contracts Program. Adjuvant chemotherapy for advanced head and neck squamous carcinoma: Final report of the Head and Neck Contracts Program. Cancer 60:301–311, 1987.
37. Jacobs C, Makuch R. Efficacy of adjuvant chemotherapy for patients with resectable head

and neck cancer: A subset analysis of the head and neck contracts program. J Clin Oncol 8:838–847, 1990.

38. Schuller DE, Metch B, Mattox D, et al. Preoperative chemotherapy in advanced resectable head and neck cancer: Final report of the Southwest Oncology Group. Laryngoscope 98:1205–1211, 1988.

39. Holoye PY, Grossman TW, Toohill RJ, et al. Randomized study of adjuvant chemotherapy for head and neck cancer. Otolaryngol Head Neck Surg 93:712–715, 1985.

40. Taylor SG, Applebaum E, Showel JL, et al. A randomized study of adjuvant chemotherapy in head and neck cancer. J Clin Oncol 3:672–679, 1985.

41. Toohil RJ, Anderson T, Byhardt RW, et al. Cisplatin and fluorouracil as neoadjuvant therapy in head and neck cancer. Arch Otolaryngol Head Neck Surg 3:758–761, 1987.

42. Martin M, Mazeron JJ, Brun B, et al. Neoadjuvant polychemotherapy of head and neck cancer: Results of a randomized study. Proc Am Soc Clin Oncol 7:152, 1988.

43. Martin M, Hazan A, Vergnes L, et al. Randomized study of 5-fluorouracil and cisplatin as neoadjuvant therapy in head and neck cancer: A preliminary report. Int J Radiat Oncol Biol Phys 19:973–975, 1990.

44. Al-Kourainy K, Kish J, Ensley J, et al. Achievement of superior survival for histologically negative versus histologically positive clinically complete responders to cisplatin combination in patients with locally advanced head and neck cancer. Cancer 59:233–238, 1987.

45. Davis RK, Stoker K, Harker G, et al. Prognostic indicators in head and neck cancer patients receiving combined therapy. Arch Otolaryngol Head Neck Surg 115:1443–1446, 1989.

46. Cognetti F, Pinnaro P, Ruggeri EM, et al. Prognostic factors for chemotherapy response and survival using combination chemotherapy as initial treatment of advanced head and neck squamous cell cancer. J Clin Oncol 7:829–837, 1989.

47. Tennvall J, Albertsson M, Biörklund A, et al. Induction chemotherapy (cisplatin + 5-fluorouracil) and radiotherapy in advanced squamous cell carcinoma of the head and neck. Acta Oncol 30:27–32, 1991.

48. Tannock IF. Neoadjuvant chemotherapy in head and neck cancer: No way to preserve a larynx [Correspondence]. J Clin Oncol 10:343–346, 1992.

49. Weaver A, Flemming S, Kish J, et al. Cis-platinum and 5-fluorouracil as induction therapy for advanced head and neck cancer. Am J Surg 144:445–448, 1982.

50. Thyss A, Schneider M, Santini J, et al. Induction chemotherapy with cis-platinum and 5-fluorouracil for squamous cell carcinoma of the head and neck. Br J Cancer 54:755–760, 1986.

51. Vikram B, Malamud S, Gold J, et al. Chemotherapy rapidly alternating with accelerated radiotherapy for advanced carcinomas of the hypopharynx and upper esophagus: A feasibility study. Head Neck 415–419, 1991.

52. Pfister DG, Strong E, Harrison L, et al. Larynx preservation with combined chemotherapy and radiation therapy in advanced but resectable head and neck cancer. J Clin Oncol 9:850–859, 1991.

53. Pfister DG, Harrison L, Strong EW, et al. Organ/function preservation in advanced oropharynx cancer: Results with induction chemotherapy and radiation. Proc Am Soc Clin Oncol 11:241, 1992.

54. Hirsch SM, Caldarelli DD, Hutchinson JC, et al. Concomitant chemotherapy and split-course radiation for cure and preservation of speech and swallowing in head and neck cancer. Laryngoscope 101:583–586, 1991.

55. Jacobs C, Goffinet DR, Goffinet L, et al. Chemotherapy as a substitute for surgery in the treatment of advanced resectable head and neck cancer. Cancer 60:1178–1183, 1987.

56. Karp DD, Vaughan CW, Carter R, et al. Larynx preservation using induction chemotherapy plus radiation therapy as an alternative to laryngectomy in advanced head and neck cancer. Am J Clin Oncol 14:273–279, 1991.

57. Urba S. Organ preservation in advanced head and neck cancer treatment with high dose

cisplatin, 5-fluorouracil, and mitoguazone followed by radiation therapy. Presented at the Third International Conference of Head and Neck Cancer, San Francisco, CA, July 26–30, 1992.

58. Urba SG, Wolf GT, McLaughlin P, et al. Neoadjuvant carboplatin, 5-fluorouracil, and radiation therapy for organ preservation in patients with resectable, advanced head and neck cancer. Presented at the Third International Conference on Head and Neck Cancer, San Francisco, CA, July 26–30, 1992.

59. Demard F, Chauvel P, Santini J, et al. Response to chemotherapy as justification for modification of the therapeutic strategy for pharyngolaryngeal carcinomas. Head Neck 12:225–231, 1990.

60. Grégoire V, Beauduin M, Humblet Y, et al. A phase I–II trial of induction chemotherapy with carboplatin and fluorouracil in locally advanced head and neck squamous cell carcinoma: A report from the UCL-Oncology Group, Belgium. J Clin Oncol 9:1385–1392, 1991.

61. Department of Veterans Affairs Laryngeal Cancer Study Group. Induction chemotherapy plus radiation compared with surgery plus radiation in patients with advanced laryngeal cancer. Ne Engl J Med 324:1685–1690, 1991.

62. Harwood AR, Rawlinson E. The quality of life of patients following treatment for laryngeal cancer. Int J Radiat Oncol Biol Phys 9:335–338, 1983.

63. Weems DH, Mendenhall WM, Parsons JT, et al. Squamous cell carcinoma of the supraglottic larynx treated with surgery and/or radiation therapy. Int J Radiat Oncol Biol Phys 13: 1483–1487, 1987.

64. Brunin F, Rodriguez J, Jaulerry C, et al. Induction chemotherapy in advanced head and neck cancer. Acta Oncol 28:62–65, 1989.

65. Basauri LDA, Pousa AL, Alba E, et al. Carboplatin, an active drug in advanced head and neck cancer. Cancer Treat Rep 70:1173–1176, 1986.

66. Volling P, Schröder M, Rauschning W, et al. Carboplatin. Arch Otolaryngol Head Neck Surg 115:695–698, 1989.

67. Gonzalez-Baron M, Vicente J, Martin G, et al. Phase II trial of carboplatin and tegafur (ftorafur) as induction therapy in squamous-cell carcinoma of the head and neck. Am J Clin Oncol 13:277–279, 1990.

68. Forastiere A, Metch B, Kappen M, et al. Randomized comparison of cisplatin + 5-fluorouracil vs. carboplatin + 5-fluorouracil vs. methotrexate in advanced squamous cell carcinoma of the head and neck. J Clin Oncol 10:1245–1251, 1992.

69. Volling P, Schröder M, Rauschning W, et al. Results of a phase II study with the new cytostatic drug carboplatin in combination with 5-fluorouracil in the primary treatment of advanced squamous cell cancers of the head and neck. Head Neck Oncol 36:452–455, 1988.

70. Lelièvre G, Gehanno P, Depondt J, et al. Induction carboplatin and 5-fluorouracil treatment versus no chemotherapy before locoregional treatment for oro and pharyngolaryngeal cancers: Preliminary results of a randomized study. Proc Am Soc Clin Oncol 11:240, 1992.

71. Spaulding MB, O'Connor B, Markowitz-Spence L, et al. Carboplatin and 5-fluorouracil in patients with advanced previously untreated head and neck cancer. Proc Am Soc Clin Oncol 11:244, 1992.

72. Urba S, Forastiere AA, Wolf GT, et al. Induction chemotherapy with intensive continuous infusion high dose cisplatin, 5-fluorouracil, and mitoguazone for advanced head and neck cancer. Proc Am Soc Clin Oncol 9:171, 1990.

73. Sickle-Santanello BJ, Farrar WB, Dobson JL, et al. Flow cytometry as a prognostic indicator in squamous cell carcinoma of the tongue. Am J Surg 152:393–395, 1986.

74. Goldsmith MM, Cresson DH, Postma DS, et al. The significance of ploidy in laryngeal cancer. Am J Surg 152:396–402, 1986.

75. Ensley J, Maciorowskiz P, Pietraszkiewicz H, et al. Prospective correlation of cytotoxic response and DNA content parameters in advanced squamous cell cancer of the head and neck. Proc Am Soc Clin Oncol 9:671, 1990.

76. Ensley JF, Maciorowski Z, Hassan M, et al. Cellular DNA content parameters in untreated and recurrent squamous cell cancers of the head and neck. Cytometry 10:334–338, 1989.
77. Truelson SM, Fisher S, Beals TE, McClatchey KD, Wolf GT. DNA content and histologic growth pattern correlate with prognosis in patients with advanced squamous cell carcinoma of the larynx. Cancer 70:56–62, 1992.
78. Gregg CM, Beals TE, Fisher SG, Wolf GT. DNA content and tumor response to induction chemotherapy in patients with advanced laryngeal squamous cell carcinoma. Otolaryngol Head Neck Surg 108:731–737, 1993.

12. Elective modified neck dissection for treatment of the clinically negative (N0) neck

David L. Callender and Randal S. Weber

Radical neck dissection was the dominant surgical procedure for treatment of metastatic head and neck cancer in the cervical lymph nodes for much of the 20th century. Proponents of radical neck dissection, such as George Crile, Sr. [1] and Hayes Martin [2], maintained the Halsteadian principle that oncologically sound surgical management of metastasis requires en bloc resection of lymph nodes and surrounding soft-tissue structures. While radical neck dissection provides effective control of regional metastasis, major cosmetic and functional deficits often accompany the procedure.

More recent trends of cosmetic and functional preservation in cancer treatment have resulted in the development of more conservative neck dissection techniques. These "modified" neck dissection procedures offer disease control comparable with radical dissection, but spare patients the undesirable morbidity associated with the classic radical dissection. Modified neck dissection techniques are particularly suited to the elective surgical treatment of the neck in patients with primary head and neck cancers at high risk for development of cervial metastasis. This chapter focuses on the rationale for modified neck dissections in elective surgical treatment of the N0 neck.

Historical perspective of neck dissections

Notable reports of attempts at surgical resection of metastatic cancer in the neck began to appear in the medical literature in the middle of the 19th century. In 1867, Warren described an attempt at resection of metastatic cancer in the neck [3]. Kocher, in 1880, reported a procedure for resection of the tongue and regional lymphatics via a submandibular approach [4]. Butlin and Spencer, in 1900, also described procedures for resection of tongue cancers and cervical lymphatics [5].

The first description of a standardized anatomic dissection of the cervical

Hong, Waun Ki and Weber, Randal S., (eds.), Head and Neck Cancer. © *1995 Kluwer Academic Publishers.*
ISBN 0-7923-3015-3. All rights reserved.

221

lymphatics is credited to George Crile, Sr. In 1906, Crile reported results of 132 cases of planned neck dissection [1]. Crile modeled the neck dissection procedure after Halstead's concept of surgical resection of primary breast carcinomas and their draining lymphatics. The rationale for these procedures was that primary cancers will first metastasize to regional lymphatics and then to distant sites. Crile felt that a radical resection of the cervical lymph nodes with surrounding soft-tissue structures, such as the internal jugular vein, sternomastoid muscle, and the spinal accessory nerve, was necessary to control cervical metastatic disease.

Following Crile's description of the radical neck dissection, controversy arose among surgeons regarding proper treatment of metastatic cancer in the neck. Many surgeons advocated a more conservative approach than the radical dissection described by Crile. Disagreement persisted over which structures required sacrifice and which could be conserved during the course of neck dissection. The routine sacrifice of cranial nerve XI, the spinal accessory nerve, during radical neck dissection was one of the early major points of contention. The functional impairment due to the loss of the cranial nerve XI is significant, and many surgeons questioned the necessity of nerve sacrifice. Blair and Brown [6], in 1933, championed resection of the spinal accessory nerve because they believed resection of the nerve allowed a more total removal of the cervical lymphatics and decreased operating time. The authors published a remarkable recurrence rate of only 2% [6].

In 1951, Hayes Martin and colleagues promoted radical neck dissection as the only acceptable procedure for suspected or obvious metastasis to the cervical lymph nodes [2]. Martin unequivocally stated that any operation attempting to preserve the spinal accessory nerve should be condemned. Dissenters, though, continued to argue that the radical dissection was not an appropriate procedure for all patients with occult or obvious metastatic neck disease. These dissenters to radical dissection reasoned that the Crile procedure was not truly an en bloc resection and argued for more conservative procedures. The principal question for surgeons favoring more conservative surgical treatment of the neck was why, from an oncologic standpoint, certain important structures, such as the carotid artery and major nerve trunks, should be spared, and yet other structures, such as the internal jugular vein and spinal accessory nerve, should not be salvaged. A number of reports of nonrandomized clinical trials emerged demonstrating spinal accessory nerve preservation and no increase in recurrence rate [7–9].

The concept of conservative, "modified," neck dissection was further expanded to encompass conserving major structures while resecting the soft tissue containing the cervical lymphatics. Bocca, in 1967, published his report of conservative neck dissection and demonstrated no significant difference in outcomes as compared to other patients who had previously undergone radical neck dissection for similar disease [10]. Jesse and co-workers likewise reported excellent results with conservative neck dissection in selected cases [9]. The rationale for these more conservative neck dissections was better preservation of neck and shoulder function, protection of the carotid artery, better patient tolerance for bilateral procedures, and decreased incidence of complications. Better cosmetic appearance of the neck and use of the procedure as a staging operation to determine the need for more extensive or additional treatment were other reasons for performing a modified neck dissection. Today, the conservative, less-than-radical neck dissection is widely accepted as an appropriate procedure for patients at risk of developing metastatic disease or those with early metastatic disease in the cervical lymphatics. Radical neck dissection continues to be an important procedure for the treatment of patients with advanced cervical metastatic disease.

Rationale for use of modified dissection in treatment of the N0 neck

An increased awareness of the impact of cancer treatment on a patient's quality of life has emerged over the past two decades. The surgeon's desire to decrease the morbidity of surgical therapy without compromising disease control has been responsible for technical modifications in neck dissection procedures [11]. Long-term morbidity of the radical neck dissection includes cosmetic deformity and potential major functional impairment. Scar bands and neck contracture commonly occur following radical neck dissection. Likewise, loss of the normal neck contour occurs through sacrifice of the sternocleidomastoid muscle, submandibular gland, and the tail of the parotid gland.

More importantly, severe functional limitation following radical dissection may be induced by the sacrifice of the spinal accessory nerve, resulting in shoulder drop with decreased abduction and decreased external rotation of the arm [12]. Additionally, denervation of the levator scapulae muscle may occur with extensive dissection. Such denervation is manifested by shoulder drop, subluxation, chronic shoulder pain, and adhesive capsulitis. Sacrifice of both jugular veins may lead to the immediate postoperative complications of bilateral blindness (from central retinal vein occlusion) and cerebral edema [13,14]. Long-term effects of jugular vein sacrifice include persistent facial and laryngeal edema.

Modifications of the radical neck dissection were developed in response to the associated morbidity. One such modification arose in cases of simultaneous bilateral radical dissection. Because of the significant morbidity that may follow synchronous bilateral internal jugular vein ligation, bilateral neck dissections began to be staged or modified to preserve one of the jugular veins. Likewise, nerve-preserving dissections emerged due to the frequently permanent shoulder morbidity associated with sacrifice of the spinal accessory nerve. Such successful modifications of the radical neck dissection further stimulated surgeons to develop oncologically sound, function-sparing procedures for treatment of cervical metastases.

Probably one of the most important indications for modification of the standard radical neck dissection occurs in the patient with an upper aerodigestive tract primary tumor without clinically apparent neck metastasis (N0). Elective neck dissection is proposed in such patients to remove the disease while still occult and contained within the lymph node capsule. Dissection of occult nodal disease may theoretically improve regional control by removing small and clinically silent metastases, thereby limiting further spread. The deleterious effect on survival of clinically apparent nodal disease with extracapsular extension is well known [15]. Likewise, elective nodal dissection may play a major role in staging and can assist in identifying patients who may benefit from combined treatment with other modalities such as radiation therapy.

On the other hand, not all patients with an N0 neck will develop clinically evident neck metastasis. Only a small percentage of patients have occult metastatic disease. The likelihood of occult disease depends on the site and size of the primary tumor. The decision to perform elective neck dissection, therefore, depends on the status of the primary cancer. To date, no studies have confirmed the utility of elective dissection in all patients at risk for the development of cervical metastasis. Elective dissection of the N0 neck is generally limited to patients undergoing surgical treatment of their primary tumor who are thought to be at high risk of developing regional nodal metastasis. While the advantage of elective versus therapeutic neck dissection in all cases is still unclear, the theoretical advantages of elective neck dissection in selected patients are very compelling.

When elective radical neck dissection is performed, a significant number of patients may incur functional and cosmetic morbidity in the absence of pathologically proven metastatic disease. Shah et al. found that two thirds of patients undergoing elective radical neck dissection for oral cavity cancers did not have metastasis present on histologic examination of the removed nodes. The remaining one third of the patients had occult metastatic disease [16]. Therefore, the majority of patients underwent a radical lymphadenectomy in the absence of metastatic disease. In the clinically N0 patient at high risk for cervical metastasis in whom an elective neck dissection is thought to be beneficial, a function-sparing procedure that removes the nodes at risk and provides adequate disease control is highly desirable. The classic radical neck dissection is no longer indicated for the patient with a squamous cell carcinoma of the upper aerodigestive tract and a clinically negative neck.

Lymphatics and metastasis

Knowledge of the nodal groups at risk for harboring metastasis is essential for performance of an appropriate neck dissection. The lymphatic pathways of the upper aerodigestive tract were carefully described by Rouviere [17] and Fisch and Sigel [18]. Additionally, Lindberg demonstrated the clinical distribution of the cervical lymph nodes most frequently involved with metastatic disease from upper aerodigestive tract mucosal primaries in a review of 1155 patients [19]. For tumors arising in the oral cavity and soft palate, a correlation was found between more advanced primary disease stage and the presence of multiple cervical metastases or fixed nodes. Importantly, this correlation did not hold for primaries of the tonsil, base of tongue, supraglottic larynx, and hypopharynx. Regardless of primary stage, carcinomas in these sites were often associated with multiple unilateral or bilateral metastases. More importantly, Lindberg noted that the risk of metastasis to the different cervical nodal stations was dependent upon the primary site. For instance, the submaxillary triangle is at risk for metastasis from primary tumors of the oral cavity but is almost never the site of isolated, clinically evident metastasis from primary tumors of the oropharynx, larynx, and hypopharynx.

Other investigators have confirmed the regional nodal metastatic patterns associated with specific primary tumor sites. Shah et al. found that the incidence of occult metastasis to lymph nodes in levels IV and V was extremely low in patients with oral cavity primary tumors [16]. The authors concluded that dissection of the level IV and V nodal groups in this clinical setting was unwarranted.

Metastasis to the posterior cervical lymph nodes is rare for primary tumors of the oral cavity and larynx. In contrast, cancers arising in the tonsil, palate, base of tongue, pharyngeal walls, and nasopharynx frequently will spread to the posterior nodes. Primary nasopharyngeal cancers also have a high incidence of metastasis to the supraclavicular nodes. Involvement of the supraclavicular nodes is rare for most other upper aerodigestive primary sites unless spread to the lower cervical nodes is present.

The predictability of patterns of cervical metastasis enables surgeons to resect nodal groups at high risk while conserving those at low risk. Furthermore, this selective dissection of high risk nodes permits sparing of important aesthetic and functional structures. The concept of predictable routes of spread does not apply in patients previously treated or in whom metastases are present. Lymphatic channels may become obstructed in these situations, leading to retrograde lymphatic flow and aberrant spread of tumor. This concept must be kept in mind when planning a modification of the standard radical neck dissection.

A modified neck dissection may be defined as any alteration of the classical radical neck dissection. This definition encompasses procedures that conserve structures such as the internal jugular vein, sternomastoid muscle, or spinal accessory nerve. Another frequent modification of the standard neck dissection is the preservation of certain nodal groups not at risk for metastasis. An example of preservable, low risk nodes would be the supraclavicular lymph nodes in a patient with early floor of mouth cancer and a clinically negative (N0) neck.

At times, resection of additional lymph node groups not normally in-cluded in the standard radical neck dissection may be indicated. Tumors arising on the pharyngeal walls, tonsil, soft palate, uvula, and base of tongue may metastasize to the retropharyngeal lymph nodes. Involvement of these lymph nodes may be heralded by a syndrome of pain radiating from the posterior neck to the supraorbital region on the side of metastasis. Ballantyne found a 44% incidence of metastasis among patients with pharyngeal primaries undergoing retropharyngeal lymph node dissection [20]. In patients with carcinomas of the laryngopharynx and cervical esophagus, the para-tracheal and Delphian lymph nodes are at significant risk for occult metastasis [19,21,22]. Though not normally removed in the standard radical neck dissection, these lymph nodes should be included for selected upper aerodigestive tract primary tumors.

Neck dissection in transition

At our institution, the transition from the standard radical neck dissection began in 1958 and gradually evolved through the 1970s. By 1978, elective radical neck dissection in the patient with a clinically negative neck was largely abandoned. Between 1978 and 1979, only 28 (17%) of the 165 neck dissections performed were of the standard radical type, with the remainder being regional or modified dissections [23].

One of the theoretical advantages of elective neck dissection is that it provides information that is useful for planning further treatment. Some patients who manifest occult nodal metastasis can benefit from combined treatment with radiotherapy. A major factor favoring the transition from the classic radical neck dissection to the modified neck dissection was the beneficial effect of combining radiation and surgery to improve disease control in the neck while at the same time preserving function. Fletcher, in 1972, reported that 5000 cGy was sufficient to sterilize subclinical microscopic disease in the neck [24]. Strong found that moderate doses of preoperative radiotherapy significantly reduced the risk of regional recurrence in stage N2 and N3 neck disease treated with a radical neck dissection [25]. Finally, Huang et al. noted a higher recurrence rate among patients with extra-capsular spread of cancer treated with surgery alone [26]. The use of modified elective neck dissection allows conservation of function with the option of combining surgery and radiation therapy for selected patients at high risk for a regional recurrence, without compromise of oncologic principles.

Previously, the terminology used to describe modified neck dissections has been confusing. Recent publications by Medina, Byers, and Robbins have attempted to standardize terminology [27–30]. In the past, any varia-tion from the classic radical neck dissection was referred to as a modified neck dissection. With current nomenclature, the phrase *modified radical*

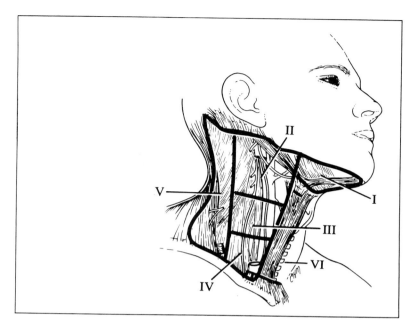

Figure 1. The level system for describing the location of lymph nodes in the neck. Level I indicates the submental and submandibular group; level II, upper jugular group; level III, middle jugular group; level IV, lower jugular group; level V, posterior triangle group; and level VI, anterior compartment group. Reprinted from Robbins et al. [30], with permission.

neck dissection refers to a procedure that spares at least one of the nonlymphatic structures in the neck. Likewise, a selective neck dissection includes those procedures that remove only lymph node groups at risk for metastasis while preserving structures usually removed with the standard radical neck dissection. The new classification system provides more precise information regarding which nodal groups were dissected and which structures were sacrificed or preserved (Figure 1).

Typically, the choice of the type of dissection performed for elective neck dissection is dictated by the histology and location of the primary tumor as well as by any prior treatment the patient has received. Once the neck dissection is completed, the specimen is oriented toward the pathologist so that any positive nodes and their location may be identified (Figure 2). Orientation for the pathologist is critical for determining which nodal groups are involved with metastasis and in assessing the need for further treatment.

Modified radical neck dissection

The phrase *modified radical neck dissection* has classically referred to procedures that remove the lymph node groups in stations I–V, the

227

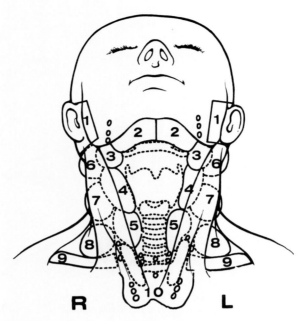

Figure 2. Diagram for orienting the contents of the neck dissection. Once the lymph nodes have been examined histologically, this information can be converted to lymph node levels I–VI. (1) parotid compartment, (2) submental-submaxillary, (3) subdigastric, (4) midjugular, (5) lower jugular, (6) upper posterior cervical, (7) mid posterior cervical, (8) lower posterior cervical, (9) supraclavicular-scalone, (10) thyroid compartments.

sternocleidomastoid muscle, and the jugular vein while sparing the spinal accessory nerve (Figure 3). More recently, modified radical neck dissection implies dissection of lymph node groups I–V with preservation of at least one of the nonlymphatic structures sacrificed in radical neck dissection [29,30]. Modified radical neck dissections may be performed for elective treatment of the N0 neck, though more selective dissections are often utilized in lieu of this more extensive procedure. In some centers this type of dissection is frequently used for the patient with a single clinically positive lymph node less than 3 cm in diameter.

At The University of Texas M. D. Anderson Cancer Center, most patients with N1 neck disease can be effectively managed with a selective neck dissection as opposed to the more radical procedure. In general, the modified radical neck dissection is reserved for patients with large, bulky metastases and/or spread to the supraclavicular lymph nodes, selected patients having failed radiotherapy, or those with multiple clinically positive nodes. With advanced regional disease, extracapsular tumor spread is frequently present and contiguous involvement of the sternocleidomastoid muscle, spinal accessory nerve, or the jugular vein is not uncommon.

228

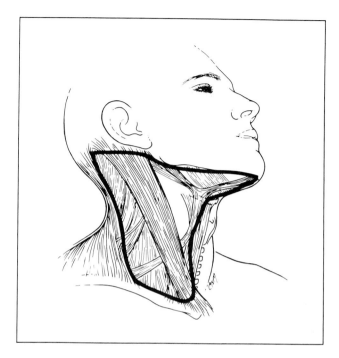

Figure 3. Area encompassed by the modified radical neck dissection. (Reprinted from Robbins et al. [30], with permission.)

Preservation of these structures is frequently impossible when extensive neck disease is present.

Regional disease control following modified radical neck dissection was examined by Molinari et al., who found a 2.5% recurrence rate for radical neck dissection in patients with an N0 neck treated with surgery alone [31]. Recurrence rate for patients treated with a more conservative neck dissection was 1.6% in this study. Among patients with histologic confirmation of metastasis, the regional recurrence rates for radical versus modified neck dissection were 9.4% and 4.5%, respectively. Lingeman et al. in 1977 reported a comparison between 337 radical neck dissections and 98 modified radical neck dissections and found no significant difference in disease control [32].

Functional neck dissection

The concept of the functional neck dissection (FND) is based on surgical removal of nodal groups I through V (as with radical neck dissection), but with preservation of the cervical structures routinely sacrificed in the radical dissection. In this sense, FND is a subclassification of the modified radical neck dissection according to present terminology [29,30]. Bocca became the principal proponent of the FND in the 1960s. Bocca defended the procedure as being as oncologically sound as radical neck dissection but without the associated functional morbidity and cosmetic defect [10].

Functional neck dissection is based on the anatomical concept of fibrofatty tissue containing lymph nodes and lymphatic vessels bounded within a complex system of fascial aponeuroses. Like the selective neck dissections, the technique of FND consists of stripping of the fascial layers containing the lymphoareolar tissue away from the surrounding vital structures. As long as nodal metastases remain confined within the nodal capsule, the lymphatics can be dissected away from the major muscles and neurovascular structures without oncologic compromise. Thus, functional neck dissection is performed only for elective dissection or for clinically positive nodes that are freely mobile.

Results from FND appear to be similar to those obtained with radical neck dissection in several retrospective series. Obviously, such studies potentially contain marked selection bias. Bocca reported a series of 1200 functional neck dissections performed in 843 patients between 1961 and 1979 [33]. He compared these cases to a group of 414 patients who underwent radical neck dissection at the same institution during the years 1948–1955. Patients in the FND group were divided into those undergoing elective dissection and those undergoing curative attempt with dissection. Six hundred and seventy-two patients had an elective FND. The recurrence rate in this group was 2.4%. Among the group of 414 patients who had undergone RND, 226 patients had elective dissection and had a recurrence rate of 6.6%. Criticisms of this study include the lack of information on the role of radiation therapy in decreasing the risk of regional recurrence and lack of data regarding the rates of surgical salvage. To date, functional neck dissection favorably compares with radical neck dissection for elective treatment of the N0 neck and for therapeutic dissection of early cervical metastasis of head and neck cancer.

The functional neck dissection is particularly useful in cases in which metastases may spread to the posterior cervical nodes or to the lower neck nodes overlying the scalene muscles and lower portion of the jugular vein. Examples of such cases are nodal metastasis from carcinoma of the thyroid, regional metastasis from metastatic melanoma, and metastasis from squamous cell carcinoma of the base of tongue, hypopharynx, and cervical esophagus. In many cases of squamous cell carcinomas from primary upper aerodigestive tract sites, a more selective dissection (such as a supraomohyoid dissection) may provide the same information regarding nodal metastasis and may be more easily accomplished than FND.

Suprahyoid neck dissection

The suprahyoid neck dissection is a selective regional neck dissection of the contents of the submental and submaxillary regions. The level I lymph nodes, submandibular gland, and surrounding fibrofatty tissues form the bulk of the surgical specimen. Suprahyoid dissections are useful in selected instances for resection of submandibular neoplasms and to provide exposure to obtain adequate margins of resection for primary tumors of the mandible when the risk of lymph node metastasis is negligible.

A suprahyoid dissection is also utilized for staging patients with lip carcinoma who present with palpable submental and submandibular lymph nodes. The incidence of pathologically proven metastasis in these patients is only 10%, and the majority of patients with palpable nodes have inflammatory enlargement rather than metastasis. Sampling of the level I lymph nodes allows determination of the need for more extensive treatment of the neck. Once the level I lymph nodes are removed, they are examined by frozen section analysis. If histologically confirmed metastasis is found, a supraomohyoid dissection is indicated.

Suprahyoid neck dissection has, at times, been advocated as a general staging procedure for all carcinomas of the oral cavity. Because of the possibility of metastases from squamous carcinomas of the oral cavity going to first echelon nodes outside the submandibular triangle, suprahyoid neck dissection should not be considered an adequate biopsy procedure in predicting metastases to lymph nodes at risk in the remainder of the neck.

Another use of the suprahyoid dissection is in patients with early superficial squamous cell carcinomas of the anterior floor of the mouth. The incidence of occult lymph node metastasis in these patients is low, and elective dissection of the neck is not usually indicated. Resection of the tumor, though, often includes the submandibular ducts and results in obstructive sialoadenitis and an indurated tender gland. On follow-up examination, the differentiation between the indurated submandibular gland and metastatic disease can be difficult. Suprahyoid dissection for resection of the gland and surrounding lymphatics at the time of the primary surgery facilitates long-term surveillance.

The isolated suprahyoid neck dissection is most consistently applied for resection of the primary neoplasm in patients with submandibular gland salivary tumors and minor salivary gland tumors of the floor of mouth. Suprahyoid dissection removes the primary tumor en bloc with the surrounding soft tissues and local draining lymphatics. For the salivary gland cancers, this procedure provides some staging information by removing the primary echelon of lymph nodes [34]. Suprahyoid dissection for removal of submandibular tumors avoids 'shelling out' of the involved gland with the accompanying high likelihood of local recurrence. Suprahyoid dissection may be easily extended to a more complete neck dissection if palpable lymph nodes are present or when the risk of occult disease in other lymph node groups is high.

Supraomohyoid neck dissection

Supraomohyoid neck dissection (SOHND) is a selective en bloc removal of the lymph node groups most likely to contain metastases in patients with squamous cell carcinomas of the oral cavity. These lymph node groups are the submental, submandibular, subdigastric, and midjugular nodes (Figure 4). Also included are the nodal groups located anterior to the cutaneous braches of the cervical plexus and superior to the omohyoid muscle. The sternomastoid muscle, spinal accessory nerve, and internal jugular vein are usually preserved.

Supraomohyoid neck dissection is utilized in the elective management of patients with T2, T3, or T4 squamous cell carcinomas of the floor of mouth, oral tongue, alveolar ridge, buccal mucosa, retromolar trigone, and faucial arch region. Bilateral supraomohyoid neck dissections are indicated for patients with cancers of the anterior tongue and floor of mouth that involve or approach the midline. Supraomohyoid neck dissection may be

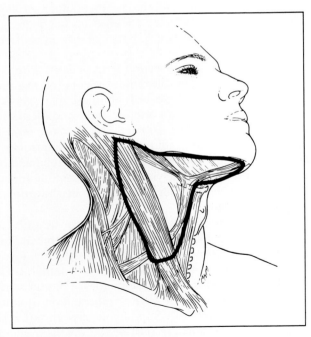

Figure 4. Supraomohyoid neck dissection. (Reprinted from Robbins et al. [30], with permission.)

performed in conjunction with parotidectomy in patients with squamous cell carcinoma, Merkel cell carcinoma, and intermediate thickness melanoma of the cheek and lateral portions of the face.

The rationale for supraomohyoid neck dissection is based on the previously described predictable distribution of cervical lymph node metastases in patients with previously untreated squamous cell carcinomas of the head and neck. Lindberg demonstrated that the subdigastric and midjugular nodes are the most frequently involved nodal groups in patients with primary oral cavity and oropharyngeal squamous cell carcinomas [19]. The author also noted that submandibular triangle nodes harbor metastatic disease in patients with buccal mucosa, oral tongue, and floor of mouth carcinomas. Likewise, these primary tumors may metastasize to both sides of the neck and may skip along the submandibular and subdigastric nodal groups, and metastasize to the midjugular nodes [35,36]. Importantly, Lindberg's study also noted that carcinomas of the oral cavity and oropharynx rarely spread to the lower jugular or posterior cervical nodes in the absence of metastases to the first echelon (submandibular, subdigastric, and midjugular) nodal groups. Studies by Skolnick [37] and Shaha et al. [38] confirm the rarity of nodal metastases to the posterior triangle (nodal group V) in patients with primary squamous cell carcinomas in the oral cavity and other sites. Supraomohyoid neck dissection is designed to provide an en bloc removal of all the lymph nodes that are most likely to contain metastases when the primary tumor is located in the oral cavity or oropharynx.

Supraomohyoid dissection provides staging information to the surgeon and may be the only therapy required for the cervical lymph nodes at risk for or containing occult metastasis. The concept of staging in the neck is important for patients with intermediate or advanced primary tumors (T2, T3, T4) who have necks clinically staged N0 or N1. The probability of lymph node metastasis is high in these patients. For oral cavity cancers the sensitivity, specificity, and overall accuracy of the clinical exam of the neck is 70%, 65%, and 68%, respectively [16]. In a study that included T1 tumors, Teichgraeber and Clairmont found occult metastasis in 37–38% of patients with cancers of the tongue and floor of mouth [39].

Neck dissection provides staging information that will determine if postoperative radiotherapy is necessary. If the lymph nodes are histologically negative, or if only microscopic foci of metastases are found in one or two lymph nodes that lie in the primary echelon drainage area, no further treatment is necessary and the patient is treated with surgery alone. If metastases spread beyond the primary echelon of nodal drainage, are present in two or more nodal echelons, or demonstrate extracapsular extension outside the nodes, postoperative radiotherapy is indicated. All the lymph nodes at risk for containing metastases must be evaluated for this decision to be made with confidence.

Supraomohyoid neck dissection for primary oral cavity cancers provides the same staging information as a radical neck dissection (RND) while sparing the patient the morbidity of radical or modified radical neck dissection, especially in bilateral cases. Cosmetic deformity is minimal upon completion of the dissection. Though neurapraxia of the spinal accessory nerve may occur after nerve retraction, prolonged dysfunction of the shoulder following supraomohyoid neck dissection is rare [40].

Radiotherapy is an alternative treatment modality to supraomohyoid neck dissection for elective treatment of the N0 neck. Several authors (Fletcher, Million, and others) feel that the risk of developing clinically positive nodes in the N0 neck can be reduced to approximately 5% with the use of comprehensive neck irradiation [24,41,42]. If indications exist for postoperative radiation of the surgically treated primary tumor site, elective irradiation of the neck should be considered when the neck has not been dissected and the risk of occult regional disease is substantial (30% or greater). Smaller tumors may be suitably treated by surgery alone. Supraomohyoid neck dissection provides staging information (regarding the need for additional treatment) in these cases and may be the only therapy necessary for occult neck disease. In such cases, supraomohyoid neck dissection can be accomplished with minimal morbidity and reduces the risk of occult disease evolving into clinically evident metastasis. The undesirable side effects of radiotherapy are avoided, and this modality is reserved for possible future treatment of second primary tumors.

Recurrence rates following supraomohyoid neck dissection compare favorably with recurrence rates following radical neck dissection. Strong reported a 6.7% incidence of recurrence in radically dissected necks that were histologically negative, a 36.5% incidence of recurrence when positive nodes were found at one level, and a 71.3% recurrence rate when positive nodes were found at multiple levels [25]. In a study by Medina and Byers, neck recurrence after supraomohyoid dissection with histologically negative nodes was 5% [28]. A 10% recurrence rate was noted when singular nodes without extracapsular node extension were found, and a 24% recurrence rate was found when multiple positive nodes or extracapsular extension were found in supraomohyoid neck dissection specimens. Postoperative radiotherapy decreased the recurrence rate to 15% in a group with multiple metastatic nodes and extracapsular extension [28].

Lateral and anterior neck dissections

The lymph nodes at risk for metastasis from primary tumors of the larynx, hypopharynx, and cervical esophagus have been described in detail by Feind [43]. The laryngeal lymphatics are compartmentalized so that ipsilateral supraglottic primaries will drain to the upper and midjugular lymph nodes on the same side. Tumors arising on or extending to the epiglottis, however, may metastasize bilaterally. The risk of regional metastasis from supraglottic cancer is somewhat stage dependent, with the overall risk of occult disease being 40–50% [43]. The glottic larynx is sparsely supplied with lymphatics; therefore, the risk of occult lymph node disease is rare for T1 and T2 primaries. For T3 tumors it ranges from approximately 3% to 10% [43]. Tumors that originate or extend into the subglottic larynx drain to the lateral cervical nodes as well as the Delphian and paratracheal lymph nodes. These latter nodes are also at risk for metastasis from cervical esophageal cancers. Occult paratracheal lymph node metastases have been implicated as an etiologic factor in peristomal recurrences following total laryngectomy [44].

Primary squamous cell carcinomas of the hypopharynx will drain to the upper and mid jugular lymph nodes. If the midjugular nodes are involved, metastases are more likely to be found in the lower jugular nodes as well. The incidence of occult metastases from primary tumors of the hypopharynx is approximately 40%. The retropharyngeal lymph nodes are also at risk for harboring metastasis from these tumors. Carcinomas of the cervical esophagus will drain to the paratracheal lymph nodes bilaterally; in addition, tumors arising in the distal cervical esophagus will metastasize to the upper mediastinal lymph nodes.

The lateral neck dissection is used electively to remove occult nodal disease for primary tumors of the larynx, hypopharynx, and cervical esoph-

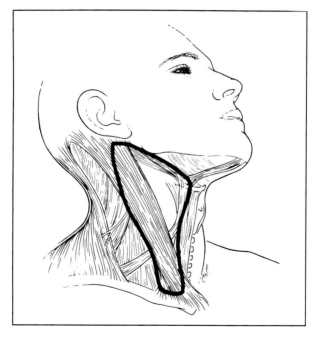

Figure 5. The lateral neck dissection that removes lymph nodes from levels II, III, and IV. (Reprinted from Robbins et al. [30], with permission.)

235

agus. Lymph nodes removed include the upper jugular (level II), middle jugular (level III), and lower jugular (level IV) nodes (Figure 5). These lateral nodal groups lie in the lateral aspect of the neck in relation to the posterior triangle, the submandibular triangle, and the anterior compartment. The rationale for the lateral neck dissection is supported by the findings of Candela et al., who noted that among 78 N0 patients undergoing 79 elective radical neck dissections for squamous cell carcinoma of the larynx, the incidence of positive lymph nodes was 37% (29/79) [45]. In their study positive level I and level V lymph nodes were seen in 5% and 2% of neck dissections, respectively. Patients who had levels I and V metastasis also had positive nodes at other levels. They concluded that dissection of levels I and V is not indicated for patients undergoing total laryngectomy in the absence of metastatic disease at other levels.

The anterior compartment neck dissection is primarily used for tumors of the larynx, hypopharynx, and cervical esophagus. This type of dissection is generally combined with lateral neck dissection for tumors arising in these sites. Among patients with thyroid cancer, the anterior dissection will remove the primary echelon nodes at risk for metastasis. When metastatic thyroid cancer is present in the lateral neck, a more comprehensive dissection is indicated to remove all of the nodal areas at risk for metastasis.

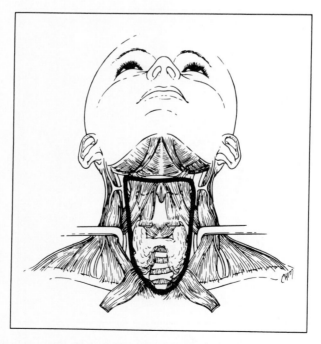

Figure 6. Anterior neck dissection for removal of level VI lymph nodes. (Reprinted from Robbins et al. [30], with permission.)

Anterior neck dissection refers to removal of the lymph nodes surrounding the midline visceral structures (level VI). The level VI nodes include the pretracheal Delphian lymph node, paratracheal, and parathyroidal nodes (Figure 6). The lateral limits are the carotid arteries, while the superior and inferior limits are the hyoid bone and the suprasternal notch, respectively. In addition to the lymph node-bearing tissue, the ipsilateral thyroid lobe (or entire gland if indicated by the site of primary tumor) is often removed (Figure 7).

Approximately 20% of patients with tumors of the larynx, hypopharynx, and cervical esophagus have occult metastatic disease in the paratracheal lymph nodes [22]. Failure to remove these nodes surgically or to sterilize

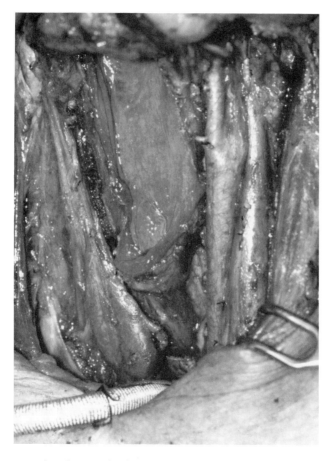

Figure 7. Intraoperative photograph of a lateral and anterior neck dissection performed for a $T_3 N_0$ glottic carcinoma. The lymph nodes in levels II, III, IV, and VI have been resected along with the left lobe of the thyroid.

Table 1. Paratracheal lymph node metastasis according to the primary site

Site	No. patients		With PTLNM (%)	
	Subtotal	Total (%)	Subtotal	Total (%)
Larynx		91 (64.5)		16 (17.6)
Glottic	39		5	
Supraglottic	19		3	
Transglottic	28		6	
Subglottic	5		2	
Hypopharynx		36 (25.5)		3 (8.3)
Cervical esophagus		14 (9.9)		10 (71.4)

PTLNM (n = 14.5) paratracheal lymph node metastasis.
Reprinted from Weber et al. [22], with permission.

them with radiotherapy may increase the risk for peristomal recurrence following total laryngectomy. Unilateral anterior compartment dissections are indicated for patients with primary tumors of the larynx or hypopharynx that are localized to one side of these anatomic regions (such as the glottic larynx or pyriform sinus). Bilateral dissections, in combination with total thyroidectomy, are indicated for patients with laryngeal tumors that have significant anterior subglottic extension, and for tumors arising in the subglottic region or cervical esophagus. In a review of central compartment neck dissections for squamous cell carcinoma of the larynx, hypopharynx, or cervical esophagus, the mean number of paratracheal lymph nodes removed was 3.9 (range, 1–30) [22]. Patients with cervical esophageal tumors had the highest incidence of paratracheal lymph node metastasis (71.4%) (Table 1). The incidence of paratracheal metastasis with supraglottic tumors was 16% in this study.

Based on these findings, our approach in the N0 patient undergoing laryngectomy with or without partial pharyngectomy is to perform a lateral neck dissection bilaterally. The anterior compartment is dissected on the side of the primary tumor to clear potential occult paratracheal lymph node metastasis and to decrease the likelihood of peristomal recurrence.

Conclusions

Modifications of the standard neck dissection procedure are an appropriate alternative to radical neck dissection for elective surgical treatment of the N0 neck. A modified dissection technique offers disease control comparable to that of the radical dissection without the accompanying morbidity. The choice of a modified neck dissection procedure for elective neck dissection is principally determined by the site and stage of the primary cancer and is

238

Table 2. Elective neck dissection for the N0 patient

Primary tumor site	Lymph node levels dissected	Type of dissection

Oral cavity
  Tongue, floor of mouth, retromolar
    trigone, alveolar ridge, buccal
    mucosa
	I, II, III	Supraomohyoid

Larynx
  Supraglottic
  Glottic
	II, III, IV, VI[a]	Lateral and anterior

Oropharynx	I, II, III, IV[c], V	Functional
Hypopharynx	II, III, IV, VI[b]	Lateral and anterior
Esophagus	II, III, IV, VI[d]	Lateral and anterior

[a] For midline supraglottic tumors, level VI nodes are not routinely removed.
[b] Level VI nodes are removed for pyriform sinus primaries but not the midline posterior pharyngeal wall.
[c] Level IV nodes are dissected when the lymph node(s) at the level of the omohyoid muscle are positive.
[d] Removal of level VI nodes bilaterally and a total thyroidectomy are indicated.

summarized in Table 2. The lymph nodes at risk for metastasis are removed while preserving the XI internal jugular vein and sternocleidomastoid muscle. Successful outcome following neck dissection depends upon appropriate selection of a procedure best suited to the individual patient's disease status and careful attention to the technical requirements of the procedure. Radical neck dissection is most appropriately reserved for the treatment of bulky cervical metastasis with marked extension to the surrounding soft tissues.

References

1. Crile G. Excision of cancer of the head and neck. JAMA 47:1780–1786, 1906.
2. Martin H, Del Valle B, Ehrlich H, et al. Neck dissection. Cancer 4:441–499, 1951.
3. Warren JM. Surgical Observations with Cases and Operations. Boston: Ticknor and Fields, 1867.
4. Kocher T. Über radicalheilung d. krebses, Deutsch Ztschr Chir 12:134, 1880.
5. Butlin HT, Spencer WG. Diseases of the Tongue. London: Cassell and Company, 1900.
6. Blair VP, Brown JB. The treatment of cancerous or potentially cancerous cervical lymph nodes. Ann Surg 98:650–651, 1933.
7. Skolnick EM, Tenta LT, Wineinger DM, et al. Preservation of XI cranial nerve in neck dissections. Laryngoscope 77:1304–1314, 1967.
8. Roy PH, Beahrs OH. Spinal accessory nerve in radical neck dissections. Am J Surg 118:800–804, 1969.
9. Jesse RH, Ballantyne AJ, Larson D. Radical or modified neck dissection: A therapeutic dilemma. Am J Surg 136:516–519, 1978.

10. Bocca E, Pignataro O. A conservation technique in radical neck dissection. Ann Otol Rhinol Laryngol 76:975–988, 1967.
11. Khafif RA, Gelbfish GA, Asase DK, et al. Modified radical neck dissection in cancer of the mouth, pharynx, and larynx. Head Neck 12:476–482, 1990.
12. Remmler D, Scheetz J, Byers R, et al. Morbidity of modified neck dissection. In: DL Larson, AJ Ballantyne, OM Guillamondegui, eds. Cancer in the Neck: Evaluation and Treatment. New York: Macmillan, 1986.
13. Schuller D. Morbidity of radical neck dissection. In: DL Larson, AJ Ballantyne, OM Guillamondegui, eds. Cancer in the Neck: Evaluation and Treatment. New York: Macmillan, 1986.
14. Torti RA, Ballantyne AJ, Berkley RG. Sudden blindness after simultaneous bilateral radical neck dissection. Arch Surg 8:271–137, 1964.
15. Johnson JT, Barnes EL, Myers EN, et al. Extracapsular spread of tumors in cervical node metastasis. Arch Otolaryngol 107:725–729, 1981.
16. Shah JP, Candela FC, Poddar AK. The patterns of cervical lymph node metastases from squamous carcinoma of the oral cavity. Cancer 66:109–113, 1990.
17. Rouviere H. Anatomy of the Human Lymphatic system, No. 2. Ann Arbor, MI: Edwards Brothers, 1938.
18. Fisch UP, Sigel ME. Cervical lymphatic system as visualized by lymphography. Ann Otol Rhinol Laryngol 73:869–882, 1964.
19. Lindberg R. Distribution of cervical lymph node metastases from squamous cell carcinoma of the upper respiratory and digestive tracts. Cancer 29:1446–1449, 1972.
20. Ballantyne AJ. Significance of retropharyngeal nodes in cancer of the head and neck. Am J Surg 108:500, 1964.
21. Olsen KD, DeSanto LW, Pearson BW. Positive Delphian lymph node: Clinical significance in laryngeal cancer. Laryngoscope 97:1033–1037, 1987.
22. Weber RS, Marvel J, Smith P, et al. Paratracheal metastastic squamous carcinoma in patients requiring total laryngectomy. Otolaryngol Head Neck Surg, 1993, in press.
23. Ballantyne AJ. Modified neck dissection. In: IT Jackson, BC Sommerlad, eds. Recent Advances in Plastic Surgery. Edinburgh: Churchill Livingstone, 1985.
24. Fletcher GH. Elective irradiation of subclinical disease in cancers of the head and neck. Cancer 29:1450–1454, 1972.
25. Strong EW. Preoperative radiation and radical neck dissection. Surg Clin North Am 49:271–276, 1969.
26. Huang DT, Johnson CR, Schmidt-Ullrich R, et al. Postoperative radiotherapy in head and neck carcinoma with extracapsular lymph node extension and/or positive resection margins: A comparative study. Int J Radiat Oncol Biol Phys 23:737–742, 1992.
27. Byers RM. Modified neck dissection: A study of 967 cases from 1970–1980. Am J Surg 150:414–421, 1985.
28. Medina JE, Byers RM. Supraomohyoid neck dissection: Rationale, indications and surgical technique. Head Neck 11:111–122, 1989.
29. Medina JE. A rational classification of neck dissections. Otolaryngol Head Neck Surg 100:169–176, 1989.
30. Robbins KT, Medina JE, Wolfe GT, Levine P, Sessions RB, Pruet CW. Standardizing neck dissection terminology. Arch Otolaryngol Head Neck Surg 117:601–605, 1991.
31. Molinari R, Chiesa F, Cantu G, et al. Retropective comparison of conservative and radical neck dissection in laryngeal cancer. Ann Otol 89:578–581, 1980.
32. Lingeman RE, Helmus C, Stephens R, et al. Neck dissection: Radical or conservative. Ann Otol 86:737–744, 1977.
33. Bocca E, Pignataro, Oldini C, et al. Functional neck dissection: An evaluation and review of 843 cases. Laryngoscope 94:942–945, 1984.
34. Weber RS, Byers RM, Petit B, Wolf P, Ang K, Luna M. Submandibular gland tumors: Adverse histologic factors and therapeutic implications. Arch Otolaryngol Head Neck Surg 116:1055–1060, 1990.

240

35. Johnson J, Leipzig B, Cummings C. Management of T_1 carcinoma of the anterior aspect of the tongue. Arch Otolaryngol 106:249–251, 1980.
36. Drouhas C, Whitehurst J. The lymphatics of the tongue in relation to cancer. Am Surg 42:670–674, 1976.
37. Skolnick EM. The posterior triangle in radical neck surgery. Arch Otolaryngol 102:1–4, 1976.
38. Shaha A, Spiro R, Shah J, et al. Squamous carcinoma of the floor of the mouth. Am J Surg 148:455–459, 1984.
39. Teichgraeber JF, Clairmont AA. The incidence of occult metastasis for cancer of the oral tongue and floor of mouth: Treatment rationale. Head Neck Surg 7:15–21, 1984.
40. Remmler D, Byers RM, Scheetz J, et al. A prospective study of shoulder disability resulting from radical and modified neck dissections. Head Neck Surg 8:280–286, 1986.
41. Million RR. Elective irradiation for T_xN_0 squamous carcinoma of the oral tongue and floor of mouth. Cancer 34:149–155, 1974.
42. Rabuzzi DD, Chung CT, Saagerman RH. Prophylactic neck irradiation. Arch Otolaryngol 106:454–455, 1980.
43. Feind CR: The head and neck. In: CD Haagensen, CR Feind, FC Hurter, CA Slantez, JA Weinberg, eds. The Lymphatics in Cancer. Philadelphia: WB Saunders, 1972, pp 59–230.
44. Harris HH, Butler E. Surgical limits in cancer. Arch Otolaryngol 87:64–67, 1968.
45. Candela FC, Shah J, Jacques DP, Shah JP. Patterns of cervical node metastasis from squamous carcinoma of the larynx. Arch Otolaryngol Head Neck Surg 116:432–435, 1990.

13. Distant metastases from head and neck squamous cancer: The role of adjuvant chemotherapy

Harlan A. Pinto and Charlotte Jacobs

The goal of adjuvant chemotherapy in the treatment of carcinomas is improved survival for patients treated with local therapy. It has been shown that adjuvant chemotherapy improves survival in a variety of animal models and in humans with breast cancer, osteosarcoma, or colorectal cancer. The central hypothesis is that chemotherapy eradicates micrometastatic or residual local disease early on.

The treatment of patients with head and neck squamous cancer is evolving. After two decades of experience using chemotherapy in the treatment of these patients, it is not yet clear what role chemotherapy should play. There is agreement that chemotherapy can provide palliation for patients with recurrent disease [1–3]. With regard to primary treatment, chemotherapy can improve outcome when used as a radiosensitizer for certain groups of patients [4–7]. In patients with advanced unresectable disease, radiation therapy and chemotherapy given in an alternating schedule improved disease-free and overall survival [8]. There is recognition that induction chemotherapy with organ preservation has a role in a curative approach to the treatment of selected patients [9,10]. Nevertheless, the use of chemotherapy in an adjuvant setting, either prior to or following standard treatment, is not well established [11–13]. Thus far, few clinical trials have shown that adjuvant chemotherapy adds to improved local control [8,14]. A recent encouraging observation, however, is the finding that early chemotherapy may reduce the incidence of distant metastases in patients with advanced disease [9,15–17].

One ethical problem in using adjuvant chemotherapy for head and neck squamous carcinoma is uncertainty about an individual patient's clinical course. In most situations adjuvant chemotherapy is given to some patients who may already be cured by surgery and/or radiotherapy. This fact prompts oncologists to develop chemotherapy programs that are well tolerated with relatively few serious side effects. This practice may com-

Hong, Waun Ki and Weber, Randal S., (eds.), Head and Neck Cancer. © 1995 Kluwer Academic Publishers. ISBN 0-7923-3015-3. All rights reserved.

promise our ability to eradicate metastasis because of a reluctance to subject patients to aggressive and toxic therapy. The ethical dilemma will become less problematic as reliable prognostic factors for the development of micrometastatic disease or tumor markers that can identify those who may benefit from adjuvant treatment become available.

Historically, most patients with head and neck cancer were either cured with aggressive local therapy or suffered local failure, and the problem of distant metastases was unrecognized or unappreciated. As local therapy has improved, prognostic information has become available regarding the likelihood of local failure and distant relapse. Clinical trials of adjuvant chemotherapy in head and neck cancer have thus far mostly included patient groups with a relatively poor prognosis and a variable probability of clinically detectable metastatic disease. Active chemotherapy combinations were not developed or integrated into combined modality programs until the early 1980s. Patients generally included in adjuvant chemotherapy trials have all had a higher risk of local failure than distant failure. With this background, adjuvant chemotherapy in head and neck cancer thus far has focused more on its potential contribution to local control rather than on its role in eradicating distant metastases. Many more clinical trials utilizing neo-adjuvant or induction chemotherapy have been reported, reflecting this reality.

Incidence of metastatic disease

Since the morbidity and mortality of head and neck squamous cancer results primarily from failure to control the primary tumor or regional metastases, little attention has been paid to the problem of distant disease. Early in this century, clinical studies supported the view that distant spread from head and neck cancer was rare, or clinically irrelevant. Crile [18,19] reported that distant metastases occurred in only 1% of patients with head and neck cancer. Crile professed that the abundant regional lymphoid tissue in the head and neck presented an almost impassable barrier to micrometastatic disease. Dorrance and McShane in 1924 [20] and Castigliano and Rominger in 1928 [21] continued this teaching because they similarly found low rates of metastases, less than 5%.

Autopsy studies published from 1930 to 1951 challenged this view. Price [22] reported an 11% incidence of distant metastases in a series of 87 patients. Distant metastases were documented in 39% of 62 autopsies by Willis [23], 23% of 284 reported by Braund and Martin [24], and 17% of 200 autopsies in the series reported by Peltier et al. [25]. Autopsy studies published since 1960 have continued to recognize a greater incidence of distant metastatic disease [26–31]. The lowest proportion of distant metastases in autopsy studies since 1960 is 37%, reported by O'Brien et al. [28]. Ju [27] reported metastases in 53% of 293 cases, and Hoye et al. [26]

Table 1. Autopsy studies of metastases in head and neck cancer

Author	Number of cases	Number with distant metastases	Percent	Percent with distant metastases only
Price [22]	87	10	11%	
Willis [23]	62	24	39%	
Braund and Martin [24]	284	65	23%	
Peltier et al. [25]	200	34	17%	
Hoye et al. [26]	42	24	57%	
Ju [27]	293	155	53%	8%
O'Brien et al. [28]	153	56	37%	
Dennington et al. [29]	64	25	39%	
Kotwall et al. [30]	832	387	47%	9%
Zbären et al. [31]	101	40	40%	5%
Total	2118	820	39%	

documented distant metastases in 57% of 42 cases. Table 1 presents the findings of 10 autopsy studies conducted since 1930.

Autopsy studies have been criticized as overestimating the incidence of distant disease because they investigate only those patients who have died, usually from disease, thus excluding treatment successes from analysis. The studies by Hoye et al. [26] and Ju [27], which report a 57% and 53% incidence of metastases, respectively, probably overestimate the incidence of distant metastases because of this bias. The study by Zbären and Lehmann [31] is instructive, however, because one quarter of the cases had no clinical evidence of disease at the time of death, and one tenth of those with local-regional recurrence had no clinical evidence of metastases at death.

Three of the autopsy studies cited in Table 1 report the proportion of patients found at autopsy to have distant metastases without regional disease. If the data from these studies are pooled, only 8% of patients are found to suffer from distant disease only, which emphasizes the problem of local and regional failure, and therefore a perception that distant metastases are less common than what is documented in postmortem examinations.

Clinical studies vary widely in their estimate of distant metastatic disease [21,32–39] (Table 2). Castigliano et al. [21] reported sequential analyses of patients treated at the Presbyterian Hospital in New York from 1930 to 1940 and again from 1940 to 1950. Distant metastases were detected in only 1% of 400 cases in the earlier decade and in 11% of those treated a decade later. Whether this represents detection bias, a biological change in the tumor or host, or is related to treatment or lack of treatment is unclear. Two studies from the early 1960s [32,33] found metastases in 21%, and two studies from the 1970s [34,35] found metastases in 12% and 11%, respectively. The clinical studies reported since 1980 all review findings in subsets of patients. Vrikam et al. [36] reported 17% of stage III or IV patients treated with combined modality therapy had distant metastases. Amdur et al. [37] found

Table 2. Clinical studies of metastases in head and neck cancer

First author	Number of patients	Number with distant metastases	Percent	Percent with distant metastases only
Castigliano and Romingh	400	4	1.0%	
[21]	121	13	11%	
Arons and Smith [32]	89	19	21%	
Rubenfeld et al. [33]	132	28	21%	
Probert et al. [34]	779	96	12%	5%
Merino et al. [35]	5019	546	11%	8%
Vrikam et al. [36][a]	114	19	17%	10%
Amdur et al. [37]	109	30	28%	
Loree and Strong [38][b]	398	36	9%	
Cerezo et al. [39][a]	492	68	14%	
Total	7653	859	11%	

[a] Stage III and IV patients only.
[b] Oral cavity carcinoma only.

that 28% of 109 patients treated with postoperative radiotherapy developed distant metastases. Loree and Strong [38] studied only those with oral cavity carcinoma and positive margins after surgery. Cerezo et al. [39] included only those with neck disease, and 14% of 492 cases developed distant metastases.

Less than 3% of patients are found to have distant metastases at presentation [40]. Given this low incidence, an extensive metastatic workup is not necessary at initial staging. A chest x-ray and liver function tests will usually suffice. Further testing should be pursued if the patient has suspicious symptoms or abnormal chemistries.

Clinical and autopsy studies report that most metastatic disease from head and neck squamous cancers develops within 2–3 years of initial treatment. Merino et al. [35] reported that 80% of distant metastases are evident within 2 years. Probert et al. [34] found that although metastatic spread can be detected later than 3 years after primary therapy, almost all distant disease is evident within 5 years. Berger and Fletcher [41] found that it took longer for patients with clinically negative necks to develop clinically detectable distant metastases; thus, they suggested that follow-up in excess of 5 years would be required to detect late distant failures in clinical studies.

The frequency of metastatic disease reported in clinical studies reflects a number of factors. The proportion of patients with early versus advanced stage disease, the specific disease sites of the patient population reported in the study, the specific treatment administered, the methods used to document metastases, and the duration of follow-up are all important. For example, patients with locally advanced disease at diagnosis are more likely to develop metastases during the course of their illness, and nearly 20% of

Table 3. Site of metastasis in 7896 cases of head and neck cancer

Metastatic site	Autopsy studies		Clinical studies		Combined totals	
	Number (n = 1966)	Percent	Number (n = 5930)	Percent	Number (n = 7896)	Percent
All sites	792	40.3	670	11.3	1462	18.5
Lung	561	70.8	361	53.9	922	63.1
Liver	283	35.7	69	10.3	352	24.1
Bone	117	14.8	150	22.4	267	18.3
Mediastinum	183	23.1	23	3.4	206	14.1
Distant lymph nodes	127	16.0	0	0.0	127	8.7
Adrenals	114	14.4	8	1.2	122	8.3
Kidney	114	14.4	6	0.9	120	8.2
Heart	105	13.3	7	1.0	112	7.7
Pleurae	92	11.6	0	0.0	92	6.3
Spleen	62	7.8	3	0.4	65	4.4
Peritoneum	56	7.0	5	0.7	61	4.2
Diaphragm	56	7.2	0	0.0	56	3.8
Pericardium	41	5.2	0	0.0	41	2.8
Soft tissue	30	3.8	6	0.9	36	2.5
Brain	24	3.0	12	1.8	36	2.5
Pancreas	34	4.3	0	0.0	34	2.3
Intestine	29	3.6	0	0.0	29	2.0
Skin	7	0.8	13	1.9	20	1.4
Pituitary	17	2.1	0	0.0	17	1.2
Thyroid	7	0.8	2	0.3	9	0.6
Bladder	5	0.6	0	0.0	5	0.3
Gallbladder	5	0.6	0	0.0	5	0.3
Esophagus	0	0.0	4	0.6	4	0.3
Stomach	4	0.5	0	0.0	4	0.3
Bone marrow	1	0.1	3	0.4	4	0.3
Spinal cord	2	0.2	0	0.0	2	0.1
Prostate	0	0.0	1	0.1	1	0.1
Middle ear	0	0.0	1	0.1	1	0.1

Data from references 24–28, 30, 31, 33–35, 38, 45, 46.

these patients will have metastases clinically detected. Early stage patients more often have their local disease eradicated, and clinical studies suggest that less than 10% of these patients will have distant metastases detected. In addition, late occurrence of distant metastases occurring in stage I and II patients can be confused with second primary cancers. Nevertheless, in approximately 10–20% of patients in clinical studies, metastases are detected. The incidence of distant spread as the only site of recurrent disease, however, is low, ranging from 5% to 10%. Clinical and autopsy studies where this has been reported appear to agree on this estimate.

The pattern of distant metastases in head and neck cancer has been well described [24–31,33–35,42] (Table 3). Autopsy studies detect distant metastases two to three times more frequently and in more sites. Nevertheless, clinical and autopsy studies recognize the lung as the predominant site of spread, occurring in 54–71%. Liver metastases are more frequently recognized at autopsy, thus accounting for only 6% of metastases in clinical studies but 26% in autopsy studies. Although clinical reports commonly recognize lung, bone, and liver as the most clinically relevant sites of distant metastasis, autopsy studies show that spread to mediastinal nodes (17%) and distant lymph nodes (11%), adrenal glands (11%), kidneys (11%), and heart (10%) to be more common than or similar in frequency to bone metastases (11%). The unusual predilection for cardiac metastases has been observed in several studies. This fact may be relevant clinically because of the varied presentation of patients with cardiac manifestations, including angina, arrhythmia, and sudden death [43,44].

Predictors of metastatic disease

In attempts to determine which patients are at greatest risk for development of metastases, several prognostic factors have been assessed. Several studies have assessed the relative risk of developing metastatic disease based on primary site [24,25,28,30,31,35,45,46] (Table 4). Brennan et al. [46] reported that distant metastases were detected in 15–17% of oral cavity primaries and 20% of oropharynx carcinomas. Marks et al. [47] found that 23% of all patients with tumors involving the pyriform sinus developed distant metastases, with 37% of those who required a total laryngectomy for initial treatment developing metastases. The highest rates of distant metastases in clinical studies are generally associated with tumors of the nasopharynx, and hypopharynx, followed by the oropharynx, oral cavity, and supraglottic larynx. The glottic larynx generally has the lowest reported incidence of distant metastases, with clinical studies reporting frequencies of under 5%. Among those with glottic cancer who die and come to autopsy, the incidence of distant disease is generally similar to that at other sites.

TNM stage at initial treatment appears to influence the subsequent development of distant metastasis [30,35,36] (Table 5). Merino et al. [35] found in a

Table 4. Site-specific metastasis rates

	Kotwall et al. [30]	Peltier et al. [25]	O'Brien et al. [28]	Braund et al. [24]	Burke [45]	Zbären and Lehmann [31]	Probert et al. [34]	Merino et al. [35]	Brennan et al. [46]
Number	832	200	153	284	88	101	779	5019	769
Minimum follow-up	Autopsy	Autopsy	Autopsy	Autopsy	Autopsy	Autopsy	5 yr	2 yr	3 yr
Oral cavity				40%		32%	14%	8%	
Floor of mouth	43%	23%	27%	6%					17%
Tongue	49%	33%	33%		25%				15%
Other	32%	13%		36%					17%
Oropharynx						34%	11%	15%	
Base of tongue	53%								20%
Tonsil	45%	13%		11%					21%
Other	47%	15%	17%	18%				7%	
Hypopharynx	60%		46%	25%	50%	35%	15%	24%	
Nasopharynx	45%		60%			100%	22%	28%	
Paranasal sinus	38%	33%	43%	35%	66%	66%		9%	
Larynx						50%			
Supraglottis	44%		65%	18%			12%	15%	
Glottis	44%		57%	12%	13%		1%	3%	

249

Table 5. Incidence of distant metastasis by stage

	Merino et al. [35]	Kotwall et al. [30]	Vrikam et al. [36]
Stage I	2%	42%	
Stage II	6%	35%	
Stage III	9%	43%	
Stage IV	20%	55%	20%

Table 6. Metastasis rate and T stage

	Merino et al. [35]	Berger and Fletcher [41]	Loree and Strong [38]	Cerezo et al. [39][a]
T1	5%	25%	15%	35%
T2	10%	20%	27%	37%
T3	13%	23%	31%	23%
T4	16%	30%	40	38%
	p < 0.05	ns	p < 0.05	ns

[a] All patients stage III or IV.

clinical study of over 5000 patients that stage was a significant predictor for subsequent metastatic spread (p < 0.05). Two percent of patients with stage I, 6% with stage II, 9% with stage III, and 20% with stage IV developed distant spread. The study had a minimum follow-up period of only 2 years and may have underestimated the true incidence of distant metastases. In contrast, the autopsy series of over 800 patients reported by Kotwall et al. [30] found no significant differences with regard to initial stage. The frequency of metastases was 35% in stage II patients, and 42%, 43%, and 55% in stages I, III, and VI patients, respectively.

Tumor and nodal status have been examined independently in several studies [37,38] (Tables 6 and 7). The clinical reports have suggested that T stage is important. Two studies found that patients presenting with larger primary tumors more often develop metastasis. Merino et al. [35] found that only 5% of T1, 10% of T2, 13% of T3, and 16% of T4 tumors developed distant metastases. The size of the study allowed for a p value of 0.05 between each T stage grouping. Loree and Strong [38] found approximately two to three times the frequency of distant metastases in a study of patients with oral cavity squamous carcinomas. Ten percent of T1, 27% of T2, 31% of T3, and 40% of T4 tumors developed metastases, and these differences were statistically significant. Two studies found no differences in metastatic rate with regard to T stage. The study by Cerezo et al. [39] included only patients with neck disease, and not surprisingly, showed that in these

Table 7. Metastasis rate and N stage

	Merino et al. [35]	Berger and Fletcher [41]	Vrikam et al. [36]	Arons and Smith [32]	Loree and Strong [38]	Kotwall et al. [30]	Zbären and Lehmann [31]
N0	5%	9%	4%	12%	3% (stage I & II) 4% (stage III & IV)	42%	24%
N1	12%	17%				18%	
N2	22%	26% (2a) 23% (2b)	25% (N1–3)	28% (N1–3)	24% (N1–3)	40% (N2–3)	34% (N1–2)
N3	27%	38% (3a) 33% (3b)					54%

patients the frequency of distant metastasis was not independently related to the size of the primary. Berger and Fletcher [41] studied only patients with tonsil, base of tongue, or nasopharynx carcinomas. Twenty percent of patients in this report had no neck involvement; however, it is possible that the disease sites or stage distribution of patients in the study made it difficult to detect a relationship to T stage.

Many studies have shown advancing neck stage to have a significant impact upon rates of distant spread [30–32,35,36,38,41] (Table 7). In the clinical studies, patients without involved cervical nodes developed distant metastasis less than 12% of the time. Approximately 25% of those with N2 disease develop distant disease, twice as often as those with N0 or N1 disease. In the autopsy study by Zbären and Lehmann [31], a clear correlation with advancing nodal status was seen: 24% of those with N0 disease developed metastases compared to 34% of those with N1–N2 and 54% of those with N3 disease. Kotwall et al. [30], in an autopsy study, found a very high incidence of distant metastases among those with N0 disease. This finding highlights the bias of some autopsy studies that focus on patients who do poorly, but also suggests that some carcinomas may spread hematogenously prior to neck involvement.

Kalnins et al. reported that increased number of nodes and extension of squamous cancer into soft tissues led to a high risk of local and regional recurrence and distant metastasis [48]. Snow et al. [49] confirmed that the finding of extracapsular lymph node extension of carcinoma put patients at a particularly high risk for recurrent disease in the neck despite neck dissection. Twenty-one percent of patients with positive nodes developed neck recurrence and 23% developed distant metastases, half of whom had all neck disease controlled. It remains controversial whether extracapsular extension also portends a higher risk of metastatic disease. Hirabayashi et al. [50] found that extracapsular extension had no impact on the development of metastatic disease in larynx cancer.

Johnson et al. [51], in a nonrandomized trial, found that adjuvant chemotherapy improved survival in patients found to have extracapsular lymph node extension. Unfortunately, whether the impact of chemotherapy derived from a reduction of local, regional, or distant metastases could not be determined with accuracy because of the number of patients and the trial design. This is an important area for further study because most patients found to have distant metastases have had local or regional recurrence, and those with extracapsular extension may turn out to be a group that can be shown to benefit from adjuvant chemotherapy secondary to improved local, regional, or micrometastatic control.

McGuirt and McCabe [52,53] reported the impact of open neck biopsy on distant metastases. In their survey of 714 patients undergoing neck dissection for cervical lymph node metastasis, those who had a biopsy of the neck mass before definitive treatment had a 39% incidence of subsequent distant metastasis compared with a 23% incidence of metastasis for those who had no biopsy or biopsy at the time of definitive treatment (p < 0.01). Rates of local recurrence and wound complications were also higher in those with an open biopsy of the cervical node. It appears that disruption of the node by open biopsy, or possibly by extracapsular spread, may contribute to metastatic spread of the disease. The performance of fine needle aspiration biopsy in the neck has not been linked systematically to adverse local or distant outcomes in head and neck cancer. Tumor spread into the needle tract and into body cavities has been reported as a consequence of needle biopsies of the chest and abdomen [54,55].

In attempts to determine better predictors of outcome, researchers have begun to investigate the usefulness of histologic grading systems, DNA ploidy, nuclear volume, and tumor markers in head and neck squamous cancer. Histopathologic grading systems [56,57] are useful but suffer from intraobserver variability. Bundegaard et al. found that quantification of DNA content and nuclear volume, using flow cytometry and image analysis techniques, was superior to histopathologic classification in determining prognosis [58]. Patients with diploid tumors survive longer than those with nondiploid tumors [59]. Truelson et al. [60] calculated an adjusted DNA index for patients with advanced laryngeal cancers. The disease-free survival and recurrence rate were significantly lower in patients with a low index. This was an independent predictor, superior to standard staging. The value of these variables thus far has looked at survival as an end point. Their specific relationship to distant metastasis has not been carefully defined.

Blood group antigens of patients and those expressed on the cell surface of cancers may play a role in cell proliferation and contact inhibition, and alterations may increase the capacity of cancer cells to metastasize [61,62]. For example, Byrne et al. [63] found that patients who are rhesus blood group negative (rh−) had shorter survival than rhesus positive (rh+) patients. Wolf et al. [64] correlated loss of blood group antigens in tumor samples with a more aggressive tumor phenotype and earlier relapse. Patients whose tumors did not express the major histocompatability complex (MHC) class I antigens were more likely to die from tumor progression [48]. Although these markers may be predictive of relapse, they do not as yet distinguish local from distant recurrence. If relapse from standard treatment can be predicted more accurately, potentially more aggressive treatment programs could be planned for selected patient groups.

Role of chemotherapy in reducing metastases

With this as background data, it is easier to evaluate reports of clinical trials that demonstrate the effect of chemotherapy on distant metastases. Trials of induction and/or adjuvant chemotherapy for head and neck cancer have predominantly enrolled patients with advanced disease. Several trials in which patients were randomized to receive standard treatment or standard

Table 8. Rates of distant metastases in randomized trials of standard therapy versus standard therapy with chemotherapy for advanced resectable head and neck cancers

Author	Number of patients	Chemotherapy	Number with distant metastases		p value
			Standard treatment	Chemotherapy	
Laramore et al. [17]	442	C, F	51 (23%)	33 (15%)	p = 0.03
VALCSG [10]	332	C, F	29 (17%)	18 (11%)	p = 0.01
HNCP [15,65]	462	C	27 (19%)	26 (19%)[a] 13 (9%)[b]	p = 0.02
Schuller et al. [16,66]	158	C, Mtx, B	17 (22%)	8 (10%)	p = 0.07
Taylor et al. [67]	82	Mtx, FA or C, D	4 (10%)	4 (10%)	ns
Fu et al. [14]	104	B, Mtx	12 (24%)	17 (38%)	ns
Rossi et al. [68]	229	Cy, A, V	20 (17%)	23 (20%)	ns
Rentschler et al. [69]	55	Mtx	5 (19%)	7 (25%)	ns
Kun et al. [70]	83	B, Cy, Mtx, F	6 (15%)	4 (9%)	ns
Arcangeli et al. [71]	134	Mtx	13 (19%)	13 (19%)	ns
Fazekas et al. [72]	337	Mtx	27 (16%)	16 (10%)	
Lo et al. [4]	112	F	6 (12%)	5 (10%)	

C = cisplatin; F = fluorouracil; B = bleomycin; Mtx = methotrexate; Cy = cyclophosphamide; V = vincristine; D = doxorubicin; FA = folinic acid.
[a] Induction chemotherapy only.
[b] Induction chemotherapy and maintenance chemotherapy.
[c] Metastasis rate among those who initially attained a complete response.

treatment plus chemotherapy have been reported in detail [4,9,14–17,65–72] (Table 8). These clinical trials have confirmed that the incidence of distant spread in patients treated with standard therapy, including surgery, radiotherapy, or both, is approximately 10–20%. Seven of these studies showed no chemotherapy-related reduction in distant metastatic rate. Most of the negative trials, however, had too few patients to detect a small difference in the frequency of distant disease. Four studies demonstrated a clear reduction in the rate of distant metastases [9,15–17,65,66,73].

In a study by the Head and Neck Intergroup, 442 patients with completely resected, advanced stage squamous cell carcinoma of the oral cavity, oropharynx, hypopharynx, or larynx were randomized to receive (1) postoperative radiation therapy or (2) three cycles of chemotherapy followed by radiation therapy [17,73]. Chemotherapy consisted of cisplatin, $100\,mg/m^2$ given on day 1, and 5-fluorouracil, $1000\,mg/m^2/day$ for 5 days, given by continuous infusion on day 1–5, repeated every 3 weeks. Chemotherapy began within 4 weeks of surgery and was generally well tolerated. No difference in survival, disease-free survival, or local control was evident at a mean time at risk of 46 months. There was, however, a difference in the overall frequency of distant metastases: 23% in the radiotherapy arm and 15% in the radiotherapy/chemotherapy arm ($p = 0.03$). The time to development of distant disease was also significantly reduced in the latter arm.

The Department of Veterans Affairs Laryngeal Cancer Study Group (VALSG) conducted a trial investigating the use of chemotherapy for organ preservation in 332 patients with advanced, resectable larynx cancer. Patients were randomized to receive (1) laryngectomy and postoperative irradiation or (2) induction chemotherapy followed by irradiation in responders [10]. The chemotherapy was the same regimen used by the Head and Neck Intergroup. Three cycles of induction chemotherapy were given to responding patients followed by radiation therapy. Salvage laryngectomy was used for non-responders and those with local recurrence in the chemotherapy arm. At a median follow-up of 33 months, there was no significant difference in the 2-year survival rate. Thirty-six percent of patients in the chemotherapy arm eventually required salvage laryngectomy. The distant metastatic rate was lower in the chemotherapy arm (11%), than in the standard treatment arm (17%; $p = 0.001$).

The Head and Neck Contracts Program (HNCP) reported on 462 patients with resectable squamous cell carcinoma of the oral cavity, hypopharynx, or larynx, randomized to treatment with (1) surgery and postoperative irradiation, (2) induction chemotherapy followed by surgery and irradiation, or (3) induction chemotherapy followed by surgery and irradiation, and then by maintenance chemotherapy [15,65]. The induction chemotherapy consisted of one cycle of cisplatin, $100\,mg/m^2$ on day 1, followed by bleomycin, $15\,mg/m^2$ IV bolus on day 3, and an infusion of bleomycin, $15\,mg/m^2/day$ for 5 days. The maintenance chemotherapy was cisplatin, $80\,mg/m^2$ given as a 24-hour infusion once every 4 weeks for an additional six treatment cycles.

Despite poor compliance with the maintenance chemotherapy arm of this study, the frequency of distant metastases was significantly reduced and the time to first distant relapse was prolonged in the maintenance chemotherapy arm. Nineteen percent of each group of patients randomized to receive standard therapy or induction chemotherapy without maintenance chemotherapy developed distant metastases. Only 9% of those treated with induction chemotherapy, surgery, radiotherapy, and maintenance chemotherapy developed metastases. This difference was statistically significant (p = 0.025), and the time to first distant relapse was also prolonged in the maintenance group. Although no overall survival or disease-fee survival benefit was documented, in a subsequent subset analysis of patients with oral cavity cancers, those on the maintenance arm had a significantly improved disease-free survival compared with the standard or induction chemotherapy arms. The same was true for patients with N1 and N2 disease on the maintenance arm.

In a study performed by the Southwest Oncology Group (SWOG) [66], 158 patients with advanced stage, resectable squamous cancers of the oral cavity, oropharynx, hypopharynx, and larynx were randomized to receive (1) surgery and postoperative radiotherapy, or (2) induction chemotherapy followed by surgery and radiotherapy. The chemotherapy used in this clinical trial was cisplatin, $50 \, mg/m^2$, methotrexate, $40 \, mg/m^2$, and vincristine, $2 \, mg$ on day 1; and bleomycin, $15 \, U/m^2$, on days 1 and 8. The chemotherapy was given every 3 weeks for a total of three cycles. With a median follow-up of approximately 5 years, there was no statistically significant difference between the two treatment groups with respect to overall survival, disease-free survival, or local failure. Distant metastases occurred in 27% of patients in the induction chemotherapy group and 52% of the standard group (p = 0.07). Almost all metastases were to the lung. Patients with hypopharyngeal primaries were most likely to have recurrences at distant sites, whereas patients with primaries of the oral cavity, oropharynx, or larynx were more likely to have local recurrences. This study was mature at its reporting, and the frequency of distant spread reported in the standard treatment group is closer to that reported in autopsy series. This longer follow-up may explain a distant recurrence rate that is higher than that seen in other trials of similar patients groups.

These four trials differ from the other trials listed in Table 8 in that at least three cycles of a cisplatini-based chemotherapy were administered. In the Intergroup study, chemotherapy followed surgery but preceded radiotherapy. In the VALCSG trial and the SWOG trial, chemotherapy preceded definitive treatment. In the HNCP study, chemotherapy preceded and followed standard therapy. From these three trials it is difficult to determine the optimal timing or duration of chemotherapy. Longer follow-up periods are needed to fully evaluate three of the studies, as 5 years is needed for a more reliable analysis of treatment failure patterns. While 3-year results are fairly accurate in patients who receive standard treatment, there is the possibility that the detection of distant disease is delayed by chemotherapy inhibiting tumor deposits at metastatic sites. The practice of increasing the time interval between follow-up visits after 2–3 years would also bias the reporting of distant failures if such events were simply delayed, but not eradicated, by chemotherapy.

Role of chemotherapy in nasopharyngeal carcinoma

Nasopharyngeal carcinoma has one of the highest rates of distant metastatic spread of the head and neck cancers [28,30,35,64–76]. The need for effective adjuvant therapy is particularly relevant because local control can be achieved with radiotherapy, even in advanced cases [77]. Nasopharyngeal carcinoma has a very high response rate to chemotherapy, with response rates to cisplatin-based regimens in the neoadjuvant setting of 80–95% [78–80] and in the recurrent disease setting of 40–70% [81,82]. These factors suggest that early systemic treatment may have an impact on the distant metastatic rate and survival.

Several uncontrolled studies have focused on improving the outcome of advanced stage patients through the use of chemotherapy [78–81,82]. Rossi et al. [68] randomized 113 patients with advanced stage disease after radiation therapy to treatment with six monthly cycles of chemotherapy with vincristine $1.2\,mg/m^2$, doxorubicin $40\,mg/m^2$, and cyclophosphamide $200\,mg/m^2$ orally on days 1–4. Fifty percent of the patients in this study developed distant metastatic disease, and there was no difference in the treatment groups. A large Intergroup trial (INT 0099, RTOG 8817, EST 2388, SWOG 8892) is underway that randomizes patients to treatment with radiotherapy alone versus three cycles of cisplatin $100\,mg/m^2$ given concurrently with radiotherapy on days 1, 21, and 43, followed by three monthly cycles of chemotherapy with cisplatin, $80\,mg/m^2$, and fluorouracil, $1000\,mg/m^2/day$, for 96 hours by infusion. With a planned accrual of over 200 patients, this trial should answer definitively whether cisplatin-based chemotherapy will decrease distant metastases in patients with advanced nasopharyngeal cancer.

Other strategies

Other strategies for reducing distant metastases include the use of biologic response modifiers, specific immunotherapy, and differentiating agents. The investigation of interferons [83,84] and interleukins [85–87] for head and neck squamous cancer has not focused on adjuvant therapy. A trial of adjuvant levamisole [88] reported a trend toward improved survival (p < 0.06) in the levamisole group due to benefit in the patient subsets with oral cavity cancer (p < 0.01) and stage II disease (p < 0.02). Adjuvant isotretinoin (13-*cis* retinoic acid) did not affect survival or distant metastasis

257

in one study [89]. Newer approaches, such as growth factor suppressors [90] and antimetastasis agents [91], may be useful in the future.

Conclusions

Randomized trials have shown that adjuvant chemotherapy is effective in reducing the incidence of distant metastases in head and neck squamous cancers. The most likely mechanism is early eradication of microscopic disease. Nevertheless, in the clinical trials conducted so far, adjuvant chemotherapy has had no impact on survival. Most deaths in this disease are attributable to local recurrence. Intercurrent diseases and second primary cancers are also responsible for a significant number of deaths. At present, cisplatin-containing chemotherapy regimens are tolerable but probably too toxic to routinely administer to patients who have a relatively low risk of developing metastatic disease. The challenge for the future will be to develop more active and better tolerated chemotherapy programs that will improve local control as well as reduce distant disease. As our understanding of the biology of carcinogenesis and metastasis improves and the investigation of poor prognostic indicators and tumor markers progresses, we may be able to more successfully identify those patients who could benefit from chemotherapy.

References

1. Leone LA, Albala MM, Rege VB. Treatment of carcinoma of the head and neck with intravenous methotrexate. Cancer 21:828–837, 1968.
2. Morton RP, Stell PM. Cytotoxic chemotherapy for patients with terminal squamous carcinoma — does it influence survival? Clin Otolaryngol 9:175–180, 1984.
3. Pinto HA, Jacobs C. Chemotherapy for recurrent and metastatic head and neck cancer. Hematol Oncol Clin North Am 5:667–686, 1991.
4. Lo TCM, Wiley AL, Ansfield FJ, Brandenburg JH, Davis HL, Gollin FF, et al. Combined radiation therapy and 5-fluorouracil for advanced squamous cell carcinoma of the oral cavity and oropharynx: A randomized study. Radiat Ther Nuclear Med 126:229–235, 1975.
5. Shanta V, Krishnamurthi S. Combined bleomycin and radiotherapy in oral cancer. Clin Radiol 31:617–620, 1980.
6. Weissberg JB, Yung HS, Papac RJ, Sasaki C, Fischer S, Lawrence R, Rockwell S, et al. Randomized trial of mitomycin-C as an adjunct to radiotherapy in head and neck cancer. Int J Radiat Oncol Biol Phys 17:3–9, 1989.
7. Marcial VA, Pajak TF, Mohiuddin M, Cooper JS, Sarraf MA, Mowry PA, et al. Concomitant cisplatin chemotherapy and radiotherapy in advanced mucosal squamous cell carcinoma of the head and neck. Cancer 66:1861–1868, 1990.
8. Merlano M, Vitale V, Rosso R, Benasso M, Corvo R, Cavallari M, et al. Treatment of advanced squamous cell carcinoma of the head and neck with alternating chemotherapy and radiotherapy. N Engl J Med 327:1115–1121, 1992.
9. Jacobs CJ, Goffinet DR, Goffinet L, Kohler M, Fee WE. Chemotherapy as a substitute for surgery in the treatment of advanced resectable head and neck cancer. A report from the Northern California Oncology Group. Cancer 60:1178–1183, 1987.

10. The Department of Veterans Affairs Laryngeal Cancer Study Group. Induction chemotherapy plus radiation compared with surgery plus radiation in patients with advanced laryngeal cancer. N Engl J Med 324:1685–1690, 1991.

11. Vokes EE, Mick R, Lester EP, Panje WR, Weichselbaum, RR. Cisplatin and fluorouracil chemotherapy does not yield long-term benefit in locally advanced head and neck cancer: Results from a single institution. J Clin Oncol 9:1376–1384, 1991.

12. Tannock I, Browman G. Lack of evidence for a role of chemotherapy in the routine management of locally advanced head and neck cancer. J Clin Oncol 4:1121–1126, 1984.

13. Jacobs CJ. Adjuvant chemotherapy for head and neck cancer. J Clin Oncol 7:823–826, 1989.

14. Fu KK, Phillips TL, Silverberg IJ, Jacobs C, Goffinet D, Chun C, et al. Combined radiotherapy and chemotherapy with bleomycin and methotrexate for advanced inoperable head and neck cancer: Update of a Northern California Oncology Group randomized trial. J Clin Oncol 5:1410–1418, 1987.

15. Head and Neck Contracts Program. Adjuvant chemotherapy for advanced head and neck squamous carcinoma: Final report of the Head and Neck Contracts Program. Cancer 60:301–311, 1987.

16. Schuller DE, Stein DW, Metch B. Analysis of treatment failure patterns. A Southwest Oncology Group study. Arch Otolaryngol Head Neck Surg 115:834–836, 1989.

17. Laramore GE, Scott CB, Al-Sarraf M, Haselow RE, Ervin TJ, Wheeler R, et al. Adjuvant chemotherapy for resectable squamous cell carcinomas of the head and neck: Report on Intergroup study 0034. Int J Radiat Oncol Biol Phys 23:705–713, 1992.

18. Crile CW. Excision of cancer of the head and neck. JAMA 47:1780–1785, 1906.

19. Crile CW. Cancer of jaws, tongue, cheeks and lips. Surg Gynecol Obstet 36:159–162, 1923.

20. Dorrance GM, McShane JK. Cancer of the tongue and floor of the mouth. Ann Surg 88:1007–1021, 1928.

21. Castigliano SG, Rominger CJ. Distant metastasis from carcinoma of the oral cavity. Am J Roentgenol 71:997–1006, 1954.

22. Price LW. Metastasis in squamous carcinoma. Am J Cancer 22:1–16, 1934.

23. Willis RA. The Spread of Tumors in the Human Body. London: JA Churchill, 1934.

24. Braund RR, Martin HE. Distant metastasis in cancer of the upper respiratory and alimentary tracts. Surg Gynecol Obstet 73:63–71, 1941.

25. Peltier LF, Thomas LB, Barclay THC, Kremen AJ. The incidence of distant metastases among patients dying with head and neck cancers. Surgery 30:827–833, 1951.

26. Hoye RC, Herrold KM, Smith RR, Thomas LB. A clinicopathological study of epidermoid carcinoma of the head and neck. Cancer 15:741–749, 1962.

27. Ju DMC. A study of the behavior of cancer of the head and neck during its late and terminal phases. Am J Surg 108:552–557, 1964.

28. O'Brien PH, Carlson R, Steubner EA, Staley CT. Distant metastases in epidermoid cell carcinoma of the head and neck. Cancer 27:304–307, 1971.

29. Dennington ML, Carter DR, Meyers AD. Distant metastases in head and neck epidermoid carcinoma. Laryngoscope 90:196–201, 1980.

30. Kotwall C, Sako K, Razack S, Rao U, Bakamjian V, Shedd DP. Metastatic patterns in squamous cell cancer of the head and neck. Am J Surg 154:439–442, 1987.

31. Zbären P, Lehmann W. Frequency and sites of distant metastases in head and neck squamous cell carcinoma. Arch Otolaryngol Head Neck Surg 113:762–764, 1987.

32. Arons MS, Smith RR. Distant metastases and local recurrence in head and neck cancer. Ann Surg 154:235–240, 1961.

33. Rubenfeld S, Kaplan G, Holder AA. Distant metastases from head and neck cancer. Am J Roentgenol 87:441–448, 1962.

34. Probert JC, Thompson RW, Bagshaw MA. Patterns of spread of distant metastases in head and neck cancer. Cancer 33:127–133, 1974.

35. Merino OR, Lindberg RD, Fletcher GH. An analysis of distant metastases from squamous cell carcinoma of the upper respiratory and digestive tracts. Cancer 40:145–151, 1977.

36. Vikram B, Strong EW, Shah JP, Spiro R. Failure at distant sites following multimodality treatment for advanced head and neck cancer. Head Neck Surg 6:730–733, 1984.
37. Amdur RJ, Parsons JT, Mendenhall WM, Million RR, Stringer SP, Cassisi NJ. Postoperative irradiation for squamous cell carcinoma of the head and neck: An analysis of treatment results and complications. Int J Radiat Oncol Biol Phys 16:25–36, 1989.
38. Loree TR, Strong EW. The significance of positive margins in oral cavity squamous carcinoma. Am J Surg 160:410–414, 1990.
39. Cerezo L, Millan I, Torre A, Aragon G, Otero J. Prognostic factors for survival and tumor control in cervical lymph node metastases from head and neck cancer. Cancer 69:1224–1234, 1991.
40. Roland NJ, Caslin AW, Nash J, Stell PM. Value of grading squamous cell carcinoma of the head and neck. Head Neck 14:224–229, 1992.
41. Berger DS, Fletcher GH. Distant metastases following local control of squamous cell carcinoma of the nasopharynx, tonsillar fossa, and base of the tongue. Radiology 10:141–143, 1971.
42. Gowen GF, DeSuto-Nagy G. The incidence and sites of distant metastases in head and neck carcinoma. Surg Gynecol Obstet 116:603–607, 1963.
43. Bisel HF, Wróblewski F, LaDue JS. Incidence and clinical manifestations of cardiac metastases. JAMA 153:712–715, 1953.
44. Hanfling SM. Metastatic cancer to the heart. Circulation 22:474–483, 1960.
45. Burke EM. Metastases in squamous cell carcinoma. Am J Cancer 30:493–503, 1937.
46. Brennan CT, Sessions DG, Spitznagel EL, Harvey JE. Surgical pathology of cancer of the oral cavity and oropharynx. Laryngoscope 101:1175–1197, 1991.
47. Marks JE, Kurnik B, Powers WE, et al. Carcinoma of the pyriform sinus: An analysis of treatment results and patterns of failure. Cancer 41:1008–1015, 1978.
48. Kalnins IK, Leonard Ag, Sako K, Pazak MS, Shedd DP. Correlation between prognosis and degree of lymph node involvement in carcinoma of the oral cavity. Am J Surg 134:450–454, 1977.
49. Snow GB, Annyas AA, Van Slooten EA, Bartelink H, Hart AAM. Prognostic factors of neck node metastasis. Clin Otolaryngol 7:185–192, 1982.
50. Hirabayashi H, Koshii K, Uno K, Ohgaki H, Nakasone Y, Fujisawa T, et al. Extracapsular spread of squamous cell carcinoma in neck nodes: Prognostic factor of laryngeal cancer. Laryngoscope 101:502–506, 1991.
51. Johnson JT, Meyers EN, Mayernik DG, Nolan TA, Sigler BA, Wagner RL. Adjuvant methotrexate-5-fluorouracil for extracapsular squamous cell carcinoma in cervical metastasis. Laryngoscope 100:590–592, 1990.
52. McGuirt WF, McCabe BF. Significance of node biopsy before definitive treatment of cervical metastatic carcinoma. Laryngoscope 88:594–597, 1978.
53. McGuirt WF. Diagnosis and management of masses in the neck, with special emphasis on metastatic malignant disease. Oncology 4:85–98, 1990.
54. Smith EH. The hazards of fine-needle aspiration biopsy. Ultrasound Med Biol 10:629–634, 1984.
55. Foussel F. Risk of metastasis during fine-needle aspiration. J Clin Pathol 43:878–879, 1990.
56. Jakobsson PA, Enroth CM, Killander D, Moberger G, Mårtenson B. Histologic classification and grading in carcinoma of the larynx. Acta Radiol Ther Phys Biol 12:1–8, 1973.
57. Crissman JD, Liu WY, Gluckman JL, Cummings G. Prognostic value of histopathologic parameters in squamous cell carcinoma of the oropharynx. Cancer 54:2995–3001, 1984.
58. Bundgaard T, Sørensen FB, Gaihede M, Søgaard H, Overgaard J. Stereologic, histolopathologic, flow cytometric, and clinical parameters in the prognostic evaluation of 74 patients with intraoral squamous cell carcinomas. Cancer 70:1–13, 1992.
59. Zatterstrom UK, Wennerberg J, Ewers SB, Willen R, Attewell R. Prognostic factors in head and neck cancer: Histologic grading, DNA ploidy, and nodal status. Head Neck 13:477–487, 1991.
60. Truelson JM, Fisher SG, Beals TE, McClatchey KD, Wolf GT. DNA content and histo-

260

logic growth pattern correlate with prognosis in patients with advanced squamous cell carcinoma of the larynx. Cancer 70:56–62, 1992.

61. Dabelsteen E, Clausen H, Mandel U. Aberrant glycosylation in oral malignant and pre-malignant lesions. J Oral Pathol Med 20:361–368, 1991.

62. Schantz SP. Experimental head and neck onocology. Curr Opin Oncol 4:478–484, 1992.

63. Byrne M, Eide GE, Lilleng R, Langmark F, Thrane PS, Dabelsteen E. A multivariate study of the prognosis of oral squamous cell carcinomas: Are blood group and hemoglobin new prognostic factors? Cancer 68:1994–1998, 1991.

64. Wolf GT, Carey TE, Schmaltz SP, McClatchey KD, Poore J, Glaser L, et al. Altered antigen expression predicts outcome in squamous cell carcinoma of the head and neck. J Natl Cancer Inst 82:1566–1572, 1990.

65. Jacobs CJ, Makuch R. Efficacy of adjuvant chemotherapy for patients with resectable head and neck cancer: A subset analysis of the Head and Neck Contracts Program. J Clin Oncol 8:838–847, 1990.

66. Schuller DE, Metch B, Stein DW, Mattox D, McCracken JD. Preoperative chemotherapy in advanced resectable head and neck cancer: Final report of the Southwest Oncology Group. Laryngoscope 98:1205–1211, 1988.

67. Taylor SG, Applebaum E, Showel JL, Norusis M, Holinger L, Hutchinson J, et al. A randomized trial of adjuvant chemotherapy in head and neck cancer. J Clin Oncol 3:672–679, 1985.

68. Rossi A, Molinari R, Boracchi P, Del Vecchio M, Marubini M, Nava M, et al. Adjuvant chemotherapy with vincristine, cyclophosphamide, and doxorubicin after radiotherapy in local-regional nasopharyngeal cancer: Results of a 4-year multicenter randomized study. J Clin Oncol 6:1401–1410, 1988.

69. Rentschler RE, Wilbur DW, Petti GH, Chonkich G, Hilliard D, Camacho E, et al. Adjuvant methotrexate escalated to toxicity for resectable stage III and IV squamous head and neck carcinomas—a prospective, randomized study. J Clin Oncol 5:278–285, 1987.

70. Kun LE, Toohill RJ, Holoye PY, Duncavage J, Byhardt R, Ritch P, et al. A randomized study of adjuvant chemotherapy for cancer of the upper aerodigestive tract. Int J Radiat Oncol Biol Phys 12:173–178, 1986.

71. Arcangeli G, Nervi C, Righini R, Creton G, Mirri A, Guerra A. Combined radiation and drugs: The effect of intra-arterial chemotherapy followed by radiotherapy in head and neck cancer. Radiother Oncol 1:101–107, 1983.

72. Fazekas JT, Sommer C, Kramer S, Concannon J, Stein J, Griem M, et al. Adjuvant intravenous methotrexate or definitive radiotherapy alone for advanced squamous cancers of the oral cavity, oropharynx, supraglottic larynx, or hypopharynx. Int J Radiat Oncol Biol Phys 6:533–541, 1980.

73. Schuller DE, Laramore G, Al-Sarraf M, Jacobs J, Pajak TF. Combined therapy for resectable head and neck cancer. A phase III intergroup study. Arch Otoloaryngol Head Neck Surg 115:364–368, 1989.

74. Ahmad A, Stefani S. Distant metastasis of nasopharyngeal carcinoma: A study of 256 male patients. J Surg Oncol 33:194–197, 1986.

75. Bedwinek JM, Perez CA, Keys D. Analysis of failures after definitive irradiation for carcinoma of the nasopharynx. Cancer 45:2725–2729, 1980.

76. Khor TH, Tan EJ, Chia KB. Distant metastases in nasopharyngeal carcinoma. Clin Radiol 29:27–30, 1978.

77. Vikram B, Mishra UB, Strong EW, Manolatos S. Patterns of failure in carcinoma of the nasopharynx: I. Failure at the primary site. Int J Radiat Oncol Biol Phys 11:1455–1459, 1985.

78. Hill BT, Price LA, MacRae KD. The promising role of safe initial non-cisplatin-containing combination chemotherapy in nasopharyngeal tumors. Cancer Invest 5:517–522, 1987.

79. Dimery IW, Legha SS, Peters LJ, Goepfert H, Oswald MJ. Adjuvant chemotherapy for advanced nasopharyngeal carcinoma. Cancer 60:943–949, 1987.

80. Cvitkovic E, Bachouchi M, Armand P. Nasopharyngeal carcinoma: Biology, natural his-

tory, and therapeutic implications. Hematol Oncol Clin North Am 5:821–838, 1991.

81. Decker D, Drelichman A, Al-Sarraf M, Crissman J, Reed ML. Chemotherapy for nasopharygeal carcinoma: A 10-year experience. Cancer 58:843–849, 1983.

82. Al-Sarraf M, Pajak TF, Cooper JS, Mohiuddin M, Herskovik A, Ager PJ. Chemo-radiotherapy in patients with locally advanced nasopharyngeal carcinoma: A Radiation Therapy Oncology Group study. J Clin Oncol 8:1342–1351, 1990.

83. Richtsmeier WJ, Koch WM, McGuire WP, Poole ME, Chang EH. Phase I–II study of advanced head and neck squamous cell carcinoma patients treated with recombinant human interferon gamma. Arch Otolaryngol Head Neck Surg 116:1271–1277, 1990.

84. Vlock DR, Johnson J, Meyers E, Day R, Gooding WE, Whiteside T, et al. Preliminary trial of nonrecombinant interferon alpha in recurrent squamous cell carcinoma of the head and neck. Head Neck 13:15–21, 1991.

85. Cortesina G, De Stefani A, Galeazzi E, Cavallo GP, Jemma C, Giovarelli M, et al. Interleukin-2 injected around tumor draining lymph nodes in head and neck cancer. Head Neck 13:125–131, 1991.

86. Vlock DR. Immunobiologic aspects of head and neck cancer. Hematol Oncol Clin North Am 5:797–820, 1991.

87. Valone FH, Gandara DR, Deisseroth AB, Perez EA, Rayner A, Aronson FR, et al. Interleukin-2, cisplatin, and 5-fluorouracil for patients with non-small cell lung and head/neck carcinomas. J Immunother 10:207–213, 1991.

88. Wanebo HJ, Hilal EY, Pinsky CM, Strong EW, Mike V, Hirshaut Y, et al. Randomized trial of levamisole in patients with squamous cancer of the head and neck: A preliminary report. Cancer Treat Rep 62:1663–1669, 1978.

89. Hong WK, Lippman SM, Itri L, Karp DD, Lee JS, Byers RM, et al. Prevention of second primary tumors with isotretinoin in squamous cell carcinoma of the head and neck. N Engl J Med 323:795–801, 1990.

90. La Rocca RV, Stein CA, Meyers CE. Suramin: Prototype of a new generation of antitumor compounds. Cancer Cells 2:106–115, 1990.

91. Kohn EC, Liotta LA. L651582: A novel antiproliferative and antimetastasis agent. J Natl Cancer Inst 82:54–60, 1990.

14. Experimental therapeutic approaches for recurrent head and neck cancer

Arlene A. Forastiere and Susan G. Urba

Patients with recurrent head and neck cancer present a challenge to physicians because of the often devastating complications of local-regional disease. Necrotic, ulcerated tumor masses can lead to disabling pain, infection, cranial nerve dysfunction, airway compromise, impairment of speech, and swallowing dysfunction with attendant dehydration and malnutrition. In addition, these patients are often rejected by family and society at large because of their cosmetic deformities and disabilities.

Forty to 60% of patient deaths are directly attributable to uncontrolled local-regional disease [1]; therefore, this is clearly a problem of significant proportions. Metastatic disease accounts for 20–30% of deaths; however, autopsy series reveal a much higher incidence of 46% on average, with a range of 32–60% depending on primary site [2]. Approximately 90% of patients with distant metastases die with uncontrolled tumor at the primary site or in the neck [2]. Thus, innovative therapies are desperately needed to palliate the large numbers of patients who will develop and die from local-regional recurrence and distant metastases.

Palliation is the term used to describe the goal of chemotherapy employed in the setting of recurrent disease that is not considered potentially curable with salvage surgery or radiotherapy. Cisplatin, carboplatin, methotrexate, 5-fluorouracil, and bleomycin are the most commonly used agents today, singly or in combination. Randomized trials comparing multi-drug regimens to single agents have been reviewed in detail in recent publications [3–5]. Some of these trials show improved overall response rates with combination chemotherapy but at a cost of increased toxicity without a survival advantage.

These results are exemplified by two recently published randomized trials comparing cisplatin and 5-fluorouracil (5-FU) to single agents (Table 1) [6,7]. Both studies accrued large numbers of patients and used standard doses and scheduling of the combinations cisplatin + 5-FU and carboplatin + 5-FU and the single agents cisplatin, 5-FU, and methotrexate. The trial

Hong, Waun Ki and Weber, Randal S., (eds.), Head and Neck Cancer. © 1995 Kluwer Academic Publishers. ISBN 0-7923-3015-3. All rights reserved.

263

Table 1. Randomized trials of cisplatin and 5-fluorouracil versus single agents

Author [ref]	Outcome	Treatment arm		
		1 CDDP/5-FU (N = 79)	2 CDDP (N = 83)	3 5-FU (N = 83)
Jacobs et al. [6]	CR + PR	32%	17%	13%
	MST (mos.)	5.5	5.0	6.1
	p values for response	arm 1 vs. 2, p = 0.035 arm 1 vs. 3, p = 0.005		
Forastiere et al. [7]		CDDP/5-FU (N = 87)	Carbo/5-FU (N = 86)	MTX (N = 88)
	CR + PR	32%	21%	10%
	MST (mos)	6.6	5.0	5.6
	p values for response	arm 1 vs. 3, p < 0.001 arm 2 vs. 3, p = 0.05		

CDDP = cisplatin; CR = complete response; PR = partial response; MST = median survival time; MTX = methotrexate.

reported by Jacobs et al. compared the combination cisplatin + 5-FU to each drug used singly [6], and the trial reported by Forastiere et al. compared the combinations cisplatin + 5-FU and carboplatin + 5-FU to single-agent methotrexate [7]. The same response rate of 32% to the cisplatin + 5-FU combination was observed in both trials. The combination regimens were statistically superior in terms of overall response rates, but median survivals were not significantly different, ranging from 5.0 to 6.6 months for all treatment arms.

Thus, treatment of recurrent squamous cell carcinoma of the head and neck with currently available cytotoxic agents provides very limited palliation. Approximately one third of patients achieve a brief response that affords transient diminution of pain and size of the tumor. Occasionally, complete response occurs that is associated with longer survival. These patients generally have an excellent performance status and small tumor burden. However, the number of patients achieving complete response is too small to impact on overall survival. Therefore, although an established role for chemotherapy in the management of head and neck cancer is the palliation of recurrent disease, investigators have not demonstrated any significant benefit for this form of treatment. All patients should, therefore, be considered for experimental therapies, which are the subject of this chapter.

New cytotoxic drugs

Piritrexim

Piritrexim is a newly developed lipid-soluble folate antagonist. It crosses the cell membrane by simple diffusion in a carrier-independent fashion because of its lipophilic nature. Its mechanism of action is the inhibition of incorporation of deoxyuridine into DNA. Uen et al. conducted a Phase II study of piritrexim in 34 patients with recurrent or unresectable head and neck cancer [8]. Patients were treated with $100 \, mg/m^2$ b.i.d. × 5 days every 2–3 weeks. Toxicity consisted of leukopenia, thrombocytopenia, and mucositis. The overall response rate was 27% (complete response = 9%, partial response = 18%). Median duration of response was 162 days. Therefore, piritrexim showed moderate activity against head and neck cancer, and because it has better cellular penetration than methotrexate, it may be effective in patients refractory to that agent.

Degardin and colleagues reported similar results in 25 heavily pretreated patients with recurrent or metastatic squamous cell carcinoma of the head and neck [9]. Piritrexim was given orally, 25 mg three times a day for 4 days each week. One complete and four partial responses were observed for a median duration of 3 months.

The activity of piritrexim sequenced with methotrexate was evaluated in 30 patients. Methotrexate, $50 \, mg/m^2$ intravenous bolus, was administered on day 1, and piritrexim, $75 \, mg/m^2$ bid, on days 8–12 [10]. Each cycle was repeated every 21 days. The response rate was disappointing, with 17% of patients achieving a partial response, and a median time to progression of 1.4 months. Thus, the response rate to antifolate chemotherapy was not enhanced by the sequential use of the two drugs. However, the use of higher doses and more rapid sequencing is under investigation.

Taxol

Taxol is a unique anticancer drug that is isolated from the bark of the Western Yew, *Taxus brevifolia*. The drug is phase specific, promoting microtubule assembly and stabilizing tubulin polymers against depolymerization in the G_2/M phase. In phase I trials, activity was observed in a number of solid tumors, including head and neck cancer. The principal toxicity was reversible neutropenia. The recommended dose for phase II trials ranged from 200 to $250 \, mg/m^2$; above $250 \, mg/m^2$ neurotoxicity was dose limiting [11]. In some solid tumors, notably overian cancer, responses were observed in heavily pretreated patients at taxol doses of $110–135 \, mg/m^2$ [12]. Therefore, the optimal dose of taxol required to achieve response is not known. To evaluate the antitumor activity of taxol in squamous carcinoma of the head and neck, the Eastern Cooperative Oncology Group conducted a phase II trial of taxol in chemotherapy-naive patients with recurrent and metastatic disease. The regimen tested was taxol 250 mg/m^2 by 24-hour continuous infusion and G-CSF 5 µg/kg/day by subcutaneous injection starting day 3. The preliminary results in 17 evaluable patients were two complete and five partial responses (41% CR + PR). The trial is ongoing and will accrue a total of 30 evaluable patients [13].

These results suggest activity for taxol in head and neck cancer. Questions that will be addressed in future trials include determining whether a dose-response effect exists for taxol and evaluating taxol in combination with cisplatin and other drugs with activity against squamous cell head and neck cancer. The maximum tolerable dose for the combination of cisplatin + taxol + G-CSF has been determined in a phase I trial in solid tumors [14]. A dose of cisplatin 75 mg/m^2 + taxol 250 mg/m^2 + G-CSF was tolerable and will be employed in subsequent evaluations of the combination in head and neck cancer.

Ifosfamide

Although ifosfamide has demonstrated antitumor activity in many solid tumors, including overian cancer, testicular cancer, sarcoma, and small cell lung cancer, its efficacy in head and neck cancer is currently under investigation. Two published trials suggest activity in head and neck cancer when ifosfamide is used in chemotherapy-naive patients [15,16]. A study from Argentina evaluated ifosfamide in patients with recurrent disease [15]. Twenty-eight patients were treated with ifosfamide, 3.5 g/m^2 as an 8-hour intravenous infusion on days 1–5, and Mesna. Cycles were repeated every 28 days for a maximum of eight cycles. Overall response to the chemotherapy was 42.7% (14.2% complete response and 28.5% partial respones). The authors concluded that this regimen had significant activity and would be further tested in the neoadjuvant setting. The second trial reported by Buesa et al. administered ifosfamide at a dose of 5 g/m^2 as a 24-hour infusion, with Mesna every 3 weeks [16]. An objective response rate of 28% (9/32) was observed. In both of these trials, prior treatment was limited to surgery and radiotherapy. A third study reported by the Rotterdam Cooperative Head and Neck Cancer Study Group [17] using the same 5 g/m^2 ifosfamide regimen resulted in only one partial response in 17 patients; however, all had previously received other chemotherapy. In the United States, a phase II trial of ifosfamide in head and neck cancer is in progress at the M. D. Anderson Cancer Center.

Chemoprotectants and biomodulators

The toxicities that commonly limit chemotherapy dosage are myelosuppression, nephrotoxicity, ototoxicity, motor and sensory peripheral neuropathy, and mucositis. The development of agents that could protect against these toxicities would result in an improved therapeutic index and the ability to safely intensify the dose. Assuming a steep dose-response curve for most cytotoxic agents with activity against carcinoma of the head and neck, the potential exists for improving complete response, duration of response, and survival.

WR-2721

WR-2721 is an aminothiol that has been of interest to investigators because preclinical studies showed selective protection of normal tissues from some of the toxicities of radiation and chemotherapy [18]. A mechanism for this selective protection is the differential absorption of the compound between normal tissue and tumors. WR-2721 rapidly concentrates in normal tissues via facilitated diffusion, but tumor cells absorb smaller amounts by passive diffusion [19]. This may be related to the hydrophilicity of the compound. At the cell membrane, it is dephosphorylated to a free sulfhydryl, which then may scavenge free radicals, repair radicals on essential molecules, and form mixed disulfides to protect normal cells [20].

Data from animal models suggested that WR-2721 could selectively protect normal tissue from cisplatin toxic effects [19,21]. Thus clinical trials have been conducted combining cisplatin and WR-2721 to determine the feasibility of administering higher doses of cisplatin. Mollman et al. treated 28 patients receiving varying doses of cisplatin with WR-2721 $740\,mg/m^2$ and compared this group to 41 patients receiving cisplatin-based combination chemotherapy [22]. Patients who received cisplatin with WR-2721 had a 25% incidence of neuropathy, while 47–100% of patients treated with the other cisplatin regimens without WR-2721 experienced neuropathy. The patients treated with WR-2721 also tolerated higher cumulative doses of cisplatin, $635\,mg/m^2$, as opposed to $383\,mg/m^2$ for the patients not treated with WR-2721.

Glover et al. treated 52 solid tumor patients with WR-2721 $740\,mg/m^2$ given prior to cisplatin, which ranged in dose from 60 to $150\,mg/m^2$ [23]. The incidence of nephrotoxicity in 161 cisplatin courses was 10%. Responses were observed in patients with melanoma, head and neck cancer, esophagus, hepatoma, and small cell lung cancer. The authors concluded that there was no evidence that WR-2721 protected against the antitumor effect of cisplatin and, compared to historic controls, there appeared to be protection against nephrotoxicity and neurotoxicity.

Kish and coworkers at Wayne State University conducted a feasibility study in 25 patients with advanced head and neck cancer, utilizing cisplatin $120\,mg/m^2$, 5-FU, and WR-2721 $740\,mg/m^2$ or $910\,mg/m^2$ [24]. Hypotensive episodes occurred during 29 of 68 courses, but study termination was required in only one patient. Ototoxicity occurred in five patients, renal failure in five, and peripheral neuropathy in four. The median cumulative dose of cisplatin in the patients experiencing neurotoxicity was $600\,mg/m^2$, similar to that reported without WR-2721. Renal failure occurred with the first course of cisplatin, and ototoxicity occurred after less than a $300\,mg/m^2$ cumulative dose of cisplatin. The investigators concluded that their results failed to show a protective effect from WR-2721 and have abandoned further study of this compound [25].

Therefore, while early testing of this agent proved promising, results have been inconsistent and disappointing. WR-2721 remains investigational.

Sodium thiosulfate

Sodium thiosulfate is a compound initially used for cyanide poisoning, but recently it was shown to protect against cisplatin nephrotoxicity. Sodium thiosulfate is rapidly cleared and concentrates in the kidneys, where it is associated with chemical inactivation of cisplatin [26]. However, there is concern that this protective agent may also attenuate the antitumor effect of cisplatin. Leeuwenkamp et al. used simple kinetic modeling to estimate the area under the concentration-time curve (AUC) of cisplatin administered with and without sodium thiosulfate [27]. They found that thiosulfate reduced tumor exposure to cisplatin by a factor of 0.87. This implied that to maintain therapeutic efficacy, the cisplatin dose would need to be escalated. With effective protection against nephrotoxicity, in theory, one could administer a large enough dose of cisplatin to obtain not only equivalent exposure but to increase the therapeutic ratio.

A phase I trial was conducted at the Memorial Sloan-Kettering Cancer Center to evaluate the toxicity of bolus high-dose cisplatin and sodium thiosulfate in 36 patients with a variety of solid tumors refractory to standard therapies [28]. The maximum tolerated dose of cisplatin with acceptable renal toxicity was $200\,mg/m^2$. However, neurotoxicity was significant and dose limiting. The overall response rate was 26%, leading the authors to conclude that there was probably no loss in antitumor activity secondary to the protective agent. Whether the response in this varied patient population was better than could be expected from cisplatin without thiosulfate was uncertain. To address this, at the same institution, Reichman and colleagues reported a phase II trial of cisplatin, $200\,mg/m^2$, and sodium thiosulfate in 11 patients with cervical carcinoma [29]. The study was closed early due to a low response rate of 27% and a short duration of response, ranging from 1 to 4 months, and considerable neurotoxicity. Nephrotoxicity was mild and transient.

In summary, sodium thiosulfate is an investigational agent that does appear to protect against cisplatin nephrotoxicity. However, trials attempting to escalate the dose of cisplatin have been limited by neurotoxicity. The potential for systemic inactivation of cisplatin and diminished antitumor effects also suggest that this compound will not prove as useful as originally anticipated.

Numerous investigators have combined leucovorin with 5-FU to modulate antitumor efficacy. Leucovorin, a reduced folate, increases 5-FU cytotoxicity by forming and maintaining a stable ternary complex with the 5-FU metabolite FdUMP and the target enzyme thymidylate synthase [30].

Dreyfuss et al. treated 35 patients with advanced, resectable head and neck cancer with two to three cycles of intensive induction chemotherapy [31]. The regimen was cisplatin $25 \, mg/m^2$ on days 1–5, 5-FU $800 \, mg/m^2$ on days 2–6, and leucovorin $500 \, mg/m^2$ on days 1–6. All drugs were given by continuous infusion. They achieved a 66% complete response rate. Ninety-four percent of patients experienced grade 2–3 mucositis. Thirty-one percent of patients required dose reductions of 5-FU and leucovorin due to toxicity.

Vokes et al. reported the results of a regimen consisting of cisplatin $100 \, mg/m^2$ on day 1, 5-FU $1000 \, mg/m^2/day \times 5$ days as continuous infusion, and oral leucovorin 100 mg every 4 hours × 5 days [32]. Thirty-one patients were treated with two cycles in the neoadjuvant setting, and a complete response rate of 29% was achieved. There were two deaths during treatment. Mucositis was the dose-limiting toxicity: 45% of patients developed grade 3 lesions, but the majority tolerated treatment when the dose of 5-FU was reduced by 20%. The authors believed that a higher complete response rate may have been achieved by administering three cycles of chemotherapy instead of two.

These results are promising, but the optimal dose and method of administration of leucovorin are still under investigation. Ultimately, a phase III trial evaluating cisplatin and 5-FU with and without leucovorin will be necessary to definitively establish superiority of the three-drug regimen. Because of the significant mucosal toxicity associated with leucovorin, only an improvement in survival would justify the routine use of this regimen.

Colony-stimulating factors

Colony-stimulating factors (CSFs) are glycoprotein hormones that regulate hematopoiesis by inducing the proliferation of progenitor cells, enhancing effector cell function, and activating other cytokines. The primary role of CSFs in high-dose chemotherapy is to stimulate early bone marrow recovery in order to reduce the duration of cytopenias and attendant risks for infection and bleeding. Hematopoietic progenitor cells and the CSFs involved in differentiation are shown in Figure 1.

G-CSF, GM-CSF, interleukin-3 (IL-3), and the GM-CSF/IL-3 fusion protein PIXY321 are CSFs that have potential utility in treating head and neck cancer patients with cytotoxic therapies. Through recombinant DNA

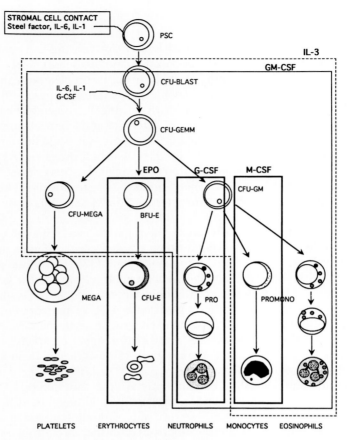

Figure 1. PSC = primitive stem cell; CFU-GEMM = colony-forming unit, granulocyte-erythrocyte-monocyte-megakaryocyte; CFU-MEGA = colony-forming unit, megakaryocyte; BFU-E = burst-forming unit, erythrocyte; CFU-GM = colony-forming unit, granulocyte, macrophage; MEGA = megakaryocyte; CFU-E = colony-forming unit, erythrocyte; PRO = promyelocyte; PROMONO = promonocyte. (Reprinted with permission from Mazanet R, Griffin JD. Hematopoietic growth factors. In: JO Armitage, KH Antman, eds. High-Dose Cancer Therapy: Pharmacology, Hematopoietins, Stem Cells. Baltimore, MD: Williams and Wilkins, 1992, pp 289–313.)

technology these proteins are now available in sufficient quantities for therapeutic evaluation.

Human granulocyte colony stimulating factor (G-CSF) accelerates the maturation time and bone marrow transit time of neutrophils. Phase III trials have shown that G-CSF decreases the duration of neutropenia and the degree of absolute neutropenia in patients treated with myelosuppressing cytotoxic regimens [33]. The end result is a decrease in the frequency of

270

febrile neutropenia and the frequency and duration of hospitalization. These effects have implications for dose intensity, potentially allowing patients to receive chemotherapy courses at full dose and on time. An example of the successful employment of G-CSF with drugs that cause primarily neutropenia are studies of taxol [11,13] and taxol + cisplatin [14] in which G-CSF support allowed repeated dosing every 3 weeks at 250 mg/m^2.

G-CSF may also act as a mucosal protectant, although the mechanism for this effect is not understood. Gabrilove et al. [34] observed a difference in mucosal toxicity in patients with bladder cancer receiving cycles of MVAC chemotherapy with and without G-CSF. Mucositis was documented in 11% of those treated with G-CSF and 44% without G-CSF. This observation has implications for head and neck cancer patients treated with 5-FU continuous infusion regimens and concomitant chemotherapy/radiotherapy. Randomized trials are in progress to objectively evaluate G-CSF as a mucosal protectant.

Granulocyte-monocyte colony-stimulating factor (GM-CSF) increases the number of circulating neutrophils, eosinophils, and monocytes. Randomized placebo-controlled trials have shown that GM-CSF can reduce the incidence of infections and shorten hospitalization time [35,36]. The primary utility for GM-CSF in the treatment of head and neck cancer patients may come from combination CSF therapy, specifically sequential or concomitant interleukin-3 (IL-3) and GM-CSF, which has been reported to stimulate megakaryocyte colony formation [37,38]. The dose-limiting toxicity of carboplatin in doses of up to 1000 mg/m^2 is myelosuppression. The ability to overcome both neutropenia and thrombocytopenia with CSF support would make this an attractive drug to test in high doses in head and neck cancer patients.

Interleukin-3 (IL-3, multi-CSF) is produced by activated helper T cells and is present in normal human bone marrow stroma. It stimulates the proliferation and differentiation of granulocyte-macrophages, eosinophils, megakaryocytes, and multipotential colony-forming cells. In the presence of erythropoietin, IL-3 also results in an increase in progenitors committed to the erythroid lineage. Preclinical studies showed that IL-3 priming of bone marrow progenitor cells followed by GM-CSF resulted in expansion of neutrophils and an increase in platelet counts [39]. Clinical trials are in progress to determine the optimal sequencing of these agents.

The GM-CSF/IL-3 fusion protein PIXY321 is a genetically engineered growth factor composed of the protein chains of human IL-3 and GM-CSF. The molecule has a three-dimensional conformation that allows binding to both cellular receptors. Preclinical studies have demonstrated enhanced leukocyte and platelet recovery after radiotherapy. PIXY appears to be a 10- to 20-fold more potent stimulator of progenitors than GM-CSF and IL-3 [40]. Phase I studies are in progress testing PIXY with high-dose carboplatin. Additional National Cancer Institute-sponsored trials are planned using PIXY with intensive chemotherapy in both solid tumors and hematologic malignancies.

In summary, genetically engineered CSFs can effectively and safely protect bone marrow against cytotoxicity and radiotherapy-related toxicity. Those that are commercially available and in development should be evaluated with high-dose therapies in head and neck cancer patients to test the question of dose intensity. Successful evaluation in patients with recurrent disease and good performance status is a first step to incorporating these therapies into primary curative treatment regimens.

Biologic response modifiers

Interleukin-2

Immunotherapy is of interest for patients with head and neck cancer because they consistently demonstrate impaired cellular immunity [41]. Interleukin-2 (IL-2), a lymphokine produced by T lymphocytes, induces the differentiation and proliferation of cytotoxic T lymphocytes. IL-2 has been shown to augment lymphokine-activated killer (LAK) cells in vitro against head and neck squamous carcinoma cell lines [42,43]. Wanebo et al. studied lymphocytes in vitro from patients with head and neck carcinoma and normal controls [44]. The addition of IL-2 to lymphocyte cultures produced a 32–35% increase of proliferative response for patients and controls, and cytotoxicity of natural killer cells was increased 2.3 times over baseline.

IL-2 has been utilized in local-regional therapy of head and neck cancer. Rivoltini injected IL-2 in the perimastoid region of 12 patients scheduled to undergo a neck dissection 7–10 days before their surgery [45]. A marked induction of cytotoxic activity against allogeneic and autologous tumor cell lines was observed in lymphocytes obtained from the cervical lymph nodes of the treated patients. The authors concluded that IL-2-activated T cells may be instrumental for targeting lymph node micrometastases in the clinical setting. Perilesional and intranodal therapy with IL-2 was studied by Snyderman et al. [46]. Thirty-six patients with unresectable disease were treated with escalating doses in a phase I study. Two partial responses were seen at very disparate doses of 20,000 units and 4 million units.

Ishikawa et al. tested the intra-arterial administration of IL-2-stimulated LAK cells in five patients with maxillary sinus cancer, and responses were reported in all patients [47]. A phase I study of intra-arterial IL-2 was conducted by Gore et al. [48]. Two of 12 patients treated with relatively low doses of IL-2, 3×10^4 IU/24 hours $\times$ 10 days, had a partial tumor response.

IL-2 has also been used in combination with chemotherapy in an attempt to improve response rate. Dimery et al. treated 25 patients with cisplatin, 5-fluorouracil, and IL-2 [49]. Toxicity was acceptable, but the response rate of 35% was not superior to that historically achieved with chemotherapy alone. Therefore, some of the early trials of immunotherapy with IL-2 hold promise for patients with head and neck cancer, but the ideal dosage and route of administration have yet to be determined.

Interferon-α

Interferon-α regulates immune function through the augmentation of natural killer activity and antiviral effects [50]. Vlock et al. administered interferon-α to 14 patients with recurrent head and neck cancer [51]. There was one complete response (greater than 30 months duration), and two patients had stabilization of disease for 8 and 12 months. The complete responder had extremely low baseline natural killer (NK) cell activity, which increased dramatically after treatment with interferon. Other patients with higher baseline levels of NK activity did not respond. Therefore, the pretreatment immunologic status of patients with head and neck cancer may predict for response to interferon therapy. However, conflicting results were reported by Teichmann et al., who demonstrated suppression of in vitro immuno-globulin synthesis, lymphocyte proliferation, and NK cell activity in five patients treated long-term with interferon [52]. Interferon dosage may be extremely important because doses that are either too high or too low may further depress the immune system. Edwards and colleagues reported that 3×10^6 U of interferon is an optimal dose for maximal stimulation of NK cells [53].

Interferon may be most effective in nasopharyngeal cancer, a tumor frequently associated with Epstein-Barr virus. Connors et al. treated 12 patients with interferon 10×10^6 units IM daily for 30 days [54]. Two patients had partial responses, two had minor responses, and three had stable disease. Although activity was modest, the patients were heavily pretreated and had poor performance status. Further testing of interferon seems warranted in patients with less advanced disease.

Interferon-α is being tested in combination with conventional chemotherapy. The Eastern Cooperative Oncology Group is conducting a randomized trial of interferon + 5-FU versus interferon + cisplatin for patients with recurrent disease. The interferon + 5-FU arm was closed due to poor response and marked toxicity, but accrual to the interferon + cisplatin arm continues [55]. Another multi-institution randomized study in progress compares cisplatin + 5-FU + interferon to cisplatin + 5-FU. These results will not be complete for several years.

IL-2 and interferon-α appear to have synergistic antitumor activity when administered in combination. Bash et al. reported that murine hepatic metastases from a colon cancer cell line responded to IL-2 and interferon after being resistant to interferon as a single agent [56]. A small pilot study of IL-2 and interferon in patients with head and neck carcinoma demonstrated a significant increase in the number of CD56 + lymphocytes and NK cell activity in responding patients [57]. Urba et al. treated 11 patients with recurrent head and neck cancer with an intensive regimen of IL-2 and interferon [58]. There were two partial responses, one of which was durable for 3 months off treatment. Toxicity was substantial and, therefore, modulation of the dose or schedule of the lymphokines would be necessary for future protocols.

Both IL-2 and interferon-α appear to have some activity in head and neck cancer. The specific role of these biologic effectors in patient management will need to be defined in current and future trials.

Retinoids

Vitamin A is necessary for normal differentiation of epithelial cells. It is required for maintenance of the mucus-secreting function of the cells of the oral cavity and upper aerodigestive tract, and its absence results in squamous metaplasia [59]. Retinoids are functionally related to vitamin A, and they can modulate the growth, maturation, and differentiation of squamous cells [60]. These cytostatic agents can prevent epithelial carcinogenesis secondary to their effect on cell differentiation. Hong et al. reported a small randomized trial showing benefit from adjuvant 13-*cis*-retinoic acid in preventing second primary cancers in patients with squamous cell carcinoma of the head and neck [61]. Several large randomized chemoprevention trials are now in progress in the United States and Europe to confirm these results in patients who have had primary treatment for early stage head and neck cancer.

Retinoids have also been studied as treatment for advanced squamous cell cancer. Lippman and colleagues reported the results of a randomized phase II study in which 40 poor prognosis patients with metastatic or recurrent disease were treated with either 13-*cis*-retinoic acid (13cRA) or methotrexate [62]. There were three objective responses (16%), including one complete response in 19 evaluable patients treated with the retinoid and no responses in the methotrexate group. The authors concluded that confirmation of these findings by other investigators would warrant studying 13cRA in combination with cytotoxic agents.

13cRA and interferon α-2a have been used in combination to treat advanced squamous cell carcinoma of the skin [63] and squamous cell carcinoma of the cervix [64]. The rationale for this regimen is based on in vitro data showing enhanced activity in hematologic and solid tumor cell lines [65,66]. Lippman et al. reported testing 13cRA 1 mg/kg/day and interferon 3 million units per day by subcutaneous injection in 28 patients with inoperable squamous cell carcinoma of the skin. There were 12 partial responses and seven complete responses, with a 68% overall response rate. Responses were observed in patients with local, regional, or distant disease and sites within previously irradiated fields. The toxic effects of the two agents were reversible and nonoverlapping; treatment duration was limited by cumulative fatigue. These results indicate that immunomodulatory agents and those that regulate malignant cell differentiation and proliferation have the potential to be highly effective therapies in advanced squamous cell cancers.

Photodynamic therapy

Photodynamic therapy utilizes a photosensitizing drug that localizes selectively in tumor. Exposure to light activates the drug and results in tumor cell death. The concept of phototherapy actually began thousands of years ago. The Egyptians applied the crushed leaves of plants containing a psoralen to depigmented skin so that exposure to sunlight resulted in sunburn [67]. In the late 1940s, Figge and Weiland demonstrated that porphyrins are preferentially taken up by rapidly dividing tissue [68]. An intravenous dose of hematoporphyrin derivate (HPD), or more recently, the more active purified dihematoporphyrin ether (DHE), incorporates into tumor cells in a higher concentration than in surrounding normal cells and fluoresces when exposed to ultraviolet light [69]. The drug is administered about 72 hours before exposure to light. A fiberoptic system delivers laser light at 630 nm wavelength, which can penetrate 5–20 mm of tissue. Light exposure activates the drug by producing energy transfer from the excited triplet hematoporphyrin to oxygen singlet molecules, causing irreversible oxidation of cellular components. Tumor blood flow is compromised by thrombosis and embolization in the microvasculature. The major toxicity of this therapy is generalized skin photosensitivity, so patients are advised to avoid direct sun exposure for 4–6 weeks after treatment.

In 1983, Dahlman et al. reported on 20 patients with head and neck cancer treated with photodynamic therapy [70]. Of 28 sites of tumor (both local recurrences and distant cutaneous metastases), the complete and partial response rate was 61%. Schuller and coworkers studied 24 patients with head and neck tumors treated with hematoporphyrin followed by exposure to argon laser [71]. While many of the tumors developed central necrosis in response to treatment, the duration of response in 15 patients was 6 weeks or less.

Wenig et al. had more encouraging results in 26 patients with early stage disease [72]. Using Photofrin II, 77% of patients achieved colmplete response, and 80% remained tumor free, with follow-up ranging from 6 to 51 months. However, these patients had relatively early disease, while large, bulky cancers and those located at the oral cavity/oropharynx junction were relatively resistant to treatment.

Because of the limitations of tissue penetration, photodynamic therapy is most useful for superficial lesions, although larger tumors have been treated with interstitial implantation of the light fibers. Optical dosimetry models based on tissue optics are being developed for improved treatment planning of larger lesions. Some patients experience impressive tumor shrinkage, but results can be unpredictable. Another group of patients who would potentially benefit from this approach are those with evidence of 'field cancerization.' These patients have multicentric superficial malignant and premalignant changes, and photodynamic therapy could theoretically treat relatively large areas of affected tissue.

At this time, the role of photodynamic therapy in the management of patients with head and neck cancer is not clear. It is likely that as experience accumulates, specific stages and sites of disease that are likely to benefit from this approach will be defined.

Monoclonal antibodies

There is considerable interest in the identification of tumor antigens in head and neck squamous carcinoma. Monoclonal antibodies directed against such antigens selectively localize in tumor cells and have potential for use in diagnosis, staging, and treatment. Fantozzi produced monoclonal antibodies to squamous carcinoma cells using standard hybridoma technology [73]. The activity of the antibody was tested in vitro against oral cavity head and neck squamous cell carcinoma and controls consisting of normal oral mucosa, hyperkeratosis, and dysplastic epithelium. Immunoperoxidase staining confirmed the binding of the monoclonal antibodies to the squamous carcinoma cells with 50–90% reactivity in most of the specimens, while there was weak or no reactivity in the control specimens. The authors concluded that these antibodies were binding to specific antigenic markers not found on the majority of normal or dysplastic cells.

Monoclonal antibodies may also be useful in identification of prognostically significant tumor cell-surface antigens. Carey et al. reported that the A9 monoclonal antibody defined an antigen expressed by squamous cell cancers [74]. The A9 antigen is found at the basement membrane of normal stratified squamous epithelium, but its expression is greatly increased in squamous carcinoma cells. This antigen is an integrin, a type of attachment molecule involved in cell binding to basement membrane laminin [75]. In 37 patients with head and neck carcinoma, the A9 antigen was associated with aggressive biologic behavior of squamous cell carcinoma cell lines in vivo and in vitro. Intense expression of A9 was also associated with the loss of A, B, and H blood-group antigens in the tumor. Patients with both of these poor prognostic indicators had statistically significantly shorter disease-free and overall survival. In a larger study of 82 previously untreated patients, Wolf and Carey again demonstrated that loss of blood-group expression and high A9 antigen expression were each directly related to increased frequency of early tumor recurrence, and the combination of both variables was significantly associated with disease-free ($p = 0.029$) and overall survival ($p = 0.05$) [76]. Therefore, immunohistologic staining holds great promise

276

as a predictor of patients at high risk for recurrence or early death from head and neck cancer.

There are limitations to the use of monoclonal antibodies. An antibody that is highly specific for one tumor may not react with another tumor because of heterogeneity of tumor cell-surface markers. Monoclonal antibodies alone are not cytotoxic. They require complement or killer effector cells to be tumoricidal. A potential use for monoclonal technology is the conjugation of such an antibody to a chemotherapeutic agent for site-specific delivery.

References

1. Tupchong L, Scott CB, Blitzer PH, Marcial VA, Lowry LD, Jacobs JR, Stetz J, Davis LW, Snow JB, Chandler R, Kramer S, Pajak TF. Randomized study of preoperative versus postoperative radiation therapy in advanced head and neck carcinoma: Long-term follow-up of RTOG Study 73-03. Int J Radiat Oncol Biol Phys 20:21–28, 1991.
2. Kotwall C, Sako K, Razack MS, Rao U, Bakamjian V, Shedd DP. Metastatic patterns in squamous cell cancer of the head and neck. Am J Surg 154:439–442, 1987.
3. Al-Sarraf M. Head and neck cancer: Chemotherapy concepts. Semin Oncol 15:70–85, 1988.
4. Urba SG, Forastiere AA. Systemic therapy of head and neck cancer: Most effective agents, areas of promise. Oncology 3:79–98, 1989.
5. Pinto HA, Jacobs CJ. Chemotherapy for recurrent and metastatic head and neck cancer. Hematol Oncol Clin North Am 5:769–783, 1991.
6. Jacobs C, Lyman G, Velez-Garcia E, Sridhar KS, Knight W, Hochster H, Goodnough LT, Mortimer JE, Einhorn LH, Schacter L, Cherng N, Dalton T, Burroughs J, Rozencweig M. A Phase III randomized study comparing cisplatin and fluorouracil as single agents and in combination for advanced squamous cell carcinoma of the head and neck. J Clin Oncol 10:257–263, 1992.
7. Forastiere AA, Metch B, Schuller DE, Ensley JF, Hutchins LF, Triozzi P, Kish JA, McClure S, VonFeldt E, Williamson SK, Von Hoff DD. Randomized comparison of cisplatin plus fluorouracil and carboplatin plus fluorouracil versus methotrexate in advanced squamous-cell carcinoma of the head and neck: A Southwest Oncology Group Study. J Clin Oncol 10:1245–1251, 1992.
8. Uen WC, Huang AT, Mennel R, et al. A Phase II study of piritrexim in patients with advanced squamous head and neck cancer. Cancer 69:1008–1011, 1992.
9. Degardin M, Demonge C, Coppelaere P, Luboinski B, Navarrete MS, Lefebure JL. Phase II piritrexim study in recurrent and/or metastatic head and neck cancer. Proc Am Soc Clin Oncol 11:244, 1992.
10. Vokes EE, Dimery IW, Jacobs CD, et al. A Phase II study of piritrexim in combination with methotrexate in recurrent and metastatic head and neck cancer. Cancer 67:2253–2257, 1991.
11. Rowinsky EK, Cazenave LA, Donehower RC. Taxol: A novel investigational antimicrotubule agent. J Natl Cancer Inst 82:1247–1259, 1990.
12. McGuire WP, Rowinsky EK, Rosenshein NB, Grumbine FC, Ettinger DS, Armstrong DK, Donehower RC. Taxol: A unique antineoplastic agent with significant activity in advanced ovarian epithelial neoplasms. Ann Intern Med 111:273–279, 1989.
13. Forastiere AA, Neuberg D, Adams G, Taylor S IV, DeConti K. Phase II trial of taxol in advanced head and neck cancer. An Eastern Cooperative Oncology Group trial. Pro-

ceedings of the Third International Conference on Head and Neck Cancer, July 26–30, 1992.

14. Forastiere AA, Rowinsky E, Chaudry V, et al. Phase I trial of taxol and cisplatin + G-CSF in solid tumors. Proc Am Soc Clin Oncol 11:289, 1992.

15. Cervellion JC, Araujo CE, Pirisi C, Francia A, Cerruti R. Ifosfamide and Mesna for the treatment of advanced squamous cell head and neck cancer. Oncology 48:89–92, 1991.

16. Buesa JM, Fernandez R, Esteban E, Estrada E, Baron FJ, Palacio I, Gracia M, Lacave AJ. Phase II trial of ifosfamide in recurrent and metastatic head and neck cancer. Ann Oncol 2:151–152, 1991.

17. Verweij J, Alexieva-Figusch J, de Boer MF, et al. Ifosfamide in advanced head and neck cancer. A Phase II study of the Rotterdam Cooperative Head and Neck Cancer Study Group. Eur J Cancer Clin Oncol 24:795–796, 1988.

18. Yuhas JM, Storer JB. Differential chemoprotection of normal and malignant tissues. J Natl Cancer Inst 42:331–335, 1969.

19. Yuhas JM. Active versus passive absorption kinetics as the basis of selective protection of normal tissues by WR-2721. Cancer Res 40:1519–1524, 1980.

20. Harris JW, Phillips TL. Radiobiological and biochemical studies of thiophosphate radioprotective compounds related to cysteamine. Radiat Res 46:362–379, 1971.

21. Yuhas JM, Spellman JM, Jordan SW. Treatment of tumors with the combination of WR-2721 and cis-dichlorodiammine platinum or cyclophosphamide. Br J Cancer 42:574–585, 1980.

22. Mollman JE, Glover DJ, Hogan WM, et al. Cisplatin neuropathy: Risk factors, prognosis, and protection by WR-2721. Cancer 61:2192–2195, 1988.

23. Glover D, Glick JH, Weiler C, et al. Phase I/II trials of WR-2721 and cis-platinum. J Radiat Oncol Biol Phys 12:1509–1512, 1986.

24. Kish JA, Ensley JF, Tapazoglou E, et al. Evaluation of the chemoprotective effect of WR-2721 in recurrent and advanced head and neck cancer patients — preliminary report. Proc Am Soc Clin Oncol 9:K697, 1990.

25. J Kish, Personal communication.

26. Pfeifle GE, Howell SB, Felthouse RD, et al. High-dose cisplatin with sodium thiosulfate protection. J Clin Oncol 3:237, 1985.

27. Leeuwenkamp OR, van der Vijgh WJF, Neijt JP, Pinedo HM. Reaction kinetics of cisplatin and its monoaquated species with the (potential) renal protecting agents (Mesna) and thiosulfate. Cancer Chemother Pharmacol 27:111–114, 1990.

28. Markman M, D'Acquisto R, Iannotti N, Kris M, Hakes T, Bajorin D, Bosl G, Reichman B, Casper E, Magill G, Budnick A. Phase-I trial of high-dose intravenous cisplatin with simultaneous intravenous sodium thiosulfate. J Cancer Res Clin Oncol 117:151–155, 1991.

29. Reichman B, Markman M, Hakes T, et al. Phase II trial of high-dose cisplatin with sodium thiosulfate nephroprotection in patients with advanced carcinoma of the uterine cervix previously untreated with chemotherapy. Gynecol Oncol 43:159–163, 1991.

30. Santi DV, McHenry CS, Sommer H. Mechanism of interaction of thymidylate synthetase with 5-fluorodeoxyuridylate. Biochemistry 13:471–481, 1974.

31. Dreyfuss AI, Clark JR, Wright JE, Norris CM, Busse PM, Lucarini JW, Fallon BG, Casey D, Anderson JW, Kelin R, Rosowsky A, Miller D, Frei E. Continuous infusion high-dose leucovorin with 5-fluorouracil and cisplatin for untreated stage IV carcinoma of the head and neck. Ann Intern Med 112:167–172, 1990.

32. Vokes EE, Schilsky RL, Weichselbaum RR, Kozloff MF, Panje WR. Induction chemotherapy with cisplatin, fluorouracil, and high-dose leucovorin for locally advanced head and neck cancer: A clinical and pharmacologic analysis. J Clin Oncol 8:241–247, 1990.

33. Crawford J, Ozer H, Stoller R, et al. Reduction by granulocyte colony-stimulating factor of fever and neutropenia induced by chemotherapy in patients with small cell lung cancer. N Engl J Med 315:164–170, 1991.

34. Gabrilove JL, Jakubowski A, Sher H, et al. Effect of granulocyte colony-stimulating factor

on neutropenia and associated morbidity due to chemotherapy for transitional-cell carcinoma of the urothelium. N Engl J Med 318:1414–1422,1988.

35. Rabinowe S, Freedman A, Demetrie G, et al. Randomized double-blinded trial of rhGM-CSF in patients with B-cell non-Hodgkin's lymphoma undergoing high-dose chemoradiotherapy and monoclonal antibody-purged autologous bone marrow transplantation. Blood 76:61, 1990.

36. Nemunaitis J, Singe JW, Buckner CD, et al. Preliminary analysis of a randomized, placebo-controlled trial of rhGM-CSF in autologous bone marrow transplantation. Proc Am Soc Clin Oncol 9:10, 1990.

37. Hoelzer D, Seipelt G, Ganser A. Interleukin-3 clone and in combination with GM-CSF in the treatment of patients with neoplastic disease. Semin Hematol 28(Suppl 2):17–24, 1991.

38. Brugger W, Bross KJ, Frisch J, et al. Combined sequential administration of IL-3 + GM-CSF after polychemotherapy with etoposide, ifosfamide and cisplatin. Blood 78(Suppl 1):162, 1991.

39. Geissler K, Valent P, Mayer P, et al. Recombinant human interleukin-3 expands the pool of circulating hematopoietic progenitor cells in primates — synergism with recombinant human granulocyte-macrophage colony-stimulating factor. Blood 75:2305–2310, 1990.

40. Williams DE, Park LS. Hematopoietic effects of a granulocyte-macrophage colony-stimulating factor/interleukin-3 fusion protein. Cancer 67:2705–2707, 1991.

41. Berlinger NT, Hilal EY, Oettgen HF, et al. Deficient cell-mediated immunity in head and neck cancer patients secondary to autologous suppressive immune cells. Laryngoscope 88:470–481, 1978.

42. Alessi DM, Hutcherson RW, Mickel RA. Production of lymphokine-activated lymphocytes. Arch Otolaryngol Head Neck Surg 115:725–730, 1989.

43. Wanebo H, Biakinton D, Weigel T, et al. Augmentation of the lymphokine-activated killer cell response in head and neck cancer patients by combination interleukin-2 and interferon-alpha. Am J Surg 162:382–387, 1991.

44. Wanebo HJ, Jones T, Pace R, et al. Immune restoration with interleukin-2 in patients with squamous cell carcinoma of the head and neck. Am J Surg 158:356–360, 1989.

45. Rivoltini L, Gambacorti-Passerini C, Squadrelli-Saraceno M, et al. In vivo interleukin-2 induced activation of lymphokine-activated killer cells and tumor cytotoxic T-cells in cervical lymph nodes of patients with head and neck tumors. Cancer Res 50:5551–5557, 1990.

46. Snyderman CH, Johnson JT, Eibling DE, et al. Phase IB trial of local/regional interleukin-2 in patients with advanced squamous cell carcinoma of the head and neck — preliminary results. Proceedings of the Third International Conference on Head and Neck Cancer, July 26–30, 1992, p 157.

47. Ishikawa T, Ikawa J, Eura M, et al. Adoptive immunotherapy for head and neck cancer with killer cells induced by stimulation of autologous or allogeneic tumor cells and recombinant interleukin-2. Acta Otolaryngol 107:340–351, 1989.

48. Gore ME, Riches P, MacLennan KA, et al. Intra-arterial interleukin-2 in squamous cell carcinoma of the head and neck. Proc Am Soc Clin Oncol 11:814, 1992.

49. Dimery I, Martin T, Bradley E, et al. Phase I trial of interleukin-2 plus cisplatin and 5-fluorouracil in recurrent or advanced squamous cell carcinoma of the head and neck. Proc Am Soc Clin Oncol 8:660, 1989.

50. Wolf GT. Tumor immunology, immune surveillance and immunotherapy of head and neck squamous carcinoma. In: Head and Neck Oncology. Boston: Martinus Nijhoff, 1984.

51. Vlock DR, Johnson J, Myers E, et al. Preliminary trial of nonrecombinant interferon alpha in recurrent squamous cell carcinoma of the head and neck. Head Neck 13:15–21, 1991.

52. Teichmann JV, Sieber G, Ludwig W, et al. Immunosuppressive effects of recombinant interferon-alpha during long-term treatment of cancer patients. Cancer 63:1990–1993, 1989.

53. Edwards BS, Merritt JA, Fuhlbrigge RC, et al. Low doses of interferon alpha result in

more effective clinical natural killer cell activation. J Clin Invest 75:1908–1913, 1985.

54. Connors JM, Andiman WA, Howarth CB, et al. Treatment of nasopharyngeal carcinoma with human leukocyte interferon. J Clin Oncol 3:813–817, 1985.

55. D. Vlock, personal communication.

56. Bash JA, Arroyo PA, Wallack MK, et al. Direct effect of alpha-interferon (IFN-A) on murine adenocarcinoma C-C36 as a basis for synergy with interleukin-2 in cytolytic lymphocyte-mediated abrogation of hepatic metastases. Proc Am Assoc Cancer Res 31: 1485, 1990.

57. Schantz SP, Clayman G, Racz T, et al. The in vivo biologic effect of interleukin 2 and interferon alpha on natural immunity in patients with head and neck cancer. Arch Otolaryngol Head Neck Surg 116:1302–1308, 1990.

58. Urba SG, Forastiere AA, Amrein PC, et al. A Phase II pilot study of concomitantly administered recombinant human interleukin-2 and roferon-A in patients with locally recurrent or metastatic head and neck cancer. Proc Am Soc Clin Oncol 10:695, 1991.

59. Poddar S, Hong WK, Thacher SM, et al. Retinoic acid suppression of squamous differentiation in human head and neck squamous carcinoma cells. Int J Cancer 48:239–247, 1991.

60. Jetten AM. Multistep process of squamous differentiation of tracheobronchial epithelial cells: Role of retinoids. Dermatologica 175:37–44, 1987.

61. Hong WK, Lippman SM, Itri LM, et al. Prevention of second primary tumors with isotretinoin in squamous-cell carcinoma of the head and neck. N Engl J Med 323:795–801, 1990.

62. Lippman SM, Kessler JF, Al-Sarraf M, et al. Advanced squamous cell carcinoma of the head and neck with isotretinoin: A Phase II randomized trial. Invest New Drugs 6:51–56, 1988.

63. Lippman SM, Parlasison DK, Itri LM, Weber RS, Schentz SP, Ota DM, Schusterman MA, Krakoff IH, Gutterman JU, Hong WK. 13-cis-retinoic acid and interferon α-2a: Effective combination therapy for advanced squamous cell carcinoma of the skin. J Natl Cancer Inst 84:235–241, 1992.

64. Lippman SM, Kavanagh JJ, Paredes-Espinoza M, Delgadillo-Madrueno F, Paredes-Casillas P, Hong WK, Holdener E, Krakoff IH. 13-cis-Retinoic acid plus interferon α-2a: Highly active systemic therapy for squamous cell carcinoma of the cervix. J Natl Cancer Inst 84:241–245, 1992.

65. Hemmi H, Breitman TR. Combinations of recombinant human interferons and retinoic acid synergistically induced differentiation of the human promyelocytic leukemia cell line HL-60. Blood 69:501–507, 1987.

66. Marth C, Daxenbichler G, Dapunt O. Synergistic antiproliferative effect of human recombinant interferons and retinoic acid in cultured breast cancer cells. J Natl Cancer Inst 77:1197–1206, 1986.

67. Gluckman JL. Photodynamic therapy for head and neck neoplasms. Otolaryngol Clin North Am 24:1559–1567, 1991.

68. Figge FJH, Weiland GS. The affinity of neoplastic, embryonic, and traumatized tissue for porphyrins and metalloporphyrins. Anat Rec 100:659, 1948.

69. Gregorie HB, Horger EO, Ward JL, et al. Hematoporphyrin derivative fluorescence in malignant neoplasms. Ann Surg 167:820–828, 1968.

70. Dahlman A, Wile AG, Burnes RG, et al. Laser photoradiation therapy of cancer. Cancer Res 43:430–434, 1983.

71. Schuller DE, McCaughan JS, Rock RP. Photodynamic therapy in head and neck cancer. Arch Otolaryngol 111:352–355, 1985.

72. Wenig BL, Kurtzman DM, Grossweiner LI, et al. Photodynamic therapy in the treatment of squamous cell carcinoma of the head and neck. Arch Otolaryngol Head Neck Surg 116:1267–1270, 1990.

73 Fantozzi RD. Development of monoclonal antibodies with specificity to oral squamous cell carcinoma. Laryngoscope 101:1076–1080, 1991.

74. Carey TE, Wolf GT, Hsu S, et al. Expression of A9 antigen and loss of blood group antigens as determinants of survival in patients with head and neck squamous carcinoma. Otolaryngol Head Neck Surg 96:221–230, 1987.
75. Van Waes C, Kozarsky KF, Warren AB, et al. The A9 antigen associated with aggressive human squamous carcinoma has structural and functional similarity to the newly defined integrin a6B4. Cancer Res 51:2395–2402, 1991.
76. Wolf GT, Carey TE. Tumor antigen phenotype, biologic staging and prognosis in head and neck squamous carcinoma. In: Biology of and Novel Therapeutic Approaches for Epithelial Cancers of the Aerodigestive Tract. National Cancer Institute Monograph no. 13, 67–74, 1992.

15. Head and neck cancer: The year 2000

Helmuth Goepfert

Most planners for health care expound as the primary goal for the future that a given disease be controlled or, better yet, eliminated. In the case of the 'cancers' of the head and neck (and there are many), this is not likely to happen in the near future. Even if prevention would become optimal, we would still have to treat established disease with today's remedies. If we accept that no significant new therapies will be available, the single most important advance should be the prescription of therapy based on scientific data rather than empirical information as we still do it today.

Cicero (106–43 BC) said, 'Physicians consider that when they have discovered the cause of disease, they have also discovered the method of treating it.' Mo-Tze (circa 5th to 4th centuries BC) said, 'The physician who is attending a patient has to know the cause of the ailment before he can cure it.' These and other statements coined centuries ago will still be true as we move into the 21st century.

It is presumptuous to believe I have a clear vision of the future and can augur how we will practice medicine in the next decade. There are many uncertainties to predicting the future; there will be change, but its degree and direction are difficult to foresee. Do we really know where we will be and how to get there from here? I don't profess to have all the answers; nevertheless, I have been asked to undertake the task of looking into the crystal ball and finding the answers to the questions clinicians and basic scientists in head and neck oncology are posting today and would like to have resolved by tomorrow. So, from the ivory towers of one of the major cancer centers of this country, having experienced the progress of oncology for nearly 30 years, I venture to leap into the future.

It is tempting to review other such predictions from the past to see how well our mentors were able to predict the advances that have occurred. The reader is urged to search through his or her personal file of references and selected readings for these predictions and be an independent judge. In all likelihood, you will find that we have never done very well in the application

Hong, Waun Ki and Weber, Randal S., (eds.), Head and Neck Cancer. © *1995 Kluwer Academic Publishers. ISBN 0-7923-3015-3. All rights reserved.*

of crystal ball technology, and there is no reason why we should be able to do a better job of forecasting today. Admitting this, the chapter could stop at this point. Nevertheless, the wealth of new information makes it compelling to continue, because there is plenty of room for optimism, in spite of the difficulties we will encounter along the way to the future.

We all would like to see change for the better, the faster, and the easier. The possibilities for significant transformation in the field of head and neck oncology within the next decade seem remote, no matter how much the scientific community forges ahead with unprecedented progress. It is likely that the stumbling blocks in the quest for a better future will be in education and cost; for both of these, the remedies are available if we collectively focus on priorities.

Budget constraints, socioeconomics, and reform in health care delivery systems

We have an interesting set of paradoxes that will require novel and original solutions if humankind is to continue to make discoveries and benefit from progress. On the one hand, we are witnessing how science and technology accelerate the pace at which new discoveries see the light of day, and how such innovations are being applied to the field of cancer care. But it seems as if this expanding knowledge of the basic biomedical sciences is butting up against a series of barriers that regulate the rate at which discoveries can be applied to the care of ailing human beings. One barrier is the regulations and monitoring systems mandated by various legislative or self-appointed agencies that either sanction or claim to monitor different steps of research from the test tube through the animal system to, finally, the human model.

By all reasonable means, precautions and safety measures are necessary, but the extent of control that such regulations exercise is often overwhelming, and some of the mandated ordinances clearly go beyond necessity. For example, the scientific bureaucracy that has been established under the justification of animal and human safety has added burden and considerable cost to every product needed for human consumption, every tool necessary to perform a task, and every drug or device that will help our patients. We have to admit that it is not just safety of a device or reasonable toxicity of a drug that is being regulated. Under the existing legal and judicial system, the liability is such a heavy burden that many innovations may not be economically viable; what seems a reasonable solution to a problem may turn prohibitively costly once the liability price tag is affixed to it. This situation is in need of revision and correction if the flow of progress is to continue.

Another barrier to 'scientific flow' is the mound of socioeconomic problems that have reached unprecedented levels and in one form or another have affected all cultures and societies on this planet. In the United States, the status of the health care system is a concern to health care professionals and citizens alike. It is likely that our failure to remedy this crisis will have a negative impact on progress in basic science, clinical research, patient care, and even teaching in the next 5–15 years. There is reason for concern. Nobody disputes the fact that the U.S. health care system is in crisis; it cannot exist for long in its present form, and somehow the stumbling blocks in the way of overall reform will have to be removed or changed into stepping stones if we are to get beyond them. The collective wisdom of experts has identified the problems, and possible solutions abound; most hang on the challenging question of whether our society is willing to work together toward a solution that will benefit all citizens.

If we admit that we can solve our health care delivery crisis and eliminate the de facto 'rationing' that the present system has established, we should be able to improve considerably the care of our patients and have a better health care system by the year 2000. To get there will require sacrifice. In a basically individualistic society that highly regards personal preferences and satisfaction, there will be a need for unbiased universal regulations that will modulate the desire for personal control of resources and destiny. It will be necessary to establish a basic health insurance system that is universal regardless of the health care status of the person and the ability of the individual and his family to pay. The system will have to be portable between jobs and locations throughout the country and must be simple to administer. The prevailing scheme of 'managed care' is perceived by most to be a fiscal drain, absorbing about one fifth of every health care dollar with little benefit to the patient. Basic health care should be available to all; supplements and amenities could be available at higher rates for those willing to pay for the extras.

Biomedical research is indispensable to progress; the financial support of our institutions and the work of their scientists is crucial to our success. Solutions to our troubled health care systems cannot address patient care only; they need to fiscally support efforts in the areas of prevention, early diagnosis, and research in basic and clinical science areas of therapy and rehabilitation. Health care budgets are shrinking, and the high cost of new technology makes it mandatory to use sophisticated measurements of economic impact when approving the application of expensive devices, treatments, and machines. Already the societal benefits of constructing and operating health care facilities are being analyzed in relation to economic costs. By the year 2000, the certificates of need for major capital investments in health care technology (imaging equipment, radiation therapy machines, operating room technology, etc.) will require documentation of carefully performed cost-utility and cost-benefit analyses. Formulas will establish the equivalency of benefits for different technologies or medical interventions, and the health economist's decision will be driven by fiscal considerations more than ever before. By the end of this decade, highly sophisticated and elaborate computer programs are expected to assist in this task.

Assuming that within the next 5 years, the U.S. health care delivery system will be reformed and improved, we should be able to streamline the steps between bench and clinical practice and ameliorate the socioeconomic pains of health care. Our patients should be better taken care of in the decades to come.

Traditionally, the implementation of new technology has followed an orderly process, undergoing careful scrutiny by the scientific community. Most of the progress has taken place at universities and research institutes. Nevertheless, in some instances, such as that of endoscopic surgery, the broad acceptance and extensive utilization of the technology move faster than what the established regulatory agencies and the peer review processes would like. The minimal access endoscopic surgery swept the country, and the academics in their ivory towers were caught unaware and had to catch up with an innovation that had come about almost entirely in communities outside of university-affiliated institutions and medical centers. This is an example of the significant influence of technology in our lives and our professions, and of the well-coordinated liaison that can occur among clinicians and the manufacturers and sellers of new technology and improved instrumentation. Whenever something appears to offer an advantage with acceptable risks, it will always sell.

How many other such paradigms will evolve in the next decade is anybody's guess. For some time, it appeared as if laser technology would take a similar rocketlike flight, but its applications in oncology have remained shy of the original predictions, and further research and development is ongoing. Improvements in laser-applied technology and refinements in energy-delivery systems and target-specific sensitizing agents are expected to allow us to identify further indications for the cancer patient. The one certainty is that the cost-utility benefit of these innovations will determine whether they are applied broadly in our specialty. If the laser beam offers an advantage in the ease of performing the task, an increased cure rate, or a reduction of morbidity, the expense of instrumentation will be justified.

Impact of prevention, early diagnosis, and intervention in communities at risk

Through public education and worldwide implementation of prevention measures, especially complete elimination of tobacco usage, it should be possible to reduce significantly the incidence of those malignant neoplasms that are caused at least in part by environmental factors and human behavior. Knowledge of the obvious benefits of smoking cessation has been slow to translate into a reduction in consumption. Enhanced public ecucation, broader implementation of smoke-free environments, and improved meth-

286

odologies for behavioral modification are in need of focused activity and support.

As we advance into the next century, populations at risk will be better defined through genetic mapping, and such groups will be enrolled in screening programs and receive intervention by appropriate molecular manipulation and removal of target tissues in the premalignant phase. The establishment of screening and detection centers is a positive trend. These centers offer a service that will become more important as we discover better means of early detection. In addition, they have a very significant educational mission for the communities they serve. There are encouraging signs that the public is being educated about the importance of prevention and early detection. Enhanced public awareness can have a significant impact on reducing the incidence, morbidity, and mortality of invasive carcinomas. History has already given us tangible examples that can be cited: The reduction of invasive uterine cervical carcinoma was achieved through mass screening of women in their reproductive years, and early detection programs and mammography have helped control breast carcinoma by treating patients at minimal tumor burden stage.

Such programs and other means for prevention and early detection that will become available in the future can have an impact only if the populations at risk are informed and, more importantly, have access to these services. The need for reforms that would make these services available to all is obvious, especially if we consider the potential financial savings resulting from prevention and early diagnosis.

A somewhat different problem will need to be faced in prevention of skin cancers, especially malignant melanoma. Although we have recognized that ultraviolet radiation is the main causative factor of this group of malignancies, the implementation of significant prevention strategies aimed at blocking the effects of damaging solar radiation is a tremendous challenge beyond the reach of medicine itself. Though we may eventually change and improve individual attitudes about self-protection from excessive sun exposure, a much bigger task is to control the adverse effects of air pollution on the protective layers of the atmosphere. It seems that the progress of industry and the development of societies create byproducts that defy our ability to prevent environmentally induced carcinogenesis, including excessive exposure to sunlight. The fruits of prosperity could be the eventual doom of future generations.

Alcohol consumption, especially in excess, has been recognized as an important cofactor in carcinogenesis of the upper aerodigestive tract. At this time, we have incomplete information on whether other dietary factors, either by excess or deficiency, have any significant influence on this process, but it is possible that in the future we will identify nutritional factors that have an influence on the development or course of malignant diseases in the head and neck region. Molecular epidemiologists are busily searching for the appropriate clues.

As research in the area of molecular epidemiology intensifies, the interaction between the genetic makeup of individuals and the influences of the environment, including dietary intake, will become clearer, and novel programs will be aimed at reversing the carcinogenetic process at the pre-invasive phase. By the year 2000, an individual's genetic code will be available as part of his or her electronic medical records, allowing identification of risk factors for which appropriate intervention technologies are available. To what extent these technologies will be applicable will depend in part on the results of the several major randomized trials in chemoprevention of squamous cell carcinoma of the upper aerodigestive tract. The results of these trials will have been tabulated and analyzed by the year 2000, and the basic science studies that were spawned by these clinical studies will have generated enough information to develop clinical protocols, not only in squamous cell carcinoma but in other tumor types as well.

Another important spin-off from chemoprevention research will come in the form of novel approaches to differentiation therapy through pharmacologic intervention in the molecular events that regulate cell cycle and tumor cell kinetics. It is not farfetched to predict that viral vectors and transfection technology will be utilized extensively to correct genetic abnormalities and influence the risk of target tissues.

'Bench to bedside' research and the impact of multidisciplinary care

We hear and read much about gene therapy, viral vectors, and the advances of genetic engineering. There has been a logarithmic expansion in the knowledge of the molecular biology of cancer and a great growth in the amount of information available on the genotypic and phenotypic characterizations of malignant tumors. The hype of news media that fuels the public's expectations and the voices of unrestrained optimism for the great solutions to cancer that these innovations seem to offer are delusory and raise false hopes. Unfortunately, progress in this area is not as fast as we would like, nor free of major logistic impediments. The answers to some questions invariably generate new questions, or to quote John A. Wheeler (Princeton University): 'We live on an island of knowledge surrounded by a sea of ignorance. As our island of knowledge grows, so does the shore of our ignorance.' Some tangible progress is occurring, however: Numerous genes and their mutations can now be identified and measured quantitatively. The analysis of genes, their mutations, translations, and expressions, is a specialty in itself and will become part of the standard armamentarium of laboratory medicine in the not-too-distant future. The genetic fingerprints of a tumor and of the host will be used to refine diagnostic capabilities, especially for the purpose of labeling prognostic factors. We can envision that it will not suffice to establish only histologic type and cytologic grade. The molecular profile of a cancer and a host will be an integral part of the information required to assign patients into certain prognostic groupings and select the most appropriate therapy. Certainly computer technology and appropriate software will assist in this task, and prospective data banks will become part of standard patient care in major research centers. We hope that the selection of therapy will be less empirical and more based on scientific observations and biologic facts.

Multidisciplinary teams and prospective planning sessions should be standard in every patient care setting by the end of this decade. There is little doubt that tumor boards and other committees of experts of various specialties that have evolved over the years are here to stay. These groups will become more complex as the provision of patient care becomes more specialized. The need for multidisciplinary care will come not only from the real scientific improvements and expanded knowledge and subspecialization, but from the often dreaded growth of rules and regulations in the practice of medicine. We can anticipate that tumor board meetings for therapy planning will have representation and input from physicians of numerous specialties, including laboratory medicine and pathology, and from dentistry, speech/language pathology, basic sciences, social work, clergy, ethics, hospital administration, insurance carriers, and possibly even legal counsel for the patient and for the practitioners of medicine. Clearly these groups will need to be steered by individuals with strong leadership abilities to keep the team focused and accomplish the final objective: multidisciplinary treatment and planning that will benefit the patient and be cost-effective. The wisdom to make the best treatment choices for patients must be valued if it is going to prevail. The still unanswered question is to what extent such proliferation of opinion and voices will bring about longer and higher quality survival while controlling strain on the patient's fiscal, physical, and emotional resources.

Questions of medical ethics and the quality of survival will have a dominant role and should be addressed with vigor for the solution of some of today's dilemmas. Prospective ethical consultations should become standard, facilitating decisions of appropriate action in the face of advanced cancer or in patients presenting with the different faces of incurable disease and terminal illness suffering. Ethical consultation for patients, their families, and the caregivers has known benefits, for it reduces tensions that all too often surface for reasons beyond what can be comprehended or solved by sophisticated technology and science.

The TNM staging system will still be in use, but with considerable modifications and improvements. In its present form, it is rudimentary and very crude, but it has withstood the test of time as a standard means of describing with consistency the extent of measurable neoplastic disease in different organ systems and anatomic locations. Biological markers will be incorporated to add refinement and objectivity to today's essentially anatomic description of cancer. Nationwide education through such organizations as the Commission on Cancer of the American College of Surgeons will play a significant role in disseminating to practitioners and health care givers the successive updated versions of the TNM staging system. By the time we advance into the next century, tumors will be characterized by location, volume, cell type, and histologic markers, and the molecular characterization of genetic material, including clonal diversity and extent of phenotypic drift of the primary tumor, will be an integral part of the patient's pretreatment evaluation. Information obtained from tumor tissue and the host will be available that will allow us to predict with reasonable accuracy the metastatic spread to regional lymph nodes and distant organs and parenchymae.

It is likely that surgery will still be an effective treatment modality for most of the solid malignant tumors. Nevertheless, except for early stage disease or minimal volume tumor burdens, additional therapies will be required, in either neoadjuvant or postsurgical contexts. At this time there is general disagreement on the merits of chemotherapy for carcinoma of the head and neck. Neither the upfront or neoadjuvant, nor the post-treatment adjuvant, therapies have proven beneficial in prolonging disease-free survival or increasing the curability of adult-onset tumors. In all likelihood, target-specific drugs and new biological modifiers will be developed. Future neoadjuvant treatment protocols will include various combinations, not only of chemotherapeutic agents but also of a variety of cytokines aimed at specific tumor cell targets whose appropriate selection will be based on laboratory analyses of the tumor and other tissues and fluids, and also of growth factors, to aid in the recovery of host parenchyma and tissues.

It is possible that for certain malignant tumors, surgical therapy will become the final rather than the first option if we can duplicate the successes that have been achieved in the management of soft-tissue sarcomas, especially rhabdomyosarcoma, in infants and children. Although this does not seem likely to occur for most squamous cell carcinomas or salivary gland tumors, new biological therapies could change the picture dramatically. Such therapies would eliminate the need for ablative surgery for certain cancers of the upper aerodigestive tract; sophisticated surgical reconstruction and functional rehabilitation would likewise become unnecessary. Again, however, as is true in the treatment of solid tumors in the preadolescent years, we could then face unwanted late sequelae of our therapeutic interventions and would have to develop the means to prevent them. Current efforts to rehabilitate major defects created by the sequelae of combined therapy are limited and mostly fall short of expectations.

Educational challenge

The practice of medicine in the 21st century will require a significant improvement in the educational background of health care professionals. This demand is significant if we consider the prevailing mediocrity of this nation's pre-college education. It is no secret that it is not unusual for high school students to be unprepared to deal with more than basics in science and math, even after 12 years of schooling. If this group is to become the qualified workforce of the year 2000, the bastions of college and graduate education, as well as the organizations responsible for the various forms of continued education, have a difficult task to carry out. The institutions of higher education and sciences have formidable laboratories, and creative research and investigation is taking place at an accelerated rate. If the cornucopia of new knowledge remains replenished throughout the beginning of the next decade, we may find ourselves without a workforce capable of putting the products of such research into practice and carrying out the work of bio-medical science and technology on a day-to-day basis.

An important mission for today's, but especially tomorrow's, generation of medical educators is to prepare the physicians of the future to make proper use of the larger amount of scientific information that will be available for patient care. The ever-rising tide of important new biological data in medicine in general and in oncology in particular calls for the utilization of new methodologies in continued medical education. This need is not unique to our time, and it was felt already over a century ago, at a time when medical knowledge progressed principally through empiricism. The 19th century German surgeon, Bernhard von Langenbeck (1810–1887) said, 'It is less important to invent new operations and new techniques of operating than to find ways and means to avoid surgery. Yet it has become increasingly difficult to keep abreast of and assimilate the investigative reports which accumulate day after day! One suffocates from exposure to the massive body of rapidly growing information.' If this was the perception of the scientific advances over a century ago by a respected leader in the field, how can what we experience today be aptly described?

It is likely that by the end of the decade all practitioners will be linked to data bases that will offer continuous updates of relevant and significant bits of information that will facilitate offering the most up-to-date diagnostic and therapeutic alternatives for each patient's specific tumor, especially in the early stages of disease. August Biel (1861–1949) said, 'There is a tremendous literature on cancer, but what we know for sure about it can be printed on a calling card.' Undoubtedly, we will be able to dismiss this statement and trade in the calling card for a series of computer disks that the practitioner will have to change every 12–18 months to keep abreast of important new information.

Mention of the significance of proper preparation of those who will take command in the field of head and neck oncology in years to come must be made. It is important to encourage and support the thorough training of young scientists and clinicians in both the clinical and basic sciences. The need for specialized training programs beyond residency in head and neck oncology, be it in surgery, medicine, or radiotherapy, has become obvious. The programs we need to prepare future leaders exist, but must be strengthened and supported. Guidelines for training and program accreditation need refinement and may benefit from some overhaul. The Joint Council for Accreditation for Advanced Training in Head and Neck Oncologic Surgery has as one of its duties to assure that training programs for the experts of the future offer a sound, solid grasp of clinical sciences. But, more important, many programs offer the opportunity for study, training, and hands-on experience in basic science. Proper mentorship in the laboratories enables the trainees not only to advance scholastically, but to build bridges that close the gap the between basic scientists and clinicians. If we expect to have molecular surgeons, we will need to offer them opportunities to become such!

Another change that is likely to take place will be the perception of cancer by physicians and the public alike. In 1926, the famous Charles H. Mayo wrote in the *Annals of Surgery* (83:357), 'While there are several chronic diseases more destructive to life than cancer, none is more feared.' Although this is true for most cancers, it is striking how often physicians and patients rush into hasty treatment decisions once the histologic diagnosis of a malignant tumor has been rendered. The fear of the illness and its consequences become vivid in their minds, and rational thinking is blocked by the shadow of devastation, pain, and impending death. Although this scenario probably will not be much different at the end of this decade, if we have made substantial discoveries and promptly developed clinical applications, the concept of cancer may change from a killer to a chronic illness that can be managed or eradicated, diminishing the fear of pain and death it harbors still today. Change will happen, and it is our collective responsibility to influence on the positive side. There should be fewer patients with head and neck cancer, and those who develop a malignancy in the tissues and anatomical sites between pleura and dura should have a better outlook for cure than they have today.

Finally, although we will make progress in many areas, it will happen only after we have taken a step backwards. History has shown that many of the great discoveries have been serendipitous, made only after well-prepared scientists have gone back to basics. Let's hope that we can continue producing those well-prepared minds who, in turn, give us the breakthroughs we can utilize tomorrow.

292

Index

294

Human papillomavirus type 32 (HPV-32), 12
Human papillomavirus type 33 (HPV-33), 2
Hungary, 199
Hydrocortisone, 178
N-4-(Hydroxycarbophenyl) retinamide, 98
N-(4-Hydroxyphenyl)-retinamide
    (fenretinide; 4HPR), 98, 99
Hydroxyurea, 175, 187, 188, 214
6-Hydroxyurea, 134
Hyopcrellin A, 160
Hyperkeratinization, 90
Hyperkeratosis, 95
Hyperplasia, 57, 90, 92
Hypocrellin A, 168
Hypopharyngeal cancer, 199, 248, 249, 255,
    256
    cigar/pipe smoking and, 74
    functional neck dissection and, 230
    lateral and anterior neck dissection and,
        234–238
    modified neck dissection and, 225
    organ preservation and, 206, 207, 207–
        208, 208, 209
    squamous cells, see Squamous cell
        carcinoma of the hypopharynx

Ifosfamide, 175, 266
Immunotherapy, 257
India, 17
Induction chemotherapy, 177
    distant metastases and, 205, 253, 255–256
    organ preservation and, 203–206, 209,
        214–215
Induction trials, for retinoids, 97–98
In situ hybridization, 14
Insulin, 47
Integrins, 125
Interferon (IFN), 3, 124, 214, 257
Interferon-α (IFN-α), 273–274
Interleukin (IL), 257
Interleukin-2 (IL-2), 272–274
Interleukin-3 (IL-3), 269, 271
Intermediate endpoint biomarkers, 103–109
Interstitial implantation, in PDT, 162, 166,
    167
Intervention, 286–288
int-2 gene, 24, 92, 124
Inverting papillomas, 12
Involucrin, 6, 8, 44, 45, 48–49, 51, 59
Iran, 145
Iron oxide, 145
Isotretinoin, see 13-Cis-retinoic acid

Japan, 161
Jugular vein, 222, 223, 225, 228, 232
jun gene, 18, 19

Kaposi's sarcoma, 163, 166–168
Keratin, 22
    HPV and, 6
    squamous cell differentiation and, 44, 45,
        46, 49–50, 51, 53, 59
Keratinizing epithelial cells, 55–56
Keratoacanthomas, 21
Keratolinin, 44
Kidney metastases, 248
Kiton Red, 161
K-ras gene, 19, 21, 22, 23, 25, 92

Laminin, 117, 121, 123, 124–125, 126, 276
Lanosterol, 44, 51
Large-cell carcinoma, 126
Laryngeal cancer, 73, 199, 225
    alcohol use and, 75
    chemoradiotherapy and, 179–180
    cigarette/cigar/pipe smoking and, 74
    diet and, 77
    distant metastases and, 249, 252, 253, 255,
        256
    int 2/hst1 genes and, 24
    lateral and anterior neck dissection and,
        234–238
    occupational risk factors and, 77
    organ preservation and, see Laryngeal
        preservation
    PDT and, 163
    radioresistance and, 135
    second primary tumors and, 105–106
    squamous cell, see Squamous cell
        carcinoma of the larynx
    verrucous, 12–13
Laryngeal papillomas, 4, 5, 6–7, 9, 11–12
Laryngeal preservation, 206, 209–211, 214–
    215
    chemoradiotherapy and, 179–180, 207,
        208, 210–211, 212–213
    chemotherapy and, 208–209, 210–211,
        215
    radiation therapy and, 200–203, 215
Laryngectomy, 210–211, 238
    adjuvant chemotherapy vs., 255
    chemoradiotherapy vs., 180, 207
    chemotherapy vs., 209
    induction chemotherapy vs., 206
    psychosocial considerations and, 199–200
    radiation therapy vs., 202
Laryngopharynx carcinoma, 226
Laryngoscopy, 144, 152
Lasers, 167
    argon ion dye pumped, 160–161, 163, 168,
        275
    carbon dioxide, 12, 165, 166
Laser surgery, 173
Latent infections, HPV, 3, 12, 15
Lateral neck dissection, 234–238

squamous cell, 206, 207–208, 233, 255, 256
    supraomohyoid neck dissection and, 233
Oropharyngeal papillomas, 11
Osteocalcin, 55
Osteosarcoma, 243
Ovarian cancer, 27, 266
Oxytocin, 55

PAI, *see* Plasminogen activator inhibitor
Palliation, 263–264
Papillomas, 22, 46
    benign, 3, 5, 11–12
    fungiform of nose, 12
    inverting, 12
    laryngeal, 4, 5, 6–7, 9, 11–12
    nasopharyngeal, 11
    oral, 12
    oropharyngeal, 11
    respiratory, 3, 12
    retinoids and, 48, 49
Paranasal sinus tumors, 249
Paranasal tumors, 190
Parathyroid tumors, 146
Parotidectomy, 233
PDGF gene, 19, *see also* Platelet-derived growth factor
PDT, *see* Photodynamic therapy
Petroleum products, 145
p53 gene, 27–28, 92–93, 94
Pharyngeal cancer, 73
    alcohol use and, 75
    chemotherapy and, 208–209
    diet and, 77
    modified neck dissection and, 225, 226
    oral hygiene and, 76
    organ preservation and, 208–209
    PDT and, 161
    snuff use and, 75
Pharyngolaryngeal carcinoma, 213
Pharyngolaryngectomy, 209
Phorbol-12-myristate-13-acetate (PMA), 124, 126
Photodynamic therapy (PDT), 159–169, 275–276
    clinical application of, 163–169
    delivery systems for, 161
    mode of action of, 161–162
    photosensitizers used in, 159–160
    technique used in, 162–163
Photofrin, 160, 162, 163, 164, 168, 275
Photosensitizers, 159–160
Physicians' Health Study, 93
Pipe smoking, 74
Piritrexim, 265
PIXY321, 269, 271
Plasmin, 121
Plasminogen activator (PA), 117, 120, 121–122

Plasminogen activator inhibitor-1 (PAI-1), 121, 122
Plasminogen activator inhibitor-2 (PAI-2), 121
Platelet-derived growth factor (PDGF), 18, 136–137
Ploidy, 26
Plumbers, 77
Plummer-Vinson syndrome, 145
Polonium-210, 75
Polyamines, 20
Polycyclic aromatic hydrocarbons (PAHs), 18, 79
Polymerase chain reaction (PCR), 14, 23–24, 78
Porfimer sodium, 160
Porphyrins, 159, 160, 275
Potentially lethal damage repair (PLDR), 132–133, 134
P0 protein, 34
p21 protein, 23, 31
p53 protein, 6, 93
Premalignant cells/lesions
    chemoprevention of, 94–95
    p53 gene and, 92
    retinoid effect on, 47–48
    retinoid effect on squamous cell differentiation in, 48–51
    squamous cell differentiation in, 45–46
Prevention, 286–288
Procollagenase IV, 121
Profilaggrin, 50–51
Proliferating-cell nuclear antigen, 91
Prophycenes, 160, 168
Prorelaxin, 44
Protease nexin, 121
Protein kinase C, 123–124, 136, 137
Proto-oncogenes, 18, 19
Psoralen, 159, 275
Psoriasis, 52
Putrescine, 20
Pyriform sinus tumors, 248

RAD 9 gene, 134
Radiation exposure, 12
Radiation injury, 131–133
Radiation therapy, 146, 173, 226, 238, *see also* Chemoradiotherapy
    distant metastases and, 246, 255–256, 257
    organ preservation and, 200–203, 205–206, 211–213, 214, 215
    PDT and, 165
    second primary tumors and, 105–106
    supraomohyoid neck dissection and, 234
    surgery and, 174
Radiation Therapy Oncology Group (RTOG), 108, 180, 186, 257
Radical lymphadenectomy, 224
Radical neck dissection, 221–222, 224, 226,

229–230, 233–234
modified, 226–229, 230, 234
Radioresistance, 131–137
Radiosensitivity, 80, 134
raf gene, 19, 135
Raf protein, 136
Randomized trials, 211–212
RARs, *see* Nuclear retinoic acid receptor
ras gene, 21, 22–24, 31, 136
Ras protein, 136
Recurrent head and neck cancer, 263–277
   biologic response modifiers and, 272–273
   biomodulators and, 266–269
   chemoprotectants and, 266–269
   CSFs and, 269–272
   IFN-α and, 273–274
   monoclonal antibodies and, 276–277
   new cytotoxic drugs for, 265–266
   PDT and, 275–276
rel gene, 19
Research, 288–290
Respiratory papillomas, 3, 12
Retinoblastoma (Rb) protein, 6
Retinoblastomas, 25
Retinoic acid, 47, 48
   β-all-*trans*, *see* β-all-*trans* retinoic acid
   9-*cis*, 47, 54, 55, 96
   13-*cis*, *see*, 13-*Cis*-retinoic acid
   HPV and, 8, 10
   squamous cell differentiation and, 49, 50, 53
Retinoic acid receptor-α (RAR-α), 54, 55, 56, 57, 58, 96
Retinoic acid receptor-β (RAR-β), 54, 55–58, 59, 96
Retinoic acid receptor-γ (RAR-γ), 54, 55, 56, 57, 58, 59, 96
Retinoic acid response elements (RAREs), 54–55, 58–59
Retinoids, 43–59, 77, *see also* specific types
   clinical trials of, 95–99
   effect on malignant/premalignant/normal cells, 47–48
   effect on squamous cell differentiation, 48–51
   lung premalignancy and, 102–103
   mechanisms involved in actions of, 51–59
   recurrent head and neck cancer and, 274–275
   second primary tumors and, 106–107, 108–110
Retinoid X receptor (RXR), 55, 96
Retinoid X receptor-α (RXR-α), 54, 55, 57, 58, 96
Retinoid X receptor-β (RXR-β), 54, 57, 96
Retinoid X receptor-γ (RXR-γ), 54, 57, 96
Retinol, 47, 104, 109
Retinyl acetate, 50
Retinyl palmitate, 100–101, 109
Retromolar trigone squamous cell

carcinoma, 232
Rhabdomyosarcoma, 290
Rhesus blood group, 253
Rhodamine, 159
Rhodamine-123, 168
Rhodamine B, 161
Rigid bronchoscopy, 151
Rigid esophagoscopy, 150
Risk factors, 73–78
RNA
   HPV, 2–3, 11, 15
   radioresistance and, 135
   ras, 23
Ro2-2985, 49
ros gene, 19
Rotterdam Cooperative Head and Neck Cancer Study Group, 266
RXR, *see* Retinoid X receptor

Salivary gland tumors, 146, 231
Sangivamycin, 136
Sarcoma, 266
Sciellin, 44
Screening, 141–153
   for bronchial cancer, 148, 150–151
   for esophageal cancer, 145, 149–150
   for nasopharyngeal cancer, 145, 151
   patient selection for, 144–146
   techniques used in, 148
   timing considerations in, 147
   for tracheal cancer, 150–151
   for upper aerodigestive tract mucosa cancer, 143–144, 148
Second primary tumors, 89–90
   field carcinogenesis and, 91, 92
   prevention of, 105–109
Sequential chemoradiotherapy, 176–180, 212–213
S2 gene, 30–34
Signal transduction, 136
Silicon naphthalocyanine, 159–160, 168
Simultaneous tumors, 143
Singapore, 199
Sinus cancer, 145, 208–209, 248, 249
ski gene, 19
Skin cancer, 287
   basal cell, 164
   PDT and, 159, 163–164
   squamous cell, 164, 274
Small cell lung cancer, 25, 50, 58, 266, 267
Smokeless tobacco, 104
   chewing, 89
   snuff, 75, 76, 99
Smoking, *see* Smoking cessation; Tobacco use
Smoking cessation, 286–287
   lung premalignancy and, 102–103
   second primary tumors and, 107–108
sno gene, 19

Warts, *see* Papillomas
Whites, 17, 73, 75
Women
   cigarette smoking and, 74
   epidemiology of cancer in, 73
   mouthwash use and, 76
   snuff use and, 75
Women's Health Study, 93
Wood dust, 77

WR-2721, 267–268

Xeroderma pigmentosum, 48, 80
X-rays, 4, 5, 136, 137, 144, 148, 150
XRCC-1 gene, 134

yes gene, 19